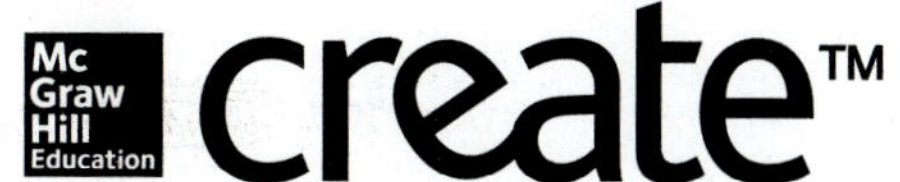

Annual Editions: Nutrition, 27/e

Edited by Janet Colson

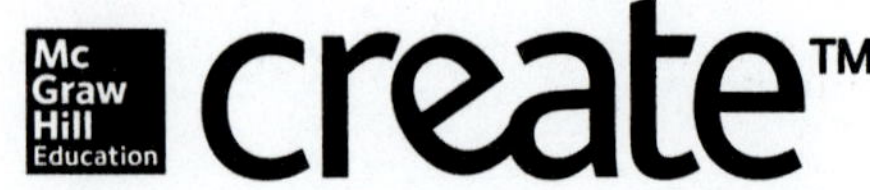

http://create.mheducation.com

ISBN-10: 1259359581 ISBN-13: 9781259359583

Contents

Preface

Annual Editions: Nutrition is a collection of articles that is updated annually and reviews latest research findings, changes in policy, and trends in nutrition-related topics. Many of the articles are based on topics identified in the *Dietary Guidelines for Americans (DGA), 2010.*

The first unit describes current trends in the field of nutrition with emphasis on how consumer demand for healthy food influences the food industry and the roles that local, state, and federal governments have in improving the health of the public.

The next unit is centered on maternal, child, and adolescent nutrition in response to the increased national emphasis on feeding and weight concerns during the early life cycle. Articles on the new guidelines for school meals and childhood obesity are the cornerstones of this unit.

Articles on a variety of nutrients follow. Sodium, added sugar, and fats are all emphasized in the *DGA* as nutrients of concern for Americans and are represented in articles in this section.

The other units include topics that focus on the relationship between nutrition, chronic diseases, and obesity. Recent research findings on the role that nutrition plays in diabetes, kidney disease, dementia, and obesity are emphasized. Several articles describe how to interpret the research findings that are often sensationalized by the media.

Food safety and technology, including information on the safety of domestic and imported food and beverages are covered next. Several articles in this section discuss genetically engineered crops, proposed FDA regulations, and technologies that facilitate food production and preservation.

The final unit focuses on sustainability of our food supply and hunger. Articles on the growing prevalence of food insecurity among all sectors of the population, including among college students, are featured.

Annual Editions: Nutrition is to be used as a companion to a standard nutrition text so that it may update, expand, or emphasize certain topics that are covered in the textbook or present totally new topics not covered in a standard textbook. Keeping up with all of the nutrition research and policy changes is a challenging task, but thanks to *Annual Editions: Nutrition,* you can easily review the latest nutrition information taken from reputable sources.

A number of features in *Annual Editions: Nutrition* have been designed to assist students in their study and expand critical thinking. Located at the beginning of each unit, Learning Outcomes outline the key concepts on which students should focus on as they are reading the article. Critical Thinking questions, located at the end of each article, allow students to test their understanding of the key concepts, and a list of recommended Internet References guides students to the best sources of additional information on a topic.

We hope that the reader will develop critical thinking and be empowered to ask questions and to seek answers from credible sources.

Your input is most valuable to improve this anthology, which is updated yearly. We would appreciate your comments.

Editor

JANET M. COLSON is a professor in the Nutrition and Food Science Program at Middle Tennessee State University. She earned her PhD in Nutrition and Food Science from Florida State University, Tallahassee, Florida. Earlier degrees include a BS in Family and Consumer Sciences Education from Mississippi College, Clinton, Mississippi, and an MS. in the same field of study from the University of Southern Mississippi.

Dr. Colson teaches maternal child nutrition and advanced nutrition classes at the undergraduate and graduate levels. She has spoken nationally on areas related to childhood obesity prevention. She edited the second edition of *Taking Sides: Clashing Views on Food and Nutrition* in addition to developing ancillaries for to accompany various publications.

Academic Advisory Board

Members of the Academic Advisory Board are instrumental in the final selection of articles for each edition of ANNUAL EDITIONS. Their review of articles for content, level, and appropriateness provides critical direction to the editors and staff. We think that you will find their careful consideration well reflected in this volume.

Sherry Best-Kai
AB-Technical Community College

Harold Borrero
Canada College

Yavuz Cakir
Benedict College

Katie Clark
University of California San Francisco

L. Nicholle Clark
College of the Desert

Brian Coble
Carroll College

Evia L. Davis
Langston University

Mark Deaton
Morehead State University

Diane Dettmore
Fairleigh Dickinson University

Jonathan Deutsch
Goodwin College

Johanna Donnenfield
Scottsdale Community College

Wilton Duncan
ASA College

Brad Engeldinger
Sierra College

Amy Frith
Ithaca College

Bernard Frye
University of Texas, Arlington

Leonard E. Gerber
University of Rhode Island

Adrienne Giuffre
Bucks County Community College

Jana Gonsalves
American River College

Aleida Gordon
California State Polytechnic University, Pomona

Megan Govindan
West Virginia University, Morgantown

Jule Anne Henstenburg
LaSalle University

Tawni Holmes
University of Central Oklahoma

Allen Jackson
Chadron State College

Barry Johnson
Davidson County Community College

Leslie Kling
Rosemont College

Laura Kruskall
University of Nevada-Las Vegas

Linda Lamont
University of Rhode Island

Xiangdong Li
New York City College of Technology

Steven Lindner
Nassau Community College

Carol MacKusick
Clayton State University

Willis McAleese
Idaho State University

Laura McArthur
East Carolina University

Mary Miller
Morehead State University

Kiran Misra
Edinboro University of Pennsylvania

Kara Montgomery
University of South Carolina

Rebecca M. Mullis
University of Georgia

Gretchen Myers-Hill
Michigan State University

Robin Ouzts
Thomas University

Sara Plaspohl
Armstrong Atlantic State University

Frankie Rabon
Grambling State University

Wendy Repovich
Eastern Washington University

Robin R. Roach
University of Memphis

Karen J. Schmitz
Madonna University

Louise E. Schneider
Loma Linda University

Joshua Searcy
Central State University

Ingrid Skoog
Oregon State University

Marta Sovyanhadi
Oakwood University

Marsha Spence
University of Tennessee, Knoxville

Diana M. Spillman
Miami University of Ohio

Marianne Stillner
University of Alaska SE, Juneau

John Stuart
Wiley College

Michael Teague
University of Iowa

Theresa Tiso
Stony Brook University

Julia VanderMolen
Davenport University

Sue Ward
Fayetteville State University

Terry Weideman
Oakland Community College

LaVern Whisenton-Davidson
Millersville University

Mustafa Yatin
Salem State University

Joseph Zielinski
State University of New York at Brockport

Unit 1

UNIT

Prepared by: Janet Colson, *Middle Tennessee State University*

Nutrition Trends

The hottest trends in nutrition today revolve around reducing the incidence of obesity/chronic disease and improving the quality of food produced, marketed, and sold in the United States. This unit addresses these current trends in nutrition with particular emphasis on the recent paradigm shift in the food industry and the role of government to ensure a healthy food supply for its citizens.

Products that are grown naturally, ethically, and safely are at increasing demand in the United States and many other developed countries. The biggest restaurant chains, food producers, and grocery chains are changing the way they do business to address the consumer sentiment for healthy food and natural ingredients. Marketing plans are changing to portray more natural, locally grown, and/or healthy foods that are, ideally, provided by family-run businesses. The words *all natural, cage free, fair trade,* and *naturally raised* are now a vital component of marketing campaigns of many food producers.

With the ease of sharing information via the Internet and social media sites, people have a venue for communicating their emotional ties to food. Food preferences are driven by emotion, and one of the strongest emotions that Americans currently have about their food is fear. Viral videos, books, and documentaries about food production in the United States are raising distrust of our industrialized food system. Whether it is concern about the use of pesticides, pink slime, growth hormones, preservatives, and antibiotics or the prevalence of *E. coli, salmonella,* or mad cow disease, Americans are vocalizing their sentiments about the U.S. food systems. American consumers' emotional attachment to food is leading the food industry to change the way it produces and markets food.

Increased attention to the ethical treatment of animals is changing the foods that are offered in popular restaurants and the nature of how some farmers raise their animals. Consumers want to feel better about how their food is raised. An example of these trends within the food industry can be seen in the changes that are occurring by fast food restaurants. McDonald's is taking strides to improve its image by offering healthier options in the United States and has changed its operations to more ethical and ecofriendly practices in Great Britain and Northern Ireland. McDonald's UK has made great strides to ensure no genetically modified foods are sold at its restaurants in Europe. Burger King promises to serve only cage-free pork and eggs by 2017.

Local, state, and federal governments are promoting programs to provide healthy foods and educate the public about proper nutrition. One of the most significant pieces of legislation that impacts the U.S. food production and supply is the Farm Bill. The Food, Conservation, and Energy Act of 2008 (i.e., "Farm Bill") is renewed every five years. The renewal often ignites conversation about the effect of the federal government's degree of financial backing for industrial growers of commodity crops in relation to the lesser support of fruit and vegetable production. The Farm Bill is a 1,770-page document that covers everything from nutrition assistance programs to land conservation. It determines agricultural subsidies and crop insurance policies in the United States. With the emphasis on increased vegetable and fruit intake in the latest *MyPlate* guidelines, many public health professionals are questioning our current agriculture policy and the role of the Farm Bill on the U.S. food supply and, secondarily, its food intake.

Lawmakers of state governments are creating initiatives that support *MyPlate.* Legislative support for improving access to locally grown fruits and vegetables, seafood, and dairy is becoming more prevalent at the state level. State governments are making attempts to have a positive impact on local economies through promotion of state agriculture. These efforts serve to improve not only the health of the states' people, but also their economies.

A recent trend in corporate wellness programs is the use of social media platforms designed to encourage employees to adopt healthy lifestyle behaviors. Social media programs can provide a venue for participants to journal, create fitness challenges, and offer support to fellow participants. It provides social support and motivating factors such as accountability and friendly competition. Many hospitals, large corporations, and state and local governments have made great progress to improve the health of their employees through a social-media-based corporate wellness program.

The articles in this unit focus on a variety of trends seen in nutrition and health environments. The selection of articles include topics that have been seen in popular media as well as trends observed within the profession of nutrition. These articles stretch across the topics commonly covered in all sections of nutrition courses.

Article

Prepared by: Janet Colson, *Middle Tennessee State University*

Have a Bite, It's Natural

Food giants are promising to use more natural, ethical ingredients, but will consumers pay?

CHRIS SORENSEN

Learning Outcomes

After reading this article, you will be able to:

- Summarize the potential impact of the higher demand for "natural" products on the food industry.
- Describe the impact of animal welfare groups on the production of eggs in the United States.

With their soft, mashed potato insides and crispy exteriors stamped in the shape of a happy face, McCain Foods' frozen Smiles are marketed as a fun-to-eat children's snack. They're not supposed to explode. And yet, that's what happened inside the Canadian food giant's laboratory in Florenceville-Bristol, N.B., as researchers attempted to "reformulate" the Smile's long list of unpronounceable ingredients, part of a company-wide strategy to make its packaged foods more natural and wholesome.

Tony Locke, McCain's director of product development, says the trouble began while trying to ditch mono- and di-glycerides, emulsifiers that help retain moisture in some packaged foods. Emboldened by previous success with frozen pizza pockets, Locke's team added a mixture of yeast, wheat gluten and flaxseed to the Smiles. "It was working very well in the lab," says Locke, referring to what was the 40th attempt to rejig the recipe. "But then when we went to scale it up, we actually had these little Smiles going down the line in the plant and coming out of the fryer and exploding. They would literally come out of the oil and burst."

And that, in the form of a combustible little potato snack, is the huge and complex challenge faced by food companies as consumers increasingly demand meals that are not only healthier, but more "natural" and therefore, it's reasoned, better for you. With the public spooked by everything from processed foods (too much salt, too many additives) to hormone-raised beef, food producers are suddenly bending over backwards to portray themselves as purveyors of local, fresh ingredients, and their suppliers as earthy, family-run outfits, as opposed to giant factory farms. The phrases "all-natural," "naturally raised" and "cage-free" are everywhere.

The latest big name to jump into the fray is Burger King. The fast-food giant recently promised to serve only "cage-free" pork and eggs at all of its 7,200 United States restaurants by 2017, marking the first time a big fast-food chain has made such a definitive pledge. McDonald's, meanwhile, has said it will work with its pork suppliers to phase out restrictive gestation crates used to house sows while they raise their piglets. And Tim Hortons is facing calls to go completely cage-free from the Humane Society of the United States, which holds a small number of shares and is proposing a shareholder vote at the company's annual meeting next week. The ethical treatment of animals is one argument driving the changes, but so too is the assertion that happier livestock translates into healthier food.

As for packaged foods, McCain is just one of several companies that's now focused on simple, easy-to-understand ingredients. Others include General Mills, with its Pillsbury Simply line of cookies, and Häagen-Dazs's Five ice cream (with just five ingredients).

But while the sudden shift in focus may seem like a welcome change, critics say it is as much about marketing as it is science. And it has left food producers faced with the prospect of spending billions to overhaul their operations, even though the new and improved approaches may, in reality, do little to improve the nutritional value of the food we eat. Everyone likes the idea of food that's "natural" and ethical, but, it must be asked, are they willing to pay the price?

For many big food companies, the pressure to change their ways intensified earlier this year. In February, Chipotle Mexican Grill (once owned by McDonald's) aired an animated ad during the Grammy Awards that became an Internet phenomenon, with some six million YouTube views. The spot depicted the evolution of factory farming over the years, starting with a farmer and his wife standing in a field with a pig and ending with hundreds of pigs being deposited by machines onto conveyor belts, where they were stuffed with pills, stamped into cubes and loaded into the back of trucks.

Then, in March, a long-simmering debate about "pink slime" (beef scraps ground into a slurry, treated with ammonia and used as hamburger filler) went from being a favourite whipping boy of celebrity chef Jamie Oliver to a mainstream public issue. By the end of the month, everyone from McDonald's to Safeway said they would no longer buy beef made with the stuff, while one of the product's major producers, Beef Products Inc., had to shut down several of its factories, and another ground beef processor, AFA Foods, filed for bankruptcy due to lack of demand.

It's against this backdrop that Burger King, under pressure from the humane society and shifting consumer sentiment, made its decision to promise to use only cage-free eggs and pork in the United States within five years (there are no immediate plans to do the same in Canada). Other companies that have offered similar promises include McDonald's, Wendy's, Subway, Costco and food giant Unilever, which makes Hellman's mayonnaise. "We're going to continue to consume beef, pork, chicken, fish, but we want to feel better about the practices," says Darren Tristano, the executive vice-president of Technomic, a food industry consulting firm in Chicago.

Driving the changes is the assertion that happier, healthier livestock translates into food that's better for you.

The idea that getting rid of cages is more "natural" comes as news to many producers. Florian Possberg, 61, has been raising hogs in Humboldt, Sask., near Saskatoon, since 1975. Possberg started out raising sows in communal pens and then eventually switched to the more restrictive gestation crates in the 1980s. Research at the time suggested it was better for the animals and consumers, decreasing the risk of disease and injury. "Sows are pretty aggressive when they live in groups," says Possberg, a director of the Canadian Pork Council. He adds that roughly half of the 5,400 sows on his farms are housed in gestation crates, while the rest are in groups, estimating that it would cost more than $1 million to switch over the rest of the operation.

It's a similar story with egg farmers, who, several decades ago, moved to caged systems because it was viewed as cleaner and helped prevent the birds from attacking and eating each other. But animal welfare groups claim the use of small "battery" cages that each house several laying hens are too cramped, preventing the birds from engaging in natural behaviours such as scratching, nesting or flapping their wings. With pressure mounting south of the border, the United Egg Producers reached a deal last year with the United States humane society to promote the use of so-called "enriched" cages, which are bigger and offer extras like perches and nesting areas. The two groups are also calling for Congress to pass laws requiring new standards in a bid to avoid a costly patchwork of state regulations, and also to ensure individual operators who make the switch aren't put at a "competitive disadvantage." Translation: if everyone has to absorb the same costs, they can more easily be passed on to consumers via higher prices.

In Canada, both pork and egg producers are looking to the National Farm Animal Care Council for guidance. The seven-year-old group devises codes of practice for the industry with input from producers, scientists, government and animal welfare groups. It's in the process of updating several of its codes, including those for hogs and poultry, although results aren't expected for a few years. "It takes a long time," says Jackie Wepruk, the council's general manager, of the typically Canadian consensus-oriented approach. "But if you look south of the border, you'll see the divisive way animal welfare is being tackled there. Most decisions are being made in a knee-jerk, reactionary sort of way."

But Peter Clarke, chairman of the Egg Farmers of Canada, says the industry may have to move more quickly depending on what happens in the United States "The major food purchasers won't accept significantly different practices on one side of the border or the other," he says, adding the cost of such an industry-wide switch would be significant.

Whether it's instant noodles or the oft-mocked Twinkie, most products that come in a bag or a box have historically been marketed based on their convenience, not provenance, and come loaded with artificial colours, flavours and other additives—all designed to maintain taste while boosting shelf life.

At McCain, the decision to reformulate its entire lineup of products (more than 80 since 2010) to include only "real" or natural ingredients represented the biggest-ever undertaking for the company's research and development team, according to Locke. The move was based on extensive customer research that suggested consumers were growing wary of additives that were synthetic-sounding. Nor was the challenge strictly limited to McCain's own operations. "We might buy a seasoning mix from a primary supplier, but of course they're getting all of the components to assemble the mix from another group of suppliers," Locke says. "So it was a complicated effort."

All of the tinkering has translated into big business for another sector of the food industry: flavour companies. Though many consumers don't realize it, many ingredients now viewed as undesirable—salt, sugar and other additives—do a lot of heavy lifting when it comes to taste. Once they're taken out, new flavours must be added to maintain a product's appeal. And not just any flavouring solution will do. Bob Eilerman, the head of science and technology at Switzerland's Givaudan, one of the biggest flavour and fragrance companies in the world, estimates that more than 50 percent of Givaudan's customers now want "natural" flavourings, as opposed to artificial ones, even though there's not much difference (other than cost). "Natural has good connotations behind it," says Eilerman. "But at the end of the day, it's all about chemicals. Whether it's a strawberry flavour that came from crushed strawberries or from one of our laboratories, the chemical composition that we're trying to create is very similar."

It raises the question of whether the current fixation on natural and ethical is ultimately worth the price. McCain seems to think so. Calla Farn, a company spokesperson, says sales of some reformulated McCain products have enjoyed gains of up to 10 percent. As for the cost, Farn admits that the new-and-improved products are more expensive to make, but says the company "worked hard to identify savings in other areas to ensure our products remained cost-neutral."

Not all companies may be so lucky. In the case of cage-free eggs, Tristano estimates that the cost per egg will go up by 25 cents to 40 cents per dozen, which threatens to squeeze the margins on a simple breakfast sandwich. That's because fast-food operators typically have a much tougher time passing on rising commodity prices than do grocery stores because of intense competition. "It's about three cents an egg on a product that sells for $2 or $3, so it doesn't seem like a lot," he says. "But when you can only increase prices by about two per cent and you're getting hit by a per cent and a half just to have cage-free, that's a big deal."

Ultimately, a bigger risk to the industry may come from the public's new heightened expectations from food companies. As they change the way food is made, there is every likelihood consumers will turn their attention to some other unappetizing aspect of the mass-production process. "Once you move forward, there's no turning back," warns Tristano. "And let's be honest: if we really cared that much, we'd all be vegetarians."

Critical Thinking

1. Summarize the potential impact of the higher demand for "natural" products on the food industry.
2. Describe the impact of animal welfare groups on the production of eggs in the United States.
3. Explain why restrictive gestation cages for pigs and cages for hens were adopted during the 1980s.
4. Critique the statement, "Happier livestock translates into healthier food."

Create Central

www.mhhe.com/createcentral

Internet References

The Academy of Nutrition and Dietetics
www.eatright.org

The Food and Drug Administration
www.fds.gov

Article

Prepared by: Janet Colson, *Middle Tennessee State University*

Go On: Eat Your Heart Out

BRUCE HOROVITZ

Learning Outcome

After reading this article, you will be able to:

- Describe how consumers' emotional attachments to food are influencing the food supply.

There are few things parents are more passionate about than the food and drink that their kids consume. So it's no accident that Honest Tea, the organic tea maker recently swallowed-up by Coca-Cola, is revamping its wildly successful Honest Kids beverage line into one that this fall will be sweetened with fruit juice instead of cane sugar. A white blaze on the front of the pouch will proclaim: Sweetened *only* with fruit juice.

"They're nutritionally the same," concedes Seth Goldman, cofounder of Honest Tea. "But parents don't want to see added sugar. They can get very emotional about this."

What Americans eat and drink has become such an emotional roller coaster for so many of us that it's utterly changing the way the nation's biggest restaurant chains, foodmakers and grocery chains do business. Food used to feed our bodies. Now it also needs to feed our brains. Our egos. Our nostalgic memories. And maybe even our social-media appetites.

"While we have always had an emotional relationship with food, what's different is we talk about it more, and the discussion is much louder," says Harry Balzer, food guru at researcher NPD Group. "Food is fashion. You wear your diet like you wear your clothes."

Talking about food has become so fashionable that we may be doing more of it than ever. Social-media chatter about food—which is where we do much of it—is up more than 13% over the past year, says Nielsen Media Incite, which tracks buzz across social networks, blogs, forums and consumer review sites. That's millions of additional social morsels just on food. The hunger for food news seems insatiable. Food Network, which had 50,000 viewers per night in the mid-'90s, now averages more than 1.1 million.

Foodmakers are listening in. They know that one of the strongest emotions that many American consumers feel toward the food they eat is fear. One week the fear is over pink slime. Then, it's about chemicals in milk. Or mad cow disease. Or too many calories stuffed into a large, sugary drink. Or even some worker's fingertip getting chopped into an Arby's roast beef sandwich.

"Every week, something raises distrust for our industrialized food system," says Gary Hirshberg, co-founder of Stonyfield Farms. "There's a real-time awareness that our food may be making us sick."

The emotional hits or misses that people feel toward the food they eat can determine everything from what Whole Foods stocks to the thickness of Stonyfield's next yogurt to the look, taste and smell of a new appetizer that Applebee's will add to its menu this fall.

Our emotional attachment to food is leading foodmakers to:

Respond to consumer concerns. Consumer research revealed to Honest Tea executives something they didn't expect: The most important word in the company's name isn't "tea." It's "honest," Goldman says. That's honest as in: We can trust what this brand stands for.

In other words, consumers just want to know what's actually in a product, and they want to know that it's beneficial to eat or drink. So, the Honest brand is looking into a better-for-you carbonated soft-drink line by next year. And it's even looking into Honest-branded foods, he says.

Consumers want to be able to look the brand straight in the eye without the brand blinking, Goldman says. They want to trust it. But that trust is always on the line. Consumers complained, for example, about a new bottle last year that was 22% lighter and which was specifically designed to create less waste. What made consumers balk was that the design change—to use less plastic—made it look like the bottle had less product. "They thought we were selling them air," says Goldman. So the bottle was quickly redesigned again to make it clear that there were no shenanigans.

Folks also want to trust the Honest brand to keep them healthy. "Fifteen years ago, people were choosing organic to save the world," Goldman says. Now, he says, they're choosing it "to save themselves—and that's a much more powerful driver."

Concoct nostalgic food. When football season begins this fall, it won't be an accident if you find this appetizer on the menu at your local Applebee's: brew pub pretzel and beer cheese dip.

"The trick for us was giving customers the sense that they were at the stadium, but in a way that would be unique," says Melissa Hunt, who has been a senior chef at Applebee's for six years. After all, she asks, what's more emotional than fall, football and gathering with friends?

So, instead of a traditional salt pretzel, Applebee's opted to rethink how to make a culinary connection between the bond at a ballpark and taste expectations at an Applebee's. That meant less salt and more pepper and herbs on the pretzel. It meant a pretzel that was crispy on the outside but soft on the inside. And, of course, what to add to the cheese dip to give it the cosmic flavor and smell of sitting in stadium seats: beer, of course.

Sell better-for-you stuff. At Panera Bread, the internal name used for its food-development team is the "lust" team, because "food is such a sensual experience," says co-founder Ron Shaich.

Shaich said Panera's basic goal is to prod consumers to "fall in love" with the restaurant: "That's what I wake up first thing in the morning thinking. If you love this place, that's all that matters. Everything else will take care of itself."

So he works on the emotional cues that hit consumers at their core: no artificial stuff, antibiotic-free meats, fully posted calorie information and intangibles, he says, such as serving food on china plates instead of paper.

The chain recently starting selling a Fuji Apple Roasted Turkey Salad with turkey meat that doesn't taste like it's from the deli. Rather, he says, it looks, feels, smells and tastes like it's from one of the most memorable spots of all: the Thanksgiving table.

"This is real turkey," says Shaich. It's cut 1/3-inch thick. It's also a hit, he says, with early sales surpassing expectations.

Cater to "mouth feel." Some 29 years ago, Gary Hirshberg started with seven cows and an idea: to make organic yogurt for the masses. His company, Stonyfield Farms, is now the nation's fourth-largest yogurt maker.

Much of his free time is spent combing yogurt aisles of stores throughout Europe, searching for the next big thing in the U.S. thicker, cheesier yogurts. Europeans, who he says are more emotional about their food than Americans, want a "thicker, creamier mouth feel" when they eat yogurt. Americans eventually will, too, which helps explain why Greek yogurt sales have grown so quickly in the United States And that's the next generation of yogurt he's searching for: thicker and cheesier than Greek.

Get more local. Whole Foods executives know there are few things folks are more passionate about than where their food comes from.

Next year it will open a store in Brooklyn, N.Y., with something none of its stores have: a 10,000-square-foot rooftop garden. "You can't get more locally grown than that," says David Lannon, executive vice president of operations.

Most recently, it took that consumer passion for all-things-local to a new store in Kailua, Hawaii. The store has a fish bar that serves locally caught, sustainably sourced fish chopped with items such as onions and soy sauce to create an "emotional connection" to what locals ate as kids, Lannon says. The store targets locals, not tourists, with three porches where folks can sit, eat and socialize. "It brings folks full circle to their memories of growing up in Hawaii."

There's also a Whole Foods in Petaluma, Calif., where eggs are sold—when available—from a local farmer whose 200 chickens are never kept inside or in cages. Never mind that the eggs cost twice as much as conventional eggs. "Customers call the store and ask if that egg delivery arrived," Lannon says. "Some decide to come based only on that."

Serve "comfort" at 30,000 feet. Then, there's British Airways. It recently realized that its first-class passengers don't want fancy-dancy desserts. Last fall, it started serving what passengers told them they wanted most: comfort food. Its Crumb Crumble cobbler was such a smash, when caterers tried to replace it on the menu with a different dessert, passengers went ballistic, says Lynn McClelland, head of catering. It's all about emotions—even the most primitive, childhood emotions, she says. When stuck high above the ground for hours in a plane, she says, "Passengers tell us what they want most is what their moms used to feed them when they were 12."

Critical Thinking

1. Describe how consumers' emotional attachment to food is influencing the U.S. food supply.
2. Explain how social media is impacting the U.S. perspective of food.
3. Interpret the following statement: "One of the strongest emotions that American consumers feel toward food is fear."

Create Central

www.mhhe.com/createcentral

Internet References

Cornucopia Institute
www.cornucopia.org

Food Institute
www.foodinstitute.com

Institute of Food Technology
www.ift.org

National Eating Disorders Association
www.nationaleatingdisorders.org

Article

Prepared by: Janet Colson, *Middle Tennessee State University*

Fresh Fruit, Hold the Insulin

While health officials wage a costly war on obesity and diabetes, taxpayers are subsidizing foods that make us fatter. It's time to rewrite the farm bill.

Learning Outcomes

After reading this article, you will be able to:

- Identify the programs and policies that are covered by the farm bill.
- Explain what could happen to the American diet if fruit and vegetable growers received the same government subsidies and insurance programs as corn growers receive.

Some years ago two nutrition experts went grocery shopping. For a dollar, Adam Drewnowski and S. E. Specter could purchase 1,200 calories of potato chips or cookies or just 250 calories worth of carrots. It was merely one example of how an unhealthy diet is cheaper than a healthy one. This price difference did not spring into existence by force of any natural laws but largely because of antiquated agricultural policies. Public money is working at cross-purposes: backing an overabundance of unhealthful calories that are flooding our supermarkets and restaurants, while also battling obesity and the myriad illnesses that go with it. It is time to align our farm policies with our health policies.

In past years farm subsidies have been a third rail of American politics—never to be touched. But their price tag, both direct and indirect, has now brought them back into the debate and created an imperative for change. Conditions such as heart disease, diabetes and arthritis are strongly correlated with excess poundage and run up medical bills of nearly $150 billion every year. The government has poured billions of dollars into dietary campaigns, from the U.S., Department of Agriculture's new MyPlate recommendation (half of daily food consumption should be fruits and vegetables) to programs aimed at providing more produce in schools and in military cafeterias.

Agricultural subsidies undercut those efforts by skewing the market in favor of unhealthful calories. Much of the food we have to choose from—and how much it costs—is determined by the 1,770-page, almost $300-billion Food, Conservation, and Energy Act of 2008 (commonly known as the "farm bill"). This piece of legislation, up for renewal this year, covers everything from nutrition assistance programs to land conservation efforts. It also determines how much money gets paid out to agricultural operations in subsidies and crop insurance programs. Federal support for agriculture, begun in earnest during the Great Depression, was originally intended as a temporary lifeline to farmers, paying them extra when crop prices were low. Nearly eight decades later the benefits flow primarily to large commodity producers of corn and soy, which are as profitable as ever.

The current bill gives some $4.9 billion a year in automatic payments to growers of such commodity crops, thus driving down prices for corn, corn-based products and corn-fed meats. Cows that are raised on corn, rather than grass, make meat that is higher in calories and contains more omega-6 fatty acids and fewer omega-3 fatty acids—a dangerous ratio that has been linked to heart disease.

Cheap corn has also become a staple in highly processed foods, from sweetened breakfast cereals to soft drinks, that have been linked to an increase in the rate of type 2 diabetes, a condition that currently affects more than one in 12 American adults. Between 1985 and 2010 the price of beverages sweetened with high-fructose corn syrup dropped 24 percent, and by 2006 American children consumed an extra 130 calories a day from these beverages. Over the same period the price of fresh fruits and vegetables rose 39 percent. For families on a budget, the price difference can be decisive in their food choices.

But fruits and vegetables do not have to be more expensive than a corn-laden chicken nugget or corn syrup-sweetened drink. One reason they are costly is that the current farm bill categorizes them as "specialty crops" that do not receive the same direct payments or crop insurance that commodity crops do.

With the government tightening its belt, some of those old subsidies finally look ready to fall. Many lawmakers across the political spectrum, including President Barack Obama and the leaders of the U.S. Senate Committee on Agriculture, Nutrition and Forestry, have recommended cutting direct commodity payments, which would save money and help us stay healthier.

There is no dearth of policy options. Research groups such as the Robert Wood Johnson Foundation in Princeton, N.J., recommend leveling the playing field by extending subsidies and insurance programs more widely to fruit and vegetable producers. The government can also use its own purchasing power, through school lunch programs and institutional buying decisions, to fill people's plates with healthy choices. The imperative, however, is clear: any new farm bill should at the very least remove the current perverse incentives for people to eat unhealthily.

Critical Thinking

1. Define the farm bill. Identify the programs and policies that are covered by this bill.
2. Identify the implications of fruits and vegetables being categorized as "specialty crops" in the farm bill.
3. Contrast the price trends of sweetened beverages and fruits/vegetables from 1985–2010.
4. Identify the original intention of agricultural subsidies. When did the subsidies begin?

Create Central

www.mhhe.com/createcentral

Internet References

Cornucopia Institute
www.cornucopia.org

Farm Bill (House Committee on Agriculture)
http://agriculture.house.gov/farmbill

My Plate
www.myplate.gov

Robert Woods Johnson Foundation
www.rwjf.org

United States Department of Agriculture (USDA)
www.USDA.gov

Article

Prepared by: Janet Colson, *Middle Tennessee State University*

The New Healthy

Lawmakers are cooking up ways to encourage better eating and cultivate local economies.

AMY WINTERFELD

Learning Outcomes

After reading this article, you will be able to:

- Describe ways local, state, and federal governments are making changes to encourage better eating among Americans.
- Explain how MyPlate can be used to improve health and the economy.

As Americans leap into the New Year, many will resolve to eat healthier to make up for holiday indulgences. New guidelines for what eating healthy means, released last year by the U.S. Department of Agriculture, include a new "MyPlate" icon: a dinner plate that divides fruits, vegetables, grains, protein and dairy into appropriate portions on a colorful place setting.

With more than 33 percent of American adults overweight or obese—resulting in medical costs of about $147 billion a year, according to 2009 study in Health Affairs—and 17 percent of children and adolescents also above a healthy weight, eating more nutritiously is paramount.

"We need to make sure we have the most nutritious food that we can," says Texas Representative Carol Alvarado. "A child who receives a healthy meal will be a better student, a healthier adult and less likely to have heart disease and diabetes."

Healthy eating is an issue many lawmakers have already tackled. Some support comes from those who want to encourage healthy choices by bringing more fruit and vegetables to their communities. Others see a silver lining in the salad plate: a lift to local economies by promoting state agriculture products.

Fill Half Your Plate with Produce

The new dietary guidelines recommend a plate half full of fruits and vegetables. Yet 32 states scored at or below the national average, in a 2011 report by the Centers for Disease Control and Prevention. The report looked at the availability of supermarkets, produce stands and farmers' markets that typically sell healthy foods such as fresh produce, whole grains and low-fat dairy products.

"My district is underserved by grocery stores and has more convenience stores that don't provide fruits and vegetables," says Alvarado. "I support community gardens—it teaches children about where food comes from and how it grows and also teaches them to take pride in their community."

State legislatures in Illinois, Louisiana, New York and Pennsylvania have supported public-private partnerships to bring healthy food sellers into urban, suburban and rural communities currently starved of produce. Not only can this help local diets, it also may give a boost to local economies. Grants, loans and tax credits are offered to grocery operators to build new full-service stores or improve existing facilities by adding refrigerated storage for fresh produce, for example. In Pennsylvania, over a five-year span, 5,000 jobs were created or retained as a result. New federal funding is available to states for these efforts.

California legislators in 2011 enacted a tax credit for farmers who donate fruits and vegetables to food banks. In 2010, Mississippi lawmakers exempted food grown or processed in Mississippi and sold at farmers' markets from the sales tax. Laws in California, Illinois, Nebraska and Washington support electronic card readers at farmers' markets to encourage public benefit recipients to use their cards to buy fresh produce.

Lawmakers have also looked at promoting healthier habits for school children while supporting local economies by purchasing local food for schools. In 2011, Michigan legislators created a school purchasing preference for food grown or produced by Michigan businesses. New Jersey lawmakers enacted a "Jersey Fresh" program that allows schools to adopt price preferences for local agricultural and farm products, improve kitchen facilities to incorporate more fresh, locally grown produce, and add information about the value of eating fresh, locally grown produce to school curricula.

"Educating our children about our state's diverse and delicious agricultural fare and the nutritious value of local and safe 'Jersey Fresh' produce will help them cultivate healthier food choices and make them aware of the importance of supporting local farmers," says New Jersey Assemblyman John McKeon.

A Rutgers University report found that $1.1 million spent in New Jersey in 2000 to promote local fare had an economic impact of $63.2 million. It also generated an increase in state and local tax revenue by $2.2 million for the year. In 2011–2012 Oregon legislators created grants to reimburse districts for buying local food products and for conducting certain food-based educational activities.

Last year, Missouri Representative Casey Guernsey sponsored legislation that established a Farm-to-Table Advisory Board to "link schools and state institutions with local and regional farms for the purchase of locally grown agricultural products; increase market opportunities for locally grown agricultural products; and assist schools and other entities to teach children and the public about nutrition, food choices, obesity, and health; and the value of having an accessible supply of locally grown food."

In Colorado and Massachusetts, lawmakers established food policy advisory councils in 2010. Massachusetts directed its council to increase local food production and state use of local products. Colorado's council is charged with fostering a healthy food supply while enhancing agricultural and natural resources, encouraging economic growth, promoting "Colorado Proud" products and improving community health.

In Texas, a "Go Texan" agricultural marketing and promotion effort by Senator Craig Estes supports programs for rural economic development, marketing and promotion of agricultural and other products grown, processed, or produced in the state. Vermont also enacted legislation in 2011 to encourage economic development by marketing state foods and products.

In 2011, legislators in at least six other states—Georgia, New Mexico, New York, South Carolina, Virginia and Washington—proposed legislation to encourage local food purchasing or "buying from the backyard" by state agencies or schools. Five of those bills carried over into 2012.

Bring on the Amber Waves

Grains cover another quarter of the USDA-recommended plate. The new dietary guidelines advise "make at least half your grains whole grains." An Oregon law enacted in 2011 puts whole grain flours on an equal footing with enriched flour. Previously, only enriched flour met health requirements for manufacturers of bread, rolls or buns.

Guidelines for healthy school foods and snacks in North Carolina and Rhode Island call for increasing whole grain and grain products. Texas has just created a grain producers indemnity fund to protect farmers from economic hardship.

Pack in the Protein

Most Americans eat enough protein, but the new guidelines encourage leaner and more varied selections of protein-rich foods. Meat, poultry, fish, beans, eggs, peanut butter and nuts or seeds all provide protein. Legislators focused on fish last year in at least two states.

Rhode Island's fishing community will benefit from a newly created Seafood Marketing Collaborative to support local fishermen and small businesses. It will be promoting the health and vitality of the state's seafood populations, identifying regulatory restrictions that inhibit local seafood businesses, and increasing consumer demand for local seafood through marketing.

Even in land-locked Nebraska, legislators appropriated funds to enhance fisheries by improving hatcheries and buying and developing fishing facilities that improve access for fishermen.

Washington appropriated $3.47 million for improving recreational fisheries. Legislators also directed state agencies to look for partnerships that will help keep fish hatcheries operating with less reliance on state money. In 2009, another New England state, Vermont, established a milk and meat pilot program to encourage purchasing local milk and meat for school meals and to provide technical assistance to schools to help them provide the most local fruits and vegetables possible.

In Arkansas and Indiana, lawmakers established liability protection for agritourism, which encourages education, entertainment or recreation on farms and ranches.

Get in the Moo-ed

MyPlate places a cool blue glass of milk next to the plate as a reminder that the dietary guidelines recommend switching to fat-free or low-fat milk. Dairy products add protein, as well as calcium, vitamins D, B12 and A, phosphorus, and potassium.

Licensed child-care facilities in California must now provide water and serve only low-fat or nonfat milk to children older than 2. Minnesota appropriated $500,000 for each of the next two years to the state's six Second Harvest food banks to purchase milk from Minnesota processors.

Massachusetts legislators, in 2010, directed the state's public health department to use scientific guidelines to set standards for school snacks and beverages that encourage greater consumption of water, low- and nonfat milk, fresh fruits and vegetables, and reduction of fat and sugar in snacks. Beverage standards set by Louisiana legislators in 2009 require high schools to serve low-fat milk or skim milk.

In New York, a Calcium Purchasing Preference Initiative is pending that would require foods and beverages that contain a higher level of calcium to be purchased for government buildings so long as they are same quality, and equal or lower in price.

Critical Thinking

1. Assess how local economies can benefit from the MyPlate guidelines.
2. Discuss the benefits of community gardens.
3. Identify five examples of how local, state, and federal government can promote the consumption of fruits and vegetables and stimulate local economies.

Create Central

www.mhhe.com/createcentral

Internet References

American Association of Community Gardens
www.communitygarden.org

Fruit and Veggies: More Matters
www.fruitsandveggiesmorematters.org

My Plate
www.myplate.gov

National Conference of State Legislators
www.ncsl.org

United States Department of Agriculture (USDA)
www.USDA.gov

Amy Winterfeld tracks nutrition issues for NCSL.

Article Prepared by: Janet Colson, *Middle Tennessee State University*

Cause + Effect

Nutrition labels might be informative, but they're not worth the package space if consumers don't understand them. One Johns Hopkins researcher explains how public policy experts could use marketers' help—and messaging prowess—to alter unhealthy consumer behaviors and develop a solution to America's obesity epidemic.

ELISABETH A. SULLIVAN

Learning Outcomes

After reading this article, you will be able to:

- Describe how the Patient Protection and Affordable Care Act of 2010 will impact restaurants and vending companies with 20 or more locations.
- Explain the premise of tracking calories using physical activity equivalents.

The link between marketing and public policy stands in stark relief against America's struggle with obesity. For years, critics have questioned the potency of marketing messages aimed at younger audiences that promote sugary cereals, high-fat and high-calorie foods or otherwise less-than-optimal consumables. At the same time, advocates have championed marketers' ability to help promote healthier consumption behaviors and encourage consumers to balance their caloric intake with more active lifestyles. Marketers wield considerable power over what consumers choose to consume—and public policy experts such as Sara Bleich want to harness that power to help alleviate the obesity problem in the United States and beyond.

Bleich, an assistant professor at Johns Hopkins' Bloomberg School of Public Health, is working to help check obesity and related diseases by researching, as her bio says, "the intersection between public policy and obesity prevention/control," including "novel environmental strategies to reduce caloric intake." Marketing, she says, plays a central role both in her research and in possible remedies to the country's obesity problem.

Late last year, Bleich and co-authors Bradley Herring, Desmond Flagg and Tiffany Gary-Webb released the results of a study that examined the effect of store signage on teens' purchase of sugary beverages. The study involved 1,600 beverage purchases made by 12- to 18-year-olds in four corner stores in Baltimore. The article, called "Reduction in Purchases of Sugar-Sweetened Beverages Among Low-Income, Black Adolescents After Exposure to Caloric Information," was published in the *American Journal of Public Health* and garnered considerable media attention, partly because it deals with the hot-button issue of obesity but mostly because it presents a noteworthy finding: that consumers' purchase decisions might be influenced by products' nutritional information that replaces the traditional calorie number with what Bleich calls the "physical activity equivalent."

Marketing News caught up with Bleich to discuss how her consumer behavior research was carried out and what the findings might mean for food and beverage marketers.

Q: Why did you decide to study the power of messaging regarding sugary, high-calorie drinks, in particular?

A: We know that people generally don't have a good understanding of the amount of calories that are in the food that they eat, and Americans typically have low numeracy skills and poor skills when it comes to calorie literacy. Basically, they don't have a good sense of what's in the foods that they eat in terms of calories and they're not good at doing mental math.

Since health reform is going to require that if you're a chain outlet with more than 20 stores, starting in the middle of this year, you're going to have to post calorie information, we thought, Well, maybe the current standard, which is calorie counts, won't be the most effective way to get people information. What we wanted to do was test three different ways of giving them information, the first being absolute calorie counts and then two others, which are much easier for people to understand without doing any mental math, and look at the effect on sugar-sweetened beverage purchases.

And we specifically focused on sugar-sweetened beverage purchases [because] when it comes to thinking about dealing with the obesity problem, there's a close link between sugar-sweetened beverage consumption and obesity. It also, in terms of a category, is very easy to isolate beverages and try to get people to consume less of them, whereas obviously food

Nutrition Tips in the Chip Aisle

In an attempt to participate in consumers' nutritional education with an industry-led initiative, several grocery store chains now feature third-party-provided nutritional ratings systems on their shelves to help guide consumers toward healthier choices within product categories. One such system, developed by Braintree, Mass.-based NuVal, takes into account more than 30 nutritional elements such as protein, calcium and vitamins, as well as sugar, sodium and cholesterol, and uses a point system to signify that higher-rated products are the healthier choices within the given category. The NuVal System currently is offered in stores such as Meijer, Kroger and Pick 'n Save, among others.

Menus Are about to Get a Whole Lot Lengthier

Nutrition-related federal legislation introduced in March 2010 is about to take effect, requiring restaurant chains—and vending machine companies—to make calorie counts and nutritional information readily available. As part of the Patient Protection and Affordable Care Act of 2010, restaurants with 20 or more locations must list calorie information for their standard menu items on all menus—including drive-through menus. Restaurants also must have other nutritional information available for consumers who request it, including a listing of the product's total calories, fat, saturated fat, cholesterol, sodium, total carbohydrates, sugars, fiber and protein.

is something where it's a little bit harder. But if you can get someone to not buy soda and maybe buy water, you can actually pull a lot of empty calories out of their diet pretty easily.

Q: How did you decide on the messaging to test?

A: We knew we wanted to do absolute calories, which is the current standard, and then two different types of relative information, so we just sat down and brainstormed and figured out, Let's do a percentage of daily intake, which is another way that we often see calories represented. And then the third was the physical activity equivalent, which is just novel and we thought that it would be more meaningful to people than both absolute calories and the percent daily value.

In terms of how we picked jogging as opposed to yoga or dancing or basketball, or a million other things that we could choose from, there's research that suggests that negative messaging is a little bit more powerful than positive messaging, so we purposefully did not pick something like dancing or basketball, which may have been attractive to our target population, which was black adolescents between the ages of 12 to 18. We chose jogging, which may be perceived as a little bit less desirable.

We calculated, for the average 110-pound adolescent, how many minutes of jogging they'd have to do to burn off a 250-calorie bottle of soda and that was about 50 minutes. And that [physical activity equivalent] sign was the most effective at reducing sugar-sweetened beverage purchasing.

[Editor's note: The study found that the signs listing the "absolute calorie" and "percentage of daily intake" information reduced the likelihood of sugar-sweetened beverage purchases by 40 percent compared with the baseline of no signage, while the "physical activity equivalent" sign reduced the likelihood of such purchases by 50 percent.]

Q: You tested this in corner stores in Baltimore. How was it logistically set up? You had the signage in there, and then did you have field researchers watching kids come in and gauging their reactions when they saw the signs? Did you have video set up or were you interviewing them?

A: I've been asked this question so many times and it's a good question. What we did is, basically, you walk into a store and you're a customer, and there are these walls of beverage cases. On the beverage cases is an 8 ½-by-11-inch sign. There's one type of sign, but there could be multiple signs if there are multiple beverage cases. But basically, it's at eye level, it's 8 ½ by 11 and it has a message on it, and it's one of three messages, which are randomized across the stores and you're only going to see one message at a time.

So you walk into the store, you go to open up the beverage case and the sign is right in front of you, and you make your selection. We had a research assistant sitting in the store in sort of an out-of-the-way place with a full, clear view of the counter and, for a random sample of adolescents who were purchasing beverages, he would record the beverage that they purchased. We purposefully did not intervene and say: 'Are you, a.) black, b.) between the ages of 12 and 18, and, c.) what did you purchase?' because we knew that the minute we started asking questions, it would mitigate the effect of information on purchasing, so we simply observed. And in the instance where an adolescent was buying two different beverages, we simply recorded the one that hit the counter first, but that was a very rare occurrence. That research assistant was consistent across all the stores and he would just observe the purchases and record them, and then we'd analyze the data later.

The other thing I should add is that to ensure that we'd get our target population, the stores had to be in zip codes that had at least 70 percent black population and they had to be located within walking distance—so less than five city blocks—of middle and high schools because that was the target age group.

Q: What was the timeline for the study?

A: It was about six months. It started in May and ended in October. It was a total of four stores and we started data collection at two of the stores first, had about a month or so of overlap time and then concluded with the second two stores. The primary reason for that was because of possible issues of seasonality because it could be that people drink differently in the summer than they do when it's a little bit colder outside, so we adjusted for all of that in the models but purposefully staggered the data collection periods.

Q: And the results were quantitative, mainly? You were really just gauging what sold after people encountered the signage?

A: Exactly. Our denominator was all purchases and we were looking at the percentage of sugar-sweetened beverage purchases.

Q: Was the researcher taking note of whether the customer looked at the signs?

A: We qualitatively talked about this. Weekly, we'd check in and he'd tell me about the signs. . . . [The research assistant] certainly said that adolescents noticed the signs, but again, we purposefully didn't stop them and say, 'Did you notice the sign and did it affect your purchasing behavior?' We simply observed the purchase.

But we have been funded to do this study again and in that, we will both be doing focus groups on the front end to ask adolescents—this time including Hispanic adolescents, too—'What sorts of things are most effective? Is it a physical activity equivalent? Is it the number of teaspoons of sugar in a can of soda?' Then on the back end, we'll do exit interviews among a sample of adolescents and ask them, 'Did you see the signs and how did it affect your behavior?'

Q: Are you also going to test whether this kind of signage or messaging would work on a label versus on a sign?

A: I think, logistically, that would be very hard because that would require a partnership with Coca-Cola or some other bottling company and I would imagine that they would be somewhat hesitant to allow us to do that. I mean, if they would, I would love to, but I think that would be somewhat tough. But it's something that would be interesting to try.

Another thing that we will look at in the follow-up study is we've [already] observed: Signs are posted and what's the immediate effect on purchasing behaviors when it comes to sugary beverages? But there could be some post-intervention effects, such that the signs come down and for three to six to nine months out, people are still being affected by what they saw previously, and we'll also test that post-intervention effect in the follow-up study.

Q: If we're going to extrapolate on these findings and guess at what kind of lasting consumer behavioral changes might take place, what do you think such signage would do? Do you think that this will increase consumers' food literacy and nutritional literacy so that they might reconsider imbibing so many sugary beverages a day? What are you hoping that this kind of educational tool will result in?

A: My sense is that this sort of information is not necessarily educating the consumer, but really it's making information more interpretable. Right now, anything that you buy that's packaged has calories on it—cookies have 200 calories, a bag of chips has 300 calories—but if you don't have a good sense of, a.) how many calories you should have in a given day and, b.) what the tradeoff is in terms of how much exercise you have to do to burn that off, I don't think people realize how much they're consuming.

What I hope this type of information will do is it will cause people to pause and say: 'I'm going to have to run for an hour and a half to burn off a bag of chips? Maybe I'll just forego the bag of chips. Maybe I'll get something that's lower-calorie instead.' By increasing the transparency around the, sort of, tradeoff between consumption and expenditure, I think it would make it easier for people to make more educated decisions about their consumption.

Q: How about from a marketplace perspective, though? Are you hoping, ultimately, that marketers will start to change their labels to be exercise-related rather than calorie-focused, or are you hoping that this will inspire more of a public service announcement approach across the industry in which this kind of educational messaging will be pumped out?

A: I think both would be wonderful. A challenge that we have in private industry is that the way that nutrition information is reported varies quite a bit by product line and by the type of item that it is. The way you see things on a can of Coke may be different than you see things on a box of sugary cereal. . . . One thing that would need to happen that's going to be really important is that assuming that we were able to provide calorie information in the form of a physical activity equivalent, it would have to be something that's standardized across the different products because if you see minutes of running in one place, minutes of yoga somewhere else and minutes of basketball in a third place, my guess is that it may lose its meaning with consumers. But if it's the same message consistently, I think that could actually have an effect.

We have to figure out, what kind of physical activity is most meaningful when it comes to changing behavior? My guess, from the literature and from this study, is that it's probably something that's more on the negative side because if you pick something that people enjoy doing, they're going to say, 'Oh, well, I'll go dancing for an hour and burn off that piece of pizza.' But if they have to run or do sit-ups or push-ups, it's not really as desirable. I guess that's the first thing.

The second is that there's obviously logistical concerns. If you're putting on a can of soda '150 or 250 calories,' that takes up a certain amount of space. If you then want to try to say, 'This is the equivalent of 50 minutes of jogging,' that'd take up a lot more space, so I think you have to figure out the best way to present this information. And if you standardized it across all of the different product lines, I think that would allow you to condense it even more because people would be used to seeing that information presented in a certain way. But I would say that, in the case of chain restaurants, the information has to be posted by the middle of this year per federal legislation, so from a public health perspective, how can we maximize something that, from a legislative perspective, is going to happen? I think that what this study tells me is that simply using calorie counts is probably not the most effective way to alter behavior.

Q: Based on studies like yours that show that exercise-related messaging could be effective, do you think that the federal government is going to step in and mandate that that sort of language be used on labels or would it be an industry-led initiative?

A: I would be surprised if there were legislation largely because I think, the industry could make the argument, which is compelling, that the information is already there and it's already required to be there. You turn this package over and it says how many calories per serving are in something. There's been a lot of industry-led initiatives when it comes to anti-obesity, anti-calorie things over the past four or five years and I think a lot of that seems to be an effort to, sort of, make sure that the heavy hand of government doesn't come down or to stay ahead of it.

Sure, I think we could see different companies thinking about ways to put information on product labeling by pulling stuff out of the bag that's supposedly useful to consumers. I would say that if you are PepsiCo, for example, maybe you could think about looking at your product line and saying: 'A bag of Fritos would be 50 minutes of running, but a bag of 'x' would be 20 minutes of running. Why don't you instead choose a bag of 'x'?' By using the substitution effect, it would be cost-neutral in the sense that you're not losing consumers; you're just driving them to a different product line.

I think the key with any of these types of studies where you're trying to change consumer behavior is that from a public health perspective, we're excited when people change what they do, but from a private industry perspective, it's got to be cost-neutral because if it's the case that I put these signs up in stores and people choose not to buy anything, then the stores aren't going to want to participate. What we found is that sugar-sweetened beverage purchases went down, but then water purchases went up. We don't know, exactly, whether or not it was perfectly cost-neutral, but what the results suggest is that if you're thirsty, you're going to buy something, but that information will sway what that something will be.

+ Food Label Literacy

59 percent of respondents to a global study conducted by Nielsen have trouble understanding nutrition labels. In the U.S., while the food label literacy rates compare favorably with that global average, more than four in 10 consumers (42 percent) still report having trouble understanding the nutritional information on packaging.

Globally, 33 percent of respondents trust calorie counts to be "always accurate" and 58 percent say that they're "sometimes accurate."

When it comes to more ambiguous nutritional claims such as "fresh," "all-natural" and "heart-healthy," approximately 80 percent of consumers doubt their veracity.

The Nielsen Global Survey of Food Labeling Trends was conducted in March and April, and August and September of 2011, and polled more than 25,000 respondents in 56 countries.

Q: What role, ideally, would marketers play in this effort to reduce consumers' caloric intake? As you're talking about here, it's a profit question and changes might impact bottom lines if Coke, for example, all of a sudden does have to put this messaging on its cans to dissuade a consumer from buying the product. That's obviously not appealing to Coke's interests, yet marketers certainly have a role to play in fostering good public health.

A: I'm one of those people who think that private industry is not the devil and that there's lots of things that public health [organizations] could do to partner with industry and think about, what are some ways that we can marry the interest in maximizing health on the public health side and the fiduciary responsibility that private industry has to maximize profits for their shareholders? How can you marry those two objectives and find things that actually work? . . .

What should happen is that these sorts of messages should be tested in a larger audience using focus groups and other sorts of mechanisms to figure out, what is the most effective way to influence people and influence different types of people? We focused on a small swath of the population, black adolescents. My sense is that this is a group who's at very high obesity risk and may or may not have strong concerns when it comes to calories and exercise and that sort of thing. If you took a swath of the population, say, middle-income white women for whom those concerns are very strong, and you gave them this sort of information, I think the effect would be much, much larger.

So I think the role that marketing could possibly play is thinking about how you take these sorts of interventions and do them on a grander scale, and then spin them in a way that's really effective. I have no background in marketing, so who knows if someone could come in that has a lot of expertise and make these signs a million times more effective by just changing a few words, or changing the colors or changing the images and that sort of thing? . . .

People are not stupid, but messages have to be simple and easily understandable in a very short amount of time when you're about to make a purchase. Where research needs to go and what marketing can possibly do is to think about how you take this complicated information, when you're combining items on a menu or having combo meals, and give it to people in easily interpretable formats. Just telling them these broad calorie numbers is not very meaningful to the average person.

Q: Is the marketer's job done when the communication has been effectively made? Corporations can change their messaging, their labeling and packaging methods, and then can they stop there? Or should they be investing in other public service or public policy initiatives to try to get people to be healthier?

A: Is it the case that you stop once you get information to consumers and you allow them to run with it? From a marketing perspective, if you have a good message, you've done your job by putting it out there. I think the bigger question is, what are you putting out there?

"It's not going to fix the problem of obesity, but more transparency about what we're eating and helping people make better decisions at the point of purchase can be effective, so I think marketing has a huge role to play."

I do think that more effort should be made to think about how you change the messages to create healthier environments. Obviously, marketing can't change the fact that there are lots of convenience stores or lots of fast-food restaurants, but marketing can change how different product lines are marketed and to whom they're targeted. Again, I strongly believe that if you are one of these big multinationals like Coca-Cola or Pepsi, you have a very diverse product line, so simply encouraging people toward the healthier side will, hopefully, not hurt your bottom line. It will just diversify what people are actually purchasing. . . . I think the key is using marketing to actually change demand—we know it's possible, that you can actually induce demand—and try to help people and steer them in the right direction when it comes to healthier eating. . . .

What's going to have to happen is to do the good public health research, we have to figure out what the most effective messaging is and that's going to come directly from marketing. That's an area where I have no expertise, so we're going to have to collaborate in terms of figuring out the most convincing way to tell people. The punch line that I try to get across is the reason that we are getting bigger as a country and across all developed countries is not because, on average, we're exercising too little. It's because we're simply eating too much. So how do you pull some calories out of the diet? I think that these messages can move us in that direction. It's not going to fix the problem of obesity, but more transparency about what we're eating and helping people make better decisions at the point of purchase can be effective, so I think marketing has a huge role to play.

Critical Thinking

1. Describe how the Patient Protection and Affordable Care Act of 2010 will impact restaurants and vending companies with 20 or more locations.
2. Explain the premise of tracking calories using physical activity equivalents.

Create Central

www.mhhe.com/createcentral

Internet References

Affordable Care Act
www.hhs.gov/healthcare/rights/law/index.html

American Marketing Association
www.marketingpower.com

California's Menu Labeling Law (CA Restaurant Association)
www.calrest.org/issues-policies/key-issues/health-nutrition/menu-labeling/overview-ca-menu-labeling-law

How to Understand and Use the Nutrition Facts Label (FDA)
www.fda.gov/Food/IngredientsPackagingLabeling/LabelingNutrition/ucm274593.htm

National Restaurant Association
www.restaurant.org/News-Research/Research

Article

Prepared by: Janet Colson, *Middle Tennessee State University*

Can Social Media Produce Wellness Results?

MICHELLE V. RAFTER

Learning Outcomes

After reading this article, you will be able to:

- Explain how a company can use "gamification" to promote workplace wellness.
- Evaluate the potential of using social media software within corporate wellness programs.

For years, *Chilton Hospital* tried to get employees to take better care of themselves.

The northwest New Jersey hospital's human resources staff launched diabetes and other disease management initiatives to improve employee well-being and reduce health care costs. But the resulting behavior changes were minor, and the programs only covered a small number of employees.

That changed, though, when Chilton switched gears to a wellness program that asked employees to get social and competitive.

In March 2011, Chilton entered a countywide fitness challenge where employees vied in teams of six against other local businesses to see who could eat the healthiest, walk the most or drop the most weight. During the 100-day challenge, competitors logged onto a private, Facebook-like social network to share results and cheer each other on. To get employees to participate, the 256-bed hospital offered $150 to each member of the winning team and $500 to the employee who shed the most pounds. All told, 56 teams signed up, about 37 percent of the staff. In the end, though, it wasn't the money that drew the workers in. It was the online camaraderie, and the challenge. "People wanted to be on the winning team," says Julie McGovern, Chilton's vice president of administration and HR.

Experiences like Chilton's are playing out across the country as companies rebuild their employee wellness programs on Internet-based social networks that are equal parts health journal, fitness challenge and online support group.

Companies hope the programs will curb escalating costs for health care benefits. In 2008, the first year American Financial Group, or AFG, ran a social media-based walking program through vendor *WalkingSpree,* the insurance company saved $9.27 in employee health care costs for every $1 spent on the program. The insurance company's health care premiums stayed flat that year because employees were healthier, according to a testimonial from AFG, which continues to use the program.

Aside from cutting costs, online-based wellness applications can help retain talent. The programs generally make employees feel better about themselves, and by extension, with the place they work, so they'll stick around longer.

"Employers are starting to recognize that incorporating elements of social media into a wellness program can boost participation and engagement and help create that buzz and culture around health and wellness that traditional engagement" methods aren't generating, says Kristie Howard, a vice president at *Longfellow Benefits,* a Boston-based benefits consultant.

Social wellness games represent a confluence of some of today's most significant online and workplace trends. One of the biggest is "gamification," or adding gamelike features to software and other business processes to make them more fun and engaging. Technology analyst Gartner Group predicts that by 2014, *70 percent* of the 2,000 largest companies in the world will use at least one "gamified" enterprise software application.

With more companies using internal social networks such as Yammer and Socialtext to improve workforce collaboration, *replace email* or streamline other aspects of work, it's easing the way for workplaces to adopt Internet-based platforms for wellness games and challenges. When wellness tech vendor *ShapeUp Inc.* polled 351 U.S. corporate wellness executives this spring, 56 percent said that they were using some type of online competition or challenge, and another 40 percent were considering it. "It's a natural migration for wellness programs," says Shawn LaVana, ShapeUp's marketing vice president.

Like other tech innovations that started out as consumer products before migrating to the world of work, many social wellness services had their roots in the personal health care apps that appeared after the iPhone and other smartphones became commonplace. Software as a service-based internal network such as ShapeUp let employees chart their progress toward losing weight or getting fit, or to record their standings in team or group challenges. Others such as Walkingspree work with pedometers or other devices that employees wear while working out, and then plug into a PC to download data to an online fitness journal.

As more employees bring smartphones to work, it has become easier for employers to offer wellness games and other social media-based content that can be accessed from a mobile device or laptop or desktop computers. But apps don't have to be that sophisticated. Employees can use ShapeUp, for example, to receive fitness-related text messages on a standard cellphone, a selling point for companies with large contingents of blue-collar workers who don't or can't use a smartphone on the job.

Enough companies are interested that industry organizations, such as the Society for Human Resource Management, are holding sessions on social media-based wellness programs at various 2012 annual conferences.

Although some companies stick to Facebook and Twitter or corporate blogs for wellness tips and to promote challenges, more employers are paying monthly or yearly subscription fees to outside vendors to run online programs for them.

To run its social wellness program, Chilton chose *Keas,* a 4-year-old online game platform co-founded by the former head of the now shuttered Google Health. The platform lets employees create profiles, share updates to a Facebook-like news feed, take online health quizzes and keep tabs on their teams and challenges. Wellness program managers use the platform to generate reports on participation, physical activity and other statistics.

During the hospital's first 100-day challenge, 336 employees used the platform to track losing an aggregate 1,230 pounds, eating 8,918 additional servings of fruit and vegetables and putting in 1,274 extra days of exercise, according to McGovern, the facility's administration and HR vice president. "It wasn't just exercise and eating better," she says. "People made a commitment to stop smoking, take stress management classes and control ongoing diseases."

The hospital's already committed to hosting two more challenges this year. But it will take time for the program to affect the hospital's bottom line. To gauge that impact, Chilton is doing free biometric screenings—height, weight, blood pressure, cholesterol and body mass index—once every six months for employees who participate in the challenges. "Because if people can keep the weight off, it will ultimately be a positive thing," for them and the company, McGovern says.

Elsewhere, reception of the new generation wellness programs has been strong. In ShapeUp's survey, 75 percent of companies offering some type of online fitness challenge said it had improved employees' perception of their corporate wellness program, and 71 percent said employees were using more wellness resources because of the programs. "It's getting people to take ownership of their health," says Fran Melmed, an employee wellness communications consultant who conducted the survey for ShapeUp.

For some companies, social wellness programs are already paying off. Sprint Nextel Corp. *estimates it saved approximately $1.1 million* through a companywide fitness challenge launched in 2011 as employees' healthier lifestyles led to fewer medical claims. In the company's first 12-week Sprint Get Fit Challenge, run by ShapeUp and benefits provider OptumHealth, about 16,000 employees in teams of up to 11 lost a collective 41,000 pounds, took more than 4.8 billion steps and logged nearly 22 million exercise minutes, according to the company.

Other employers and social wellness vendors are still calculating the return on investment such products can have. Traditional wellness programs such as Weight Watchers have a head start because of their longevity, Melmed says, but new vendors are taking steps to quantify how well their programs work. ShapeUp and Healthways Inc.'s *MeYou Health,* for example, are doing studies to compile hard data, she says.

A weight-loss study that ShapeUp conducted in 2009 is one of the first analyses of online-based employee-wellness programs to be published in a peer-reviewed medical or scientific journal. The results are based on data from 3,330 overweight or obese people in 987 teams that completed a 12-week online challenge. The results, published online in March by *Obesity,* a research journal, support the theory that online programs that let people work out with teammates can help workers lose weight, according to the report.

Despite the advantages social wellness programs offer, some employees worry about their personal information being compromised, says Howard of Longfellow Benefits who helped start the *Worksite Wellness Council of Massachusetts* last year. Howard isn't aware of any breaches, "but due to the potential for issues with HIPAA privacy, social media is an area employers and wellness vendors should approach cautiously," she says. Also to avoid privacy issues, social wellness product vendors are being careful to use their platforms to share health and wellness information but not dispense personalized health care advice, Howard says.

Melmed agrees. "Employers should look to insurers and other third parties to help them expand their programs with sensors or devices," she says. "That way the employer gets a better sense of movement, activity or engagement but doesn't get into how many steps Suzy or Jack took today. It makes for an easier, cleaner message to the employee as well."

It may be easy to get employees excited about an eight- or 10-week weight-loss challenge or a one-time companywide biometric screening. But for long-term success, social media-based programs need to be part of a larger commitment, wellness experts say.

In addition to online challenges, a wellness program has to foster ongoing discussion of healthy lifestyles, whether through a digital network, blog, e-newsletter or old-fashioned print materials, says Jennifer Benz, founder of a San Francisco-based employee wellness communications consultancy. Companies also need to offer a healthy work environment, one with fitness facilities, nutritious options in the cafeteria and a culture that doesn't prize overtime at the expense of its employees' well-being, says Benz, who partnered with wellness application vendor Limeade on a wellness app platform called *Limeade GreenLine.* "You have to address all those structure things that get in the way of people achieving their optimal health," she says.

Chilton Hospital has taken that advice to heart. Since that first 100-day challenge a year ago, the hospital put a walking path around campus and organized walking groups and a hiking club. McGovern scaled back the prizes she's offering for signups and winners because workers no longer need as much persuading.

McGovern says she believes that the combination of the online wellness challenge, biometric screenings and running a separate disease management program will eventually help the hospital cut health care costs. The social media wellness campaign is a major part of that, especially because so many of the facility's employees who don't sit at a desk all day can use it. And they are—everyone from nurses to the cleaning crew and cafeteria staff. "They're finding ways to use it on their breaks, or on their smartphones at home," she says. "To have so many people participating, it shows you how much they want to do it."

Critical Thinking

1. Evaluate the potential of using social media software to encourage weight loss and the adoption of healthy lifestyles.
2. Define gamification. Explain how gamification can be used in corporate wellness programs.
3. Summarize the wellness program developed by Chilton Hospital in New Jersey.

Create Central

www.mhhe.com/createcentral

Internet References

Center for Disease Control and Prevention. National Healthy Workplace Wellness Program
www.cdc.gov/nationalhealthyworksite/index.html

National Coalition of Promoting Physical Activity
www.ncppa.org/membership

U.S. Department of Labor and the U.S. Department of Health and Human Services.Workplace Wellness Study, 2013
www.dol.gov/ebsa/pdf/workplacewellnessstudyfinal.pdf

Michelle V. Rafter is a *Workforce Management* contributing editor.

Article

Prepared by: Janet Colson, *Middle Tennessee State University*

Tea's Good for the Heart: Studies Show a Few Cups a Day Keep Heart Disease at Bay

LORI ZANTESON

Learning Outcomes

After reading this article, you will be able to:

- Describe the five types of tea.
- Recognize the health-promoting substance found in various types of tea and the possible benefits of each.

There's nothing like having a hot cup of tea to jump-start your morning or a tall glass of iced tea to cool you off in the summertime.

For more than 5,000 years, various peoples and cultures across the globe have enjoyed drinking tea, making it the most consumed beverage second only to water. Fortunately, our tea-drinking ancestors had the wisdom to recognize its value and the foresight to continue the tradition of enjoying this elixir that we now know has powerful health benefits. One of the many known benefits uncovered by modern research: High tea consumption leads to a healthier heart.

Upbeat Findings

According to data published in 2012 in *Food & Function,* black and green tea may reduce the risk of coronary heart disease and stroke by 10% to 20%.[1] Two years before, one of the largest studies on the impact of tea drinking on heart health was published in *Arteriosclerosis, Thrombosis and Vascular Biology.* The study followed more than 37,000 people in the Netherlands for 13 years and found that people who drink plenty of tea are less likely to die of heart disease than people who don't drink tea. Study participants who drank three to six cups of tea per day were 45% less likely to die from heart disease than those who drank less than one cup, and drinking more than six cups of tea per day was associated with a 36% lower risk of developing heart disease than drinking less than one cup.[2]

Tea Defined

While all four types of tea known as true teas—white, green, oolong, and black—offer myriad health benefits, most studies show that black and green teas are the heart-health leaders. Each tea type is made from the leaves of the evergreen shrub *Camellia sinensis,* but the differences between them are due to the ways in which they're processed into individual varieties.

White tea is the least processed and is made from buds and certain leaves of the *Camellia sinensis* plant, which are steamed and dried. Green tea is produced from freshly harvested leaves, which immediately are steamed to prevent oxidation or oxygen exposure. Oolong tea is allowed to oxidize for a short period, and black tea is completely oxidized. The results of the varying degrees of oxidation affect the health-promoting components, which make each type of tea unique.

Go Green

The steaming process of green tea destroys the enzymes that break down the color pigments in the leaves, allowing them to maintain their green color. The leaves then are rolled and dried, preserving their natural polyphenols, the potent antioxidants.

Most of the polyphenols in green tea are in the form of flavonoids, specifically known as catechins, the plant chemicals responsible for green tea's heart-healthy properties. Because of the differences in processing, green tea contains the most catechins of the other tea varieties. Of the six types of catechins in green tea, epigallocatechin-3-gallate (EGCG) is the most studied and most bioactive for heart benefits.

Several recently published studies, such as one in the July 2012 issue of *Pharmacological Reports,* show that the powerful antioxidants in green tea, particularly EGCG, may help prevent atherosclerosis, specifically coronary artery disease, because of their anti-inflammatory effects on plaque buildup in the bloodstream and arterial walls, which can lead to heart disease and stroke.[3]

Green tea catechins also work together to lower cholesterol. A systematic review and meta-analysis in the November 2011 issue of the Journal of the American Dietetic Association reported that of the 20 randomized controlled trials evaluated, "the consumption of green tea catechins is associated with a statistically significant reduction in total and LDL cholesterol levels."[4]

In addition to lowering inflammation in the bloodstream and reducing LDL cholesterol, tea protects LDL particles from becoming oxidized, which causes plaque buildup in the arteries and can lead to atherosclerosis, according to Janet Bond Brill, PhD, RD, LDN, CSSD, an expert on food and fitness for heart health and the author of several books, including the forthcoming *Blood Pressure Down: The 10-Step Plan to Lower Your Blood Pressure in 4 Weeks Without Prescription Drugs.*

In the Black

Black tea may not have as many polyphenols as its green counterpart, but the changes in its polyphenols during the oxidation process produce a set of unique compounds that have their own heart-health benefits. In fact, a 2012 study published in *Preventive Medicine* found that drinking three cups of black tea per day for 12 weeks led to significant reductions in blood sugar levels and triglycerides, an increase in HDL cholesterol levels, and increased blood levels of antioxidants, which can protect against oxidative stress and inflammation.[5]

Other research, such as a 2012 study reported in *Archives of Internal Medicine,* has shown black tea improves endothelial function and blood pressure. This study found that drinking three cups of black tea per day for six months lowered both systolic and diastolic blood pressure, which the report said could reduce the risk of cardiovascular disease.[6]

Herbal Teas

Even though green, white, oolong, and black teas pack the most powerful antioxidant punch, herbal teas still are a healthful option, according to Emily Bailey, RD, LD, who oversees the corporate wellness program for the Republic of Tea and is director of nutrition coaching at NutriFormance-Fitness, Therapy, and Performance in St Louis. "Herbal teas have lower concentrations of antioxidants because the chemical composition varies widely among the different plants" from which they're made, she explains. Rooibos, or red tea, made from the South African plant *Aspalathus linearis,* has been shown to have heart benefits, such as in a 2011 study where volunteers drank six cups of rooibos tea per day for six weeks and experienced reduced LDL cholesterol and significantly increased HDL cholesterol, both associated with a lower risk of developing cardiovascular disease.[7]

A common ingredient in many herbal tea blends, hibiscus tea (or tisane) also may be good for the heart. A 2010 study showed that six weeks of drinking hibiscus tea each day lowered blood pressure in pre- and mildly hypertensive adults, which may make it a heart-healthy dietary addition for this group of people.[8]

Herbal teas may be especially relevant for those who don't like green or black teas; the key is to drink it frequently. "The jury is still out on how much tea should be consumed, but adding any to your typical intake can be very beneficial," Bailey says. Whether you steep it yourself—*Consumer Reports* found that tea steeped from bags had the highest antioxidant levels—or choose bottled varieties, Bailey says it's important to choose the "whole, real food first."

"As an RD, the body of research supports eating the food rather than the supplement," Brill says. "The bulk of research supports the people who drink quite a bit of tea." Popping tea supplements may be tempting if the thought of drinking tea all day seems impossible, but frequency, a little creativity, and variety is all it takes, she says.

Steep Often

To maximize the beneficial effects of tea, Brill recommends enjoying it throughout the day. "It functions as an antioxidant, so keep a high level in your bloodstream," she explains. Studies support that timing is important to reap green tea's benefits. A 2004 study in *Circulation* found that when mice were fed a high cholesterol diet and then were injected with green tea extract, they had 55% less plaque in their arteries after three weeks and 73% less after six weeks.[9] A 2008 Greek study found that when people drank green tea they had better blood vessel function just 30 minutes later, which helps prevent atherosclerosis.[10]

Drink tea "several times a day and learn to do it in different ways," Brill says, "[for example] instead of water, drink iced tea." Hot or cold, the benefits are the same, but she suggests drinking it without milk, which can blunt the favorable effect on the arteries. On the other hand, feel free to add a squeeze of lemon juice, which is a source of vitamin C, to add an extra health boost to your cup.

References

1. Bøhn SK, Ward NC, Hodgson JM, Croft KD. Effects of tea and coffee on cardiovascular disease risk. *Food Funct.* 2012;3(6):575–591.
2. de Koning Gans JM, Uiterwaal CS, van der Schouw YT, et al. Tea and coffee consumption and cardiovascular morbidity and mortality. *Arterioscler Thromb Vasc Bio.* 2010;30(8):1665–1671.
3. Li M, Liu JT, Pang XM, Han CJ, Mao JJ. Epigallocatechin-3-gallate inhibits angiotensin II and interleukin-6-induced C-reactive protein production in macrophages. *Pharmacol Rep.* 2012;64(4):912–918.
4. Kim A, Chiu A, Barone MK, et al. Green tea catechins decrease total and low-density lipoprotein cholesterol: a systematic review and meta-analysis. *J Am Diet Assoc.* 2011;111(11):1720–1729.
5. Bahorun T, Luximon-Ramma A, Neergheen-Bhujun VS, et al. The effect of black tea on risk factors of cardiovascular disease in a normal population. *Prev Med.* 2012;54 Suppl:S98–S102.
6. Hodgson JM, Puddey IB, Woodman RJ, et al. Effects of black tea on blood pressure: a randomized controlled trial. *Arch Intern Med.* 2012;172(2):186–188.

7. Marnewick JL, Rautenbach F, Venter I, et al. Effects of rooibos (Aspalathus linearis) on oxidative stress and biochemical parameters in adults at risk for cardiovascular disease. *J Ethnopharmacol.* 2011;133(1):46–52.
8. McKay DL, Chen CY, Saltzman E, Blumberg JB. Hibiscus sabdariffa L. tea (tisane) lowers blood pressure in prehypertensive and mildly hypertensive adults. *J Nutr.* 2010;140(2):298–303.
9. Chyu KY, Babbidge SM, Zhao X, et al. Differential effects of green tea–derived catechin on developing versus established atherosclerosis in apolipoprotein E-null mice. *Circulation.* 2004;109(20):2448–2453.
10. Alexopoulos N, Vlachopoulos C, Aznaouridis K, et al. The acute effect of green tea consumption on endothelial function in healthy individuals. *Eur J Cardiovasc Prev Rehabil.* 2008;15(3):300–305.

Critical Thinking

1. Describe the differences between white, green, and black teas.
2. Compare the polyphenol content of green tea to the content of black tea.
3. Identify the type of tea that is most beneficial to lower each of the following: blood pressure, serum LDL cholesterol, serum tryglyceride, and blood glucose.
4. Look at the various types of tea in your grocery store. Which teas have a health claim? Based on the article, are the claims substantiated?
5. How do the tea-related health benefits suggested in this article compare to the claims approved by the FDA? (See FDA website below.)

Create Central

www.mhhe.com/createcentral

Internet References

Tea Association of the USA
www.teausa.org

United Kingdom Tea Council
www.tea.co.uk

Summary of Qualified Health Claims Subject to Enforcement Discretion (FDA)
www.fda.gov/Food/IngredientsPackagingLabeling/LabelingNutrition/ucm073992.htm#gtea

---

Lori Zanteson is a freelance food, nutrition, and health writer and editor based in southern California.

Article

Prepared by: Janet Colson, *Middle Tennessee State University*

FDA to Investigate Added Caffeine

MICHAEL R. TAYLOR

Learning Outcomes

After reading this article, you will be able to:

- Explain why FDA is concerned about the trend of adding caffeine to foods.
- Outline the current FDA regulations regarding caffeine content of foods and beverages.

The Food and Drug Administration (FDA) has announced that, in response to a trend in which caffeine is being added to a growing number of products, the agency will investigate the safety of caffeine in food products, particularly its effects on children and adolescents.

Q: The announcement comes just as Wrigley's (a subsidiary of Mars) is promoting a new pack of gum with eight pieces, each containing as much caffeine as half a cup of coffee. Is the timing coincidental?

A: The gum is just one more unfortunate example of the trend to add caffeine to food. Our concern is about caffeine appearing in a range of new products, including ones that may be attractive and readily available to children and adolescents, without careful consideration of their cumulative impact.

One pack of this gum is like having four cups of coffee in your pocket. Caffeine is even being added to jelly beans, marshmallows, sunflower seeds and other snacks for its stimulant effect.

Meanwhile, "energy drinks" with caffeine are being aggressively marketed, including to young people. An instant oatmeal on the market boasts that one serving has as much caffeine as a cup of coffee, and then there are similar products, such as a so-called "wired" waffle and "wired" syrup with added caffeine.

The proliferation of these products in the marketplace is very disturbing to us.

Q: What is your first step in this process?

A: We have to address the fundamental question of the potential consequences of all these caffeinated products in the food supply to children and to some adults who may be at risk from excess caffeine consumption. We need to better understand caffeine consumption and use patterns and determine what is a safe level for total consumption of caffeine. Importantly, we need to address the types of products that are appropriate for the addition of caffeine, especially considering the potential for consumption by young children and adolescents.

We've already met with some companies to hear their rationale for adding caffeine to varied products and to express our concern. We've also reached out to the American Beverage Association, which represents the non-alcoholic beverage industry, and the Grocery Manufacturers Association, which represents food, beverage and consumer-products companies.

Q: What is currently considered a safe amount of daily caffeine?

A: For healthy adults FDA has cited 400 milligrams a day—that's about four or five cups of coffee—as an amount not generally associated with dangerous, negative effects. FDA has not set a level for children, but the American Academy of Pediatrics discourages the consumption of caffeine and other stimulants by children and adolescents. We need to continue to look at what are acceptable levels.

We're particularly concerned about children and adolescents and the responsibility FDA and the food industry have to protect public health and respect social norms that suggest we shouldn't be marketing stimulants, such as caffeine, to our children.

Q: What currently are FDA requirements concerning caffeine being added to foods?

A: Manufacturers can add it to products if they decide it meets the relevant safety standards, and if they include it on the ingredient list. While various uses may meet federal food safety standards, the only time FDA explicitly approved adding caffeine was for colas in the 1950s. Existing rules never anticipated the current proliferation of caffeinated products.

Q: Is it possible that FDA would set age restrictions for purchase?

A: We have to be practical; enforcing age restrictions would be challenging. For me, the more fundamental questions are whether it is appropriate to use foods that may be inherently attractive and accessible to children as the vehicle to deliver the stimulant caffeine and whether we should place limits on the amount of caffeine in certain products.

Q: Have you taken any actions on other caffeinated products?

A: In 2010, we brought about the withdrawal from the market of caffeinated alcoholic beverages, primarily malt beverages, in part because of studies indicating that combined ingestion of caffeine and alcohol may lead to hazardous and life-threatening situations. Caffeine can mask some of the sensory cues that people might normally rely on to determine their level of intoxication.

Q: Don't new regulations take a lot of resources and time?

A: They do. But we believe that some in the food industry are on a dubious, potentially dangerous path. If necessary, and if the science indicates that it is warranted, we are prepared to go through the regulatory process to establish clear boundaries and conditions on caffeine use. We are also prepared to consider enforcement action against individual products as appropriate.

However, we hope this can be a turning point for all to prevent the irresponsible addition of caffeine to food and beverages. Together, we should be immediately looking at what voluntary restraint can be used by industry as FDA gets the right regulatory boundaries and conditions in place.

I'm hopeful that industry will step up.

Critical Thinking

1. Why would a company like Wrigley's decide to add caffeine to chewing gums?
2. Explain why FDA is concerned about adding caffeine to chewing gums.
3. Cola products were granted approval to add caffeine in the 1950s. In your opinion, why did the soft drink industry request approval to add caffeine and what has caused the proliferation in beverages and foods that contain added caffeine in recent years?
4. Locate a website for a company that produces foods that add caffeine such as Wired Waffle. Outline the history of the caffeinated food and determine if the company has FDA approval of its caffeinated product.

Create Central

www.mhhe.com/createcentral

Internet References

American Beverage Association
www.ameribev.org

Food and Drug Administration
www.fda.gov

National Grocer's Association
www.nationalgrocers.org

Wired Waffle
www.wiredwaffles.com

Michael R. Taylor, deputy commissioner for foods and veterinary medicine at FDA, answers questions about his concerns and possible FDA actions.

Article

Prepared by: Janet Colson, *Middle Tennessee State University*

The Extraordinary Science of Addictive Junk Food

MICHAEL MOSS

Learning Outcomes

After reading this article, you will be able to:

- Explain why typical processed snack foods are high in salt, sugar, and fat.
- Describe the steps that the food industry takes to develop and test a new product.

On the evening of April 8, 1999, a long line of Town Cars and taxis pulled up to the Minneapolis headquarters of Pillsbury and discharged 11 men who controlled America's largest food companies. Nestlé was in attendance, as were Kraft and Nabisco, General Mills and Procter & Gamble, Coca-Cola and Mars. Rivals any other day, the C.E.O.'s and company presidents had come together for a rare, private meeting. On the agenda was one item: the emerging obesity epidemic and how to deal with it. While the atmosphere was cordial, the men assembled were hardly friends. Their stature was defined by their skill in fighting one another for what they called "stomach share"—the amount of digestive space that any one company's brand can grab from the competition.

James Behnke, a 55-year-old executive at Pillsbury, greeted the men as they arrived. He was anxious but also hopeful about the plan that he and a few other food-company executives had devised to engage the C.E.O.'s on America's growing weight problem. "We were very concerned, and rightfully so, that obesity was becoming a major issue," Behnke recalled. "People were starting to talk about sugar taxes, and there was a lot of pressure on food companies." Getting the company chiefs in the same room to talk about anything, much less a sensitive issue like this, was a tricky business, so Behnke and his fellow organizers had scripted the meeting carefully, honing the message to its barest essentials. "C.E.O.'s in the food industry are typically not technical guys, and they're uncomfortable going to meetings where technical people talk in technical terms about technical things," Behnke said. "They don't want to be embarrassed. They don't want to make commitments. They want to maintain their aloofness and autonomy."

A chemist by training with a doctoral degree in food science, Behnke became Pillsbury's chief technical officer in 1979 and was instrumental in creating a long line of hit products, including microwavable popcorn. He deeply admired Pillsbury but in recent years had grown troubled by pictures of obese children suffering from diabetes and the earliest signs of hypertension and heart disease. In the months leading up to the C.E.O. meeting, he was engaged in conversation with a group of food-science experts who were painting an increasingly grim picture of the public's ability to cope with the industry's formulations—from the body's fragile controls on overeating to the hidden power of some processed foods to make people feel hungrier still. It was time, he and a handful of others felt, to warn the C.E.O.'s that their companies may have gone too far in creating and marketing products that posed the greatest health concerns.

The discussion took place in Pillsbury's auditorium. The first speaker was a vice president of Kraft named Michael Mudd. "I very much appreciate this opportunity to talk to you about childhood obesity and the growing challenge it presents for us all," Mudd began. "Let me say right at the start, this is not an easy subject. There are no easy answers—for what the public health community must do to bring this problem under control or for what the industry should do as others seek to hold it accountable for what has happened. But this much is clear: For those of us who've looked hard at this issue, whether they're public health professionals or staff specialists in your own companies, we feel sure that the one thing we shouldn't do is nothing."

As he spoke, Mudd clicked through a deck of slides—114 in all—projected on a large screen behind him. The figures were staggering. More than half of American adults were now considered overweight, with nearly one-quarter of the adult population—40 million people—clinically defined as obese. Among children, the rates had more than doubled since 1980, and the number of kids considered obese had shot past 12 million. (This was still only 1999; the nation's obesity rates would climb much higher.) Food manufacturers were now being blamed for the problem from all sides—academia, the Centers for Disease Control and Prevention, the American Heart Association and the American Cancer Society. The secretary of agriculture, over whom the industry had long held sway, had recently called obesity a "national epidemic."

Mudd then did the unthinkable. He drew a connection to the last thing in the world the C.E.O.'s wanted linked to their products: cigarettes. First came a quote from a Yale University professor of psychology and public health, Kelly Brownell, who was an especially vocal proponent of the view that the processed-food industry should be seen as a public health menace: "As a culture, we've become upset by the tobacco companies advertising to children, but we sit idly by while the food companies do the very same thing. And we could make a claim that the toll taken on the public health by a poor diet rivals that taken by tobacco."

"If anyone in the food industry ever doubted there was a slippery slope out there," Mudd said, "I imagine they are beginning to experience a distinct sliding sensation right about now."

Mudd then presented the plan he and others had devised to address the obesity problem. Merely getting the executives to acknowledge some culpability was an important first step, he knew, so his plan would start off with a small but crucial move: the industry should use the expertise of scientists—its own and others—to gain a deeper understanding of what was driving Americans to overeat. Once this was achieved, the effort could unfold on several fronts. To be sure, there would be no getting around the role that packaged foods and drinks play in overconsumption. They would have to pull back on their use of salt, sugar and fat, perhaps by imposing industrywide limits. But it wasn't just a matter of these three ingredients; the schemes they used to advertise and market their products were critical, too. Mudd proposed creating a "code to guide the nutritional aspects of food marketing, especially to children."

"We are saying that the industry should make a sincere effort to be part of the solution," Mudd concluded. "And that by doing so, we can help to defuse the criticism that's building against us."

What happened next was not written down. But according to three participants, when Mudd stopped talking, the one C.E.O. whose recent exploits in the grocery store had awed the rest of the industry stood up to speak. His name was Stephen Sanger, and he was also the person—as head of General Mills—who had the most to lose when it came to dealing with obesity. Under his leadership, General Mills had overtaken not just the cereal aisle but other sections of the grocery store. The company's Yoplait brand had transformed traditional unsweetened breakfast yogurt into a veritable dessert. It now had twice as much sugar per serving as General Mills' marshmallow cereal Lucky Charms. And yet, because of yogurt's well-tended image as a wholesome snack, sales of Yoplait were soaring, with annual revenue topping $500 million. Emboldened by the success, the company's development wing pushed even harder, inventing a Yoplait variation that came in a squeezable tube—perfect for kids. They called it Go-Gurt and rolled it out nationally in the weeks before the C.E.O. meeting. (By year's end, it would hit $100 million in sales.)

According to the sources I spoke with, Sanger began by reminding the group that consumers were "fickle." (Sanger declined to be interviewed.) Sometimes they worried about sugar, other times fat. General Mills, he said, acted responsibly to both the public and shareholders by offering products to satisfy dieters and other concerned shoppers, from low sugar to added whole grains. But most often, he said, people bought what they liked, and they liked what tasted good. "Don't talk to me about nutrition," he reportedly said, taking on the voice of the typical consumer. "Talk to me about taste, and if this stuff tastes better, don't run around trying to sell stuff that doesn't taste good."

To react to the critics, Sanger said, would jeopardize the sanctity of the recipes that had made his products so successful. General Mills would not pull back. He would push his people onward, and he urged his peers to do the same. Sanger's response effectively ended the meeting.

"What can I say?" James Behnke told me years later. "It didn't work. These guys weren't as receptive as we thought they would be." Behnke chose his words deliberately. He wanted to be fair. "Sanger was trying to say, 'Look, we're not going to screw around with the company jewels here and change the formulations because a bunch of guys in white coats are worried about obesity.'"

The meeting was remarkable, first, for the insider admissions of guilt. But I was also struck by how prescient the organizers of the sit-down had been. Today, one in three adults is considered clinically obese, along with one in five kids, and 24 million Americans are afflicted by type 2 diabetes, often caused by poor diet, with another 79 million people having pre-diabetes. Even gout, a painful form of arthritis once known as "the rich man's disease" for its associations with gluttony, now afflicts eight million Americans.

The public and the food companies have known for decades now—or at the very least since this meeting—that sugary, salty, fatty foods are not good for us in the quantities that we consume them. So why are the diabetes and obesity and hypertension numbers still spiraling out of control? It's not just a matter of poor willpower on the part of the consumer and a give-the-people-what-they-want attitude on the part of the food manufacturers. What I found, over four years of research and reporting, was a conscious effort—taking place in labs and marketing meetings and grocery-store aisles—to get people hooked on foods that are convenient and inexpensive. I talked to more than 300 people in or formerly employed by the processed-food industry, from scientists to marketers to C.E.O.'s. Some were willing whistle-blowers, while others spoke reluctantly when presented with some of the thousands of pages of secret memos that I obtained from inside the food industry's operations. What follows is a series of small case studies of a handful of characters whose work then, and perspective now, sheds light on how the foods are created and sold to people who, while not powerless, are extremely vulnerable to the intensity of these companies' industrial formulations and selling campaigns.

I. 'In This Field, I'm a Game Changer'

John Lennon couldn't find it in England, so he had cases of it shipped from New York to fuel the "Imagine" sessions. The Beach Boys, ZZ Top and Cher all stipulated in their contract riders that it be put in their dressing rooms when they toured. Hillary Clinton asked for it when she traveled as first lady, and ever after her hotel suites were dutifully stocked.

What they all wanted was Dr Pepper, which until 2001 occupied a comfortable third-place spot in the soda aisle behind Coca-Cola and Pepsi. But then a flood of spinoffs from the two soda giants showed up on the shelves—lemons and limes, vanillas and coffees, raspberries and oranges, whites and blues and clears—what in food-industry lingo are known as "line extensions," and Dr Pepper started to lose its market share.

Responding to this pressure, Cadbury Schweppes created its first spinoff, other than a diet version, in the soda's 115-year history, a bright red soda with a very un-Dr Pepper name: Red Fusion. "If we are to re-establish Dr Pepper back to its historic growth rates, we have to add more excitement," the company's president, Jack Kilduff, said. One particularly promising market, Kilduff pointed out, was the "rapidly growing Hispanic and African-American communities."

But consumers hated Red Fusion. "Dr Pepper is my all-time favorite drink, so I was curious about the Red Fusion," a California mother of three wrote on a blog to warn other Peppers away. "It's disgusting. Gagging. Never again."

Stung by the rejection, Cadbury Schweppes in 2004 turned to a food-industry legend named Howard Moskowitz. Moskowitz, who studied mathematics and holds a Ph.D. in experimental psychology from Harvard, runs a consulting firm in White Plains, where for more than three decades he has "optimized" a variety of products for Campbell Soup, General Foods, Kraft and PepsiCo. "I've optimized soups," Moskowitz told me. "I've optimized pizzas. I've optimized salad dressings and pickles. In this field, I'm a game changer."

In the process of product optimization, food engineers alter a litany of variables with the sole intent of finding the most perfect version (or versions) of a product. Ordinary consumers are paid to spend hours sitting in rooms where they touch, feel, sip, smell, swirl and taste whatever product is in question. Their opinions are dumped into a computer, and the data are sifted and sorted through a statistical method called conjoint analysis, which determines what features will be most attractive to consumers. Moskowitz likes to imagine that his computer is divided into silos, in which each of the attributes is stacked. But it's not simply a matter of comparing Color 23 with Color 24. In the most complicated projects, Color 23 must be combined with Syrup 11 and Packaging 6, and on and on, in seemingly infinite combinations. Even for jobs in which the only concern is taste and the variables are limited to the ingredients, endless charts and graphs will come spewing out of Moskowitz's computer. "The mathematical model maps out the ingredients to the sensory perceptions these ingredients create," he told me, "so I can just dial a new product. This is the engineering approach."

Moskowitz's work on Prego spaghetti sauce was memorialized in a 2004 presentation by the author Malcolm Gladwell at the TED conference in Monterey, Calif.: "After . . . months and months, he had a mountain of data about how the American people feel about spaghetti sauce. . . . And sure enough, if you sit down and you analyze all this data on spaghetti sauce, you realize that all Americans fall into one of three groups. There are people who like their spaghetti sauce plain. There are people who like their spaghetti sauce spicy. And there are people who like it extra-chunky. And of those three facts, the third one was the most significant, because at the time, in the early 1980s, if you went to a supermarket, you would not find extra-chunky spaghetti sauce. And Prego turned to Howard, and they said, 'Are you telling me that one-third of Americans crave extra-chunky spaghetti sauce, and yet no one is servicing their needs?' And he said, 'Yes.' And Prego then went back and completely reformulated their spaghetti sauce and came out with a line of extra-chunky that immediately and completely took over the spaghetti-sauce business in this country. . . . That is Howard's gift to the American people. . . . He fundamentally changed the way the food industry thinks about making you happy."

Well, yes and no. One thing Gladwell didn't mention is that the food industry already knew some things about making people happy—and it started with sugar. Many of the Prego sauces—whether cheesy, chunky or light—have one feature in common: The largest ingredient, after tomatoes, is sugar. A mere half-cup of Prego Traditional, for instance, has the equivalent of more than two teaspoons of sugar, as much as two-plus Oreo cookies. It also delivers one-third of the sodium recommended for a majority of American adults for an entire day. In making these sauces, Campbell supplied the ingredients, including the salt, sugar and, for some versions, fat, while Moskowitz supplied the optimization. "More is not necessarily better," Moskowitz wrote in his own account of the Prego project. "As the sensory intensity (say, of sweetness) increases, consumers first say that they like the product more, but eventually, with a middle level of sweetness, consumers like the product the most (this is their optimum, or 'bliss,' point)."

I first met Moskowitz on a crisp day in the spring of 2010 at the Harvard Club in Midtown Manhattan. As we talked, he made clear that while he has worked on numerous projects aimed at creating more healthful foods and insists the industry could be doing far more to curb obesity, he had no qualms about his own pioneering work on discovering what industry insiders now regularly refer to as "the bliss point" or any of the other systems that helped food companies create the greatest amount of crave. "There's no moral issue for me," he said. "I did the best science I could. I was struggling to survive and didn't have the luxury of being a moral creature. As a researcher, I was ahead of my time."

Moskowitz's path to mastering the bliss point began in earnest not at Harvard but a few months after graduation, 16 miles from Cambridge, in the town of Natick, where the U.S. Army hired him to work in its research labs. The military has long been in a peculiar bind when it comes to food: how to get soldiers to eat more rations when they are in the field. They know that over time, soldiers would gradually find their meals-ready-to-eat so boring that they would toss them away, half-eaten, and not get all the calories they needed. But what was causing this M.R.E.-fatigue was a mystery. "So I started asking soldiers how frequently they would like to eat this or that, trying to figure out which products they would find boring," Moskowitz said. The answers he got were inconsistent. "They liked flavorful foods like turkey tetrazzini, but only at first; they quickly grew tired of them. On the other hand, mundane foods like white bread would never get them too excited, but they could eat lots and lots of it without feeling they'd had enough."

This contradiction is known as "sensory-specific satiety." In lay terms, it is the tendency for big, distinct flavors to overwhelm the brain, which responds by depressing your desire to have more. Sensory-specific satiety also became a guiding principle for the processed-food industry. The biggest hits—be they Coca-Cola or Doritos—owe their success to complex formulas that pique the taste buds enough to be alluring but don't have a distinct, overriding single flavor that tells the brain to stop eating.

Thirty-two years after he began experimenting with the bliss point, Moskowitz got the call from Cadbury Schweppes asking him to create a good line extension for Dr Pepper. I spent an afternoon in his White Plains offices as he and his vice president for research, Michele Reisner, walked me through the Dr Pepper campaign. Cadbury wanted its new flavor to have cherry and vanilla on top of the basic Dr Pepper taste. Thus, there were three main components to play with. A sweet cherry flavoring, a sweet vanilla flavoring and a sweet syrup known as "Dr Pepper flavoring."

Finding the bliss point required the preparation of 61 subtly distinct formulas—31 for the regular version and 30 for diet. The formulas were then subjected to 3,904 tastings organized in Los Angeles, Dallas, Chicago and Philadelphia. The Dr Pepper tasters began working through their samples, resting five minutes between each sip to restore their taste buds. After each sample, they gave numerically ranked answers to a set of questions: How much did they like it overall? How strong is the taste? How do they feel about the taste? How would they describe the quality of this product? How likely would they be to purchase this product?

Moskowitz's data—compiled in a 135-page report for the soda maker—is tremendously fine-grained, showing how different people and groups of people feel about a strong vanilla taste versus weak, various aspects of aroma and the powerful sensory force that food scientists call "mouth feel." This is the way a product interacts with the mouth, as defined more specifically by a host of related sensations, from dryness to gumminess to moisture release. These are terms more familiar to sommeliers, but the mouth feel of soda and many other food items, especially those high in fat, is second only to the bliss point in its ability to predict how much craving a product will induce.

In addition to taste, the consumers were also tested on their response to color, which proved to be highly sensitive. "When we increased the level of the Dr Pepper flavoring, it gets darker and liking goes off," Reisner said. These preferences can also be cross-referenced by age, sex and race.

On Page 83 of the report, a thin blue line represents the amount of Dr Pepper flavoring needed to generate maximum appeal. The line is shaped like an upside-down U, just like the bliss-point curve that Moskowitz studied 30 years earlier in his Army lab. And at the top of the arc, there is not a single sweet spot but instead a sweet range, within which "bliss" was achievable. This meant that Cadbury could edge back on its key ingredient, the sugary Dr Pepper syrup, without falling out of the range and losing the bliss. Instead of using 2 milliliters of the flavoring, for instance, they could use 1.69 milliliters and achieve the same effect. The potential savings is merely a few percentage points, and it won't mean much to individual consumers who are counting calories or grams of sugar. But for Dr Pepper, it adds up to colossal savings. "That looks like nothing," Reisner said. "But it's a lot of money. A lot of money. Millions."

The soda that emerged from all of Moskowitz's variations became known as Cherry Vanilla Dr Pepper, and it proved successful beyond anything Cadbury imagined. In 2008, Cadbury split off its soft-drinks business, which included Snapple and 7-Up. The Dr Pepper Snapple Group has since been valued in excess of $11 billion.

II. 'Lunchtime Is All Yours'

Sometimes innovations within the food industry happen in the lab, with scientists dialing in specific ingredients to achieve the greatest allure. And sometimes, as in the case of Oscar Mayer's bologna crisis, the innovation involves putting old products in new packages.

The 1980s were tough times for Oscar Mayer. Red-meat consumption fell more than 10 percent as fat became synonymous with cholesterol, clogged arteries, heart attacks and strokes. Anxiety set in at the company's headquarters in Madison, Wis., where executives worried about their future and the pressure they faced from their new bosses at Philip Morris.

Bob Drane was the company's vice president for new business strategy and development when Oscar Mayer tapped him to try to find some way to reposition bologna and other troubled meats that were declining in popularity and sales. I met Drane at his home in Madison and went through the records he had kept on the birth of what would become much more than his solution to the company's meat problem. In 1985, when Drane began working on the project, his orders were to "figure out how to contemporize what we've got."

Drane's first move was to try to zero in not on what Americans felt about processed meat but on what Americans felt about lunch. He organized focus-group sessions with the people most responsible for buying bologna—mothers—and as they talked, he realized the most pressing issue for them was time. Working moms strove to provide healthful food, of course, but they spoke with real passion and at length about the morning crush, that nightmarish dash to get breakfast on the table and lunch packed and kids out the door. He summed up their remarks for me like this: "It's awful. I am scrambling around. My kids are asking me for stuff. I'm trying to get myself ready to go to the office. I go to pack these lunches, and I don't know what I've got." What the moms revealed to him, Drane said, was "a gold mine of disappointments and problems."

He assembled a team of about 15 people with varied skills, from design to food science to advertising, to create something completely new—a convenient prepackaged lunch that would have as its main building block the company's sliced bologna and ham. They wanted to add bread, naturally, because who ate bologna without it? But this presented a problem: There was no way bread could stay fresh for the two months their product needed to sit in warehouses or in grocery coolers. Crackers, however, could—so they added a handful of cracker rounds to the package. Using cheese was the next obvious move, given its increased presence in processed foods. But what kind of cheese would work? Natural Cheddar, which they started off with, crumbled and didn't slice very well, so they moved on to processed varieties, which could bend and be sliced and would last forever, or they could knock another two cents off per unit by using an even lesser product called "cheese food," which had lower scores than processed cheese in taste tests. The cost dilemma was solved when Oscar Mayer merged with Kraft in 1989 and the company didn't have to shop for cheese anymore; it got all the processed cheese it wanted from its new sister company, and at cost.

Drane's team moved into a nearby hotel, where they set out to find the right mix of components and container. They gathered around tables where bagfuls of meat, cheese, crackers and all sorts of wrapping material had been dumped, and they let their imaginations run. After snipping and taping their way through a host of failures, the model they fell back on was the American TV dinner—and after some brainstorming about names (Lunch Kits? Go-Packs? Fun Mealz?), Lunchables were born.

The trays flew off the grocery-store shelves. Sales hit a phenomenal $218 million in the first 12 months, more than anyone was prepared for. This only brought Drane his next crisis. The production costs were so high that they were losing money with each tray they produced. So Drane flew to New York, where he met with Philip Morris officials who promised to give him the money he needed to keep it going. "The hard thing is to figure out something that will sell," he was told. "You'll figure out how to get the cost right." Projected to lose $6 million in 1991, the trays instead broke even; the next year, they earned $8 million.

With production costs trimmed and profits coming in, the next question was how to expand the franchise, which they did by turning to one of the cardinal rules in processed food: When in doubt, add sugar. "Lunchables With Dessert is a logical extension," an Oscar Mayer official reported to Philip Morris executives in early 1991. The "target" remained the same as it was for regular Lunchables—"busy mothers" and "working women," ages 25 to 49—and the "enhanced taste" would attract shoppers who had grown bored with the current trays. A year later, the dessert Lunchable morphed into the Fun Pack, which would come with a Snickers bar, a package of M&M's or a Reese's Peanut Butter Cup, as well as a sugary drink. The Lunchables team started by using Kool-Aid and cola and then Capri Sun after Philip Morris added that drink to its stable of brands.

Eventually, a line of the trays, appropriately called Maxed Out, was released that had as many as nine grams of saturated fat, or nearly an entire day's recommended maximum for kids, with up to two-thirds of the max for sodium and 13 teaspoons of sugar.

When I asked Geoffrey Bible, former C.E.O. of Philip Morris, about this shift toward more salt, sugar and fat in meals for kids, he smiled and noted that even in its earliest incarnation, Lunchables was held up for criticism. "One article said something like, 'If you take Lunchables apart, the most healthy item in it is the napkin.' "

Well, they did have a good bit of fat, I offered. "You bet," he said. "Plus cookies."

The prevailing attitude among the company's food managers—through the 1990s, at least, before obesity became a more pressing concern—was one of supply and demand. "People could point to these things and say, 'They've got too much sugar, they've got too much salt,' " Bible said. "Well, that's what the consumer wants, and we're not putting a gun to their head to eat it. That's what they want. If we give them less, they'll buy less, and the competitor will get our market. So you're sort of trapped." (Bible would later press Kraft to reconsider its reliance on salt, sugar and fat.)

When it came to Lunchables, they did try to add more healthful ingredients. Back at the start, Drane experimented with fresh carrots but quickly gave up on that, since fresh components didn't work within the constraints of the processed-food system, which typically required weeks or months of transport and storage before the food arrived at the grocery store. Later, a low-fat version of the trays was developed, using meats and cheese and crackers that were formulated with less fat, but it tasted inferior, sold poorly and was quickly scrapped.

When I met with Kraft officials in 2011 to discuss their products and policies on nutrition, they had dropped the Maxed Out line and were trying to improve the nutritional profile of Lunchables through smaller, incremental changes that were less noticeable to consumers. Across the Lunchables line, they said they had reduced the salt, sugar and fat by about 10 percent, and new versions, featuring mandarin-orange and pineapple slices, were in development. These would be promoted as more healthful versions, with "fresh fruit," but their list of ingredients—containing upward of 70 items, with sucrose, corn syrup, high-fructose corn syrup and fruit concentrate all in the same tray—have been met with intense criticism from outside the industry.

One of the company's responses to criticism is that kids don't eat the Lunchables every day—on top of which, when it came to trying to feed them more healthful foods, kids themselves were unreliable. When their parents packed fresh carrots, apples and water, they couldn't be trusted to eat them. Once in school, they often trashed the healthful stuff in their brown bags to get right to the sweets.

This idea—that kids are in control—would become a key concept in the evolving marketing campaigns for the trays. In what would prove to be their greatest achievement of all, the Lunchables team would delve into adolescent psychology to discover that it wasn't the food in the trays that excited the kids; it was the feeling of power it brought to their lives. As Bob Eckert, then the C.E.O. of Kraft, put it in 1999: "Lunchables aren't about lunch. It's about kids being able to put together what they want to eat, anytime, anywhere."

Kraft's early Lunchables campaign targeted mothers. They might be too distracted by work to make a lunch, but they loved their kids enough to offer them this prepackaged gift. But as the focus swung toward kids, Saturday-morning cartoons started carrying an ad that offered a different message: "All day, you gotta do what they say," the ads said. "But lunchtime is all yours."

With this marketing strategy in place and pizza Lunchables—the crust in one compartment, the cheese, pepperoni and sauce in others—proving to be a runaway success, the entire world of fast food suddenly opened up for Kraft to pursue. They came out with a Mexican-themed Lunchables called Beef Taco Wraps; a Mini Burgers Lunchables; a Mini Hot Dog Lunchable, which also happened to provide a way for Oscar Mayer to sell its wieners. By 1999, pancakes—which included syrup, icing, Lifesavers candy and Tang, for a whopping 76 grams of sugar—and waffles were, for a time, part of the Lunchables franchise as well.

Annual sales kept climbing, past $500 million, past $800 million; at last count, including sales in Britain, they were approaching the $1 billion mark. Lunchables was more than a hit; it was now its own category. Eventually, more than 60 varieties of Lunchables and other brands of trays would show up in the grocery stores. In 2007, Kraft even tried a Lunchables Jr. for 3- to 5-year-olds.

In the trove of records that document the rise of the Lunchables and the sweeping change it brought to lunchtime habits, I came across a photograph of Bob Drane's daughter, which he had slipped into the Lunchables presentation he showed to food developers. The picture was taken on Monica Drane's wedding day in 1989, and she was standing outside the family's home in Madison, a beautiful bride in a white wedding dress, holding one of the brand-new yellow trays.

During the course of reporting, I finally had a chance to ask her about it. Was she really that much of a fan? "There must have been some in the fridge," she told me. "I probably just took one out before we went to the church. My mom had joked that it was really like their fourth child, my dad invested so much time and energy on it."

Monica Drane had three of her own children by the time we spoke, ages 10, 14 and 17. "I don't think my kids have ever eaten a Lunchable," she told me. "They know they exist and that Grandpa Bob invented them. But we eat very healthfully."

Drane himself paused only briefly when I asked him if, looking back, he was proud of creating the trays. "Lots of things are trade-offs," he said. "And I do believe it's easy to rationalize anything. In the end, I wish that the nutritional profile of the thing could have been better, but I don't view the entire project as anything but a positive contribution to people's lives."

Today Bob Drane is still talking to kids about what they like to eat, but his approach has changed. He volunteers with a nonprofit organization that seeks to build better communications between school kids and their parents, and right in the mix of their problems, alongside the academic struggles, is childhood obesity. Drane has also prepared a précis on the food industry that he used with medical students at the University of Wisconsin. And while he does not name his Lunchables in this document, and cites numerous causes for the obesity epidemic, he holds the entire industry accountable. "What do University of Wisconsin M.B.A.'s learn about how to succeed in marketing?" his presentation to the med students asks. "Discover what consumers want to buy and give it to them with both barrels. Sell more, keep your job! How do marketers often translate these 'rules' into action on food? Our limbic brains love sugar, fat, salt. . . . So formulate products to deliver these. Perhaps add low-cost ingredients to boost profit margins. Then 'supersize' to sell more. . . . And advertise/promote to lock in 'heavy users.' Plenty of guilt to go around here!"

III. 'It's Called Vanishing Caloric Density'

At a symposium for nutrition scientists in Los Angeles on Feb. 15, 1985, a professor of pharmacology from Helsinki named Heikki Karppanen told the remarkable story of Finland's effort to address its salt habit. In the late 1970s, the Finns were consuming huge amounts of sodium, eating on average more than two teaspoons of salt a day. As a result, the country had developed significant issues with high blood pressure, and men in the eastern part of Finland had the highest rate of fatal cardiovascular disease in the world. Research showed that this plague was not just a quirk of genetics or a result of a sedentary lifestyle—it was also owing to processed foods. So when Finnish authorities moved to address the problem, they went right after the manufacturers. (The Finnish response worked. Every grocery item that was heavy in salt would come to be marked prominently with the warning "High Salt Content." By 2007, Finland's per capita consumption of salt had dropped by a third, and this shift—along with improved medical care—was accompanied by a 75 percent to 80 percent decline in the number of deaths from strokes and heart disease.)

Karppanen's presentation was met with applause, but one man in the crowd seemed particularly intrigued by the presentation, and as Karppanen left the stage, the man intercepted him and asked if they could talk more over dinner. Their conversation later that night was not at all what Karppanen was expecting. His host did indeed have an interest in salt, but from quite a different vantage point: the man's name was Robert I-San Lin, and from 1974 to 1982, he worked as the chief scientist for Frito-Lay, the nearly $3-billion-a-year manufacturer of Lay's, Doritos, Cheetos and Fritos.

Lin's time at Frito-Lay coincided with the first attacks by nutrition advocates on salty foods and the first calls for federal regulators to reclassify salt as a "risky" food additive, which could have subjected it to severe controls. No company took this threat more seriously—or more personally—than Frito-Lay, Lin explained to Karppanen over their dinner. Three years after he left Frito-Lay, he was still anguished over his inability to effectively change the company's recipes and practices.

By chance, I ran across a letter that Lin sent to Karppanen three weeks after that dinner, buried in some files to which I had gained access. Attached to the letter was a memo written when Lin was at Frito-Lay, which detailed some of the company's efforts in defending salt. I tracked Lin down in Irvine, Calif., where we spent several days going through the internal company memos, strategy papers and handwritten notes he had kept. The documents were evidence of the concern that Lin had for consumers and of the company's intent on using science not to address the health concerns but to thwart them. While at Frito-Lay, Lin and other company scientists spoke openly about the country's excessive consumption of sodium and the fact that, as Lin said to me on more than one occasion, "people get addicted to salt."

Not much had changed by 1986, except Frito-Lay found itself on a rare cold streak. The company had introduced a series of high-profile products that failed miserably. Toppels, a cracker with cheese topping; Stuffers, a shell with a variety of fillings; Rumbles, a bite-size granola snack—they all came and went in a blink, and the company took a $52 million hit. Around that time, the marketing team was joined by Dwight Riskey, an expert on cravings who had been a fellow at the Monell Chemical Senses Center in Philadelphia, where he was part of a team of scientists that found that people could beat their salt habits simply by refraining from salty foods long enough for their taste buds to return to a normal level of sensitivity. He had also done work on the bliss point, showing how a product's allure is contextual, shaped partly by the other foods a person is eating, and that it changes as people age. This seemed to help explain why Frito-Lay was having so much trouble selling new snacks. The largest single block of customers, the baby boomers, had begun hitting middle age. According to the research, this suggested that their liking for salty snacks—both in the concentration of salt and how much they ate—would be tapering off. Along with the rest of the snack-food industry, Frito-Lay anticipated lower sales because of an aging population, and marketing plans were adjusted to focus even more intently on younger consumers.

Except that snack sales didn't decline as everyone had projected, Frito-Lay's doomed product launches notwithstanding. Poring over data one day in his home office, trying to understand just who was consuming all the snack food, Riskey realized that he and his colleagues had been misreading things all along. They had been measuring the snacking habits of different age groups and were seeing what they expected to see, that older consumers ate less than those in their 20s. But what they weren't measuring, Riskey realized, is how those snacking habits of the boomers compared to *themselves* when they were in their 20s. When he called up a new set of sales data and performed what's called a cohort study, following a single group over time, a far more encouraging picture—for Frito-Lay, anyway—emerged. The baby boomers were not eating fewer salty snacks as they aged. "In fact, as those people aged, their consumption of all those segments—the cookies, the crackers, the candy, the chips—was going up," Riskey said. "They were not only eating what they ate when they were younger, they were eating more of it." In fact, everyone in the country, on average, was eating more salty snacks than they used to. The rate of consumption was edging up about one-third of a pound every year, with the average intake of snacks like chips and cheese crackers pushing past 12 pounds a year.

Riskey had a theory about what caused this surge: Eating real meals had become a thing of the past. Baby boomers, especially, seemed to have greatly cut down on regular meals. They were skipping breakfast when they had early-morning meetings. They skipped lunch when they then needed to catch up on work because of those meetings. They skipped dinner when their kids stayed out late or grew up and moved out of the house. And when they skipped these meals, they replaced them with snacks. "We looked at this behavior, and said, 'Oh, my gosh, people were skipping meals right and left,' " Riskey told me. "It was amazing." This led to the next realization, that baby boomers did not represent "a category that is mature, with no growth. This is a category that has huge growth potential."

The food technicians stopped worrying about inventing new products and instead embraced the industry's most reliable method for getting consumers to buy more: the line extension. The classic Lay's potato chips were joined by Salt & Vinegar, Salt & Pepper and Cheddar & Sour Cream. They put out Chili-Cheese-flavored Fritos, and Cheetos were transformed into 21 varieties. Frito-Lay had a formidable research complex near Dallas, where nearly 500 chemists, psychologists and technicians conducted research that cost up to $30 million a year, and the science corps focused intense amounts of resources on questions of crunch, mouth feel and aroma for each of these items. Their tools included a $40,000 device that simulated a chewing mouth to test and perfect the chips, discovering things like the perfect break point: people like a chip that snaps with about four pounds of pressure per square inch.

To get a better feel for their work, I called on Steven Witherly, a food scientist who wrote a fascinating guide for industry insiders titled, "Why Humans Like Junk Food." I brought him two shopping bags filled with a variety of chips to taste. He zeroed right in on the Cheetos. "This," Witherly said, "is one of the most marvelously constructed foods on the planet, in terms of pure pleasure." He ticked off a dozen attributes of the Cheetos that make the brain say more. But the one he focused on most was the puff's uncanny ability to melt in the mouth. "It's called vanishing caloric density," Witherly said. "If something melts down quickly, your brain thinks that there's no calories in it . . . you can just keep eating it forever."

As for their marketing troubles, in a March 2010 meeting, Frito-Lay executives hastened to tell their Wall Street investors that the 1.4 billion boomers worldwide weren't being neglected; they were redoubling their efforts to understand exactly what it was that boomers most wanted in a snack chip. Which was basically everything: great taste, maximum bliss but minimal guilt about health and more maturity than puffs. "They snack a lot," Frito-Lay's chief marketing officer, Ann Mukherjee, told the investors. "But what they're looking for is very different. They're looking for new experiences, real food experiences." Frito-Lay acquired Stacy's Pita Chip Company, which was started by a Massachusetts couple who made food-cart sandwiches and started serving pita chips to their customers in the mid-1990s. In Frito-Lay's hands, the pita chips averaged 270 milligrams of sodium—nearly one-fifth a whole day's recommended maximum for most American adults—and were a huge hit among boomers.

The Frito-Lay executives also spoke of the company's ongoing pursuit of a "designer sodium," which they hoped, in the near future, would take their sodium loads down by 40 percent. No need to worry about lost sales there, the company's C.E.O., Al Carey, assured their investors. The boomers would see less salt as the green light to snack like never before.

There's a paradox at work here. On the one hand, reduction of sodium in snack foods is commendable. On the other, these changes may well result in consumers eating more. "The big thing that will happen here is removing the barriers for boomers and giving them permission to snack," Carey said. The prospects for lower-salt snacks were so amazing, he added, that the company had set its sights on using the designer salt to conquer the toughest market of all for snacks: schools. He cited, for example, the school-food initiative championed by Bill Clinton and the American Heart Association, which is seeking to improve the nutrition of school food by limiting its load of salt, sugar and fat. "Imagine this," Carey said. "A potato chip that tastes great and qualifies for the Clinton-A.H.A. alliance for schools. . . . We think we have ways to do all of this on a potato chip, and imagine getting that product into schools, where children can have this product and grow up with it and feel good about eating it."

Carey's quote reminded me of something I read in the early stages of my reporting, a 24-page report prepared for Frito-Lay in 1957 by a psychologist named Ernest Dichter. The company's chips, he wrote, were not selling as well as they could for one simple reason: "While people like and enjoy potato chips, they feel guilty about liking them. . . . Unconsciously, people expect to be punished for 'letting themselves go' and enjoying them." Dichter listed seven "fears and resistances" to the chips: "You can't stop eating them; they're fattening; they're not good for you; they're greasy and messy to eat; they're too expensive; it's hard to store the leftovers; and they're bad for children." He spent the rest of his memo laying out his prescriptions, which in time would become widely used not just by Frito-Lay but also by the entire industry. Dichter suggested that Frito-Lay avoid using the word "fried" in referring to its chips and adopt instead the more healthful-sounding term "toasted." To counteract the "fear of letting oneself go," he suggested repacking the chips into smaller bags. "The more-anxious consumers, the ones who have the deepest fears about their capacity to control their appetite, will tend to sense the function of the new pack and select it," he said.

Dichter advised Frito-Lay to move its chips out of the realm of between-meals snacking and turn them into an ever-present item in the American diet. "The increased use of potato chips and other Lay's products as a part of the regular fare served by restaurants and sandwich bars should be encouraged in a concentrated way," Dichter said, citing a string of examples: "potato chips with soup, with fruit or vegetable juice appetizers; potato chips served as a vegetable on the main dish; potato chips with salad; potato chips with egg dishes for breakfast; potato chips with sandwich orders."

In 2011, *The New England Journal of Medicine* published a study that shed new light on America's weight gain. The subjects—120,877 women and men—were all professionals in the health field, and were likely to be more conscious about nutrition, so the findings might well understate the overall trend. Using data back to 1986, the researchers monitored everything the participants ate, as well as their physical activity and smoking. They found that every four years, the participants exercised less, watched TV more and gained an average of 3.35 pounds. The researchers parsed the data by the caloric content of the foods being eaten, and found the top contributors to weight gain included red meat and processed meats, sugar-sweetened beverages and potatoes, including mashed and French fries. But the largest weight-inducing food was the potato chip. The coating of salt, the fat content that rewards the brain with instant feelings of pleasure, the sugar that exists not as an additive but in the starch of the potato itself—all of this combines to make it the perfect addictive food. "The starch is readily absorbed," Eric Rimm, an associate professor of epidemiology and nutrition at the Harvard School of Public Health and one of the study's authors, told me. "More quickly even than a similar amount of sugar. The starch, in turn, causes the glucose levels in the blood to spike"—which can result in a craving for more.

If Americans snacked only occasionally, and in small amounts, this would not present the enormous problem that it does. But because so much money and effort has been invested over decades in engineering and then relentlessly selling these products, the effects are seemingly impossible to unwind. More than 30 years have passed since Robert Lin first tangled with Frito-Lay on the imperative of the company to deal with the formulation of its snacks, but as we sat at his dining-room table, sifting through his records, the feelings of regret still played on his face. In his view, three decades had been lost, time that he and a lot of other smart scientists could have spent searching for ways to ease the addiction to salt, sugar and fat. "I couldn't do much about it," he told me. "I feel so sorry for the public."

IV. 'These People Need a Lot of Things, but They Don't Need a Coke'

The growing attention Americans are paying to what they put into their mouths has touched off a new scramble by the processed-food companies to address health concerns. Pressed by the Obama administration and consumers, Kraft, Nestlé, Pepsi, Campbell and General Mills, among others, have begun to trim the loads of salt, sugar and fat in many products. And with consumer advocates pushing for more government intervention, Coca-Cola made headlines in January by releasing ads that promoted its bottled water and low-calorie drinks as a way to counter obesity. Predictably, the ads drew a new volley of scorn from critics who pointed to the company's continuing drive to sell sugary Coke.

One of the other executives I spoke with at length was Jeffrey Dunn, who, in 2001, at age 44, was directing more than half of Coca-Cola's $20 billion in annual sales as president and chief operating officer in both North and South America. In an effort to control as much market share as possible, Coke extended its aggressive marketing to especially poor or vulnerable areas of the U.S., like New Orleans—where people were drinking twice as much Coke as the national average—or Rome, Ga., where the per capita intake was nearly three Cokes a day. In Coke's headquarters in Atlanta, the biggest consumers were referred to as "heavy users." "The other model we use was called 'drinks and drinkers,' " Dunn said. "How many drinkers do I have? And how many drinks do they drink? If you lost one of those heavy users, if somebody just decided to stop drinking Coke, how many drinkers would you have to get, at low velocity, to make up for that heavy user? The answer is a lot. It's more efficient to get my existing users to drink more."

One of Dunn's lieutenants, Todd Putman, who worked at Coca-Cola from 1997 to 2001, said the goal became much larger than merely beating the rival brands; Coca-Cola strove to outsell every other thing people drank, including milk and water. The marketing division's efforts boiled down to one question, Putman said: "How can we drive more ounces into more bodies more often?" (In response to Putman's remarks, Coke said its goals have changed and that it now focuses on providing consumers with more low- or no-calorie products.)

In his capacity, Dunn was making frequent trips to Brazil, where the company had recently begun a push to increase consumption of Coke among the many Brazilians living in *favelas.* The company's strategy was to repackage Coke into smaller, more affordable 6.7-ounce bottles, just 20 cents each. Coke was not alone in seeing Brazil as a potential boon; Nestlé began deploying battalions of women to travel poor neighborhoods, hawking American-style processed foods door to door. But Coke was Dunn's concern, and on one trip, as he walked through one of the impoverished areas, he had an epiphany. "A voice in my head says, 'These people need a lot of things, but they don't need a Coke.' I almost threw up."

Dunn returned to Atlanta, determined to make some changes. He didn't want to abandon the soda business, but he did want to try to steer the company into a more healthful mode, and one of the things he pushed for was to stop marketing Coke in public schools. The independent companies that bottled Coke viewed his plans as reactionary. A director of one bottler wrote a letter to Coke's chief executive and board asking for Dunn's head. "He said what I had done was the worst thing he had seen in 50 years in the business," Dunn said. "Just to placate these crazy leftist school districts who were trying to keep people from having their Coke. He said I was an embarrassment to the company, and I should be fired." In February 2004, he was.

Dunn told me that talking about Coke's business today was by no means easy and, because he continues to work in the food business, not without risk. "You really don't want them mad at you," he said. "And I don't mean that, like, I'm going to end up at the bottom of the bay. But they don't have a sense of humor when it comes to this stuff. They're a very, very aggressive company."

When I met with Dunn, he told me not just about his years at Coke but also about his new marketing venture. In April 2010, he met with three executives from Madison Dearborn Partners, a private-equity firm based in Chicago with a wide-ranging portfolio of investments. They recently hired Dunn to run one of their newest acquisitions—a food producer in the San Joaquin Valley. As they sat in the hotel's meeting room, the men listened to Dunn's marketing pitch. He talked about giving the product a personality that was bold and irreverent, conveying the idea that this was the ultimate snack food. He went into detail on how he would target a special segment of the 146 million Americans who are regular snackers—mothers, children, young professionals—people, he said, who "keep their snacking ritual fresh by trying a new food product when it catches their attention."

He explained how he would deploy strategic storytelling in the ad campaign for this snack, using a key phrase that had been developed with much calculation: "Eat 'Em Like Junk Food."

After 45 minutes, Dunn clicked off the last slide and thanked the men for coming. Madison's portfolio contained the largest Burger King franchise in the world, the Ruth's Chris Steak House chain and a processed-food maker called AdvancePierre whose lineup includes the Jamwich, a peanut-butter-and-jelly contrivance that comes frozen, crustless and embedded with four kinds of sugars.

The snack that Dunn was proposing to sell: carrots. Plain, fresh carrots. No added sugar. No creamy sauce or dips. No salt. Just baby carrots, washed, bagged, then sold into the deadly dull produce aisle.

"We act like a snack, not a vegetable," he told the investors. "We exploit the rules of junk food to fuel the baby-carrot conversation. We are pro-junk-food behavior but anti-junk-food establishment."

The investors were thinking only about sales. They had already bought one of the two biggest farm producers of baby carrots in the country, and they'd hired Dunn to run the whole operation. Now, after his pitch, they were relieved. Dunn had figured out that using the industry's own marketing ploys would work better than anything else. He drew from the bag of tricks that he mastered in his 20 years at Coca-Cola, where he learned one of the most critical rules in processed food: The selling of food matters as much as the food itself.

Later, describing his new line of work, Dunn told me he was doing penance for his Coca-Cola years. "I'm paying my karmic debt," he said.

Critical Thinking

1. Explain the relationships between obesity and the snack food and sugar-sweetened beverage industry.
2. How did Oscar Mayer "contemporize" bologna during the 1980s? Describe changes other food manufacturers have made in their snack foods and beverages.
3. List three processed foods or beverages that were introduced last year that are no longer available in grocery stores. Explain why the foods are removed from the market.
4. Describe the courses a student could take at your university and the type of work experience a college student could have that will prepare him or her to work in the processed food industry.
5. Obesity, hypertension, and type 2 diabetes are nutrition-related problems common in all developed countries. What one change in the food supply will have the strongest effect to reduce the prevalence of these conditions? Explain how the change can be accomplished and why you think it will have a strong effect.

Create Central

www.mhhe.com/createcentral

Internet References

American Beverage Association
www.ameribev.org

General Mills
www.generalmills.com

Kraft Foods
www.kraftfoodsgroup.com

Nabisco
http://brands.nabisco.com

Pepsico (Pepsi products plus a variety of snacks)
www.pepsico.com

Michael Moss is an investigative reporter for *New York.* He won a Pulitzer Prize in 2010 for his reporting on the meat industry.

Unit 2

UNIT

Prepared by: Janet Colson, *Middle Tennessee State University*

Maternal, Child, and Adolescent Nutrition

Let's Move! is a comprehensive initiative designed to solve the problem of obesity and improve health within a generation. Hopefully, children born in this decade will grow up healthier than children in previous generations. The initiative recognizes we must all work together to take actions that will improve the health of our nation's children. Efforts should begin during pregnancy and continue throughout childhood and the teen years. Families, schools, the government, healthcare, restaurants, and entire communities must work together to produce a healthy future.

Childhood obesity continues to be a problem. According to the Centers for Disease Control, childhood obesity has more than tripled in the past 30 years. In the United States, 17.7 percent of 6- to 11-year-olds and 20.5 percent of 12- to 19-year-olds are considered obese and 31.8 percent of U.S. children are considered overweight. Because of this, childhood obesity has gained much needed attention in the media and in health and political arenas.

Recent data from the National Health and Nutrition Examination Survey (NHANES) indicate that the typical diet eaten by youth is below recommendations for vitamins and minerals and above recommendations for added sugar and saturated fat. Foods that are commonly marketed to children are often high in calories with low nutrient density. Excess calories contribute to obesity and diets that are low in nutrient density may impede learning, affect behavior, reduce resistance to infections, and promote dental caries.

Data from 2008 NHANES indicate that 90 percent of children over 8 years old do not eat the recommended servings of vegetables and 75 percent consume less than recommended amounts of fruit. Over 50 percent of boys aged 9–18 years and 90 percent of girls do not consume the recommended amount of dairy. The outcome of this results in diets low in calcium, potassium, fiber, and vitamins A, C, D, and E among many other micronutrients.

Major changes in the diets of American children and teens were first noticed in the 1977 NHANES data. Shifts in beverage consumption from milk to sugar-sweetened beverages, higher daily consumption of calories, snacking on "junk food," and more food eaten outside of the home have steadily increased over the last 35 years.

Overweight and obese children often mature into unhealthy adults who are plagued by obesity-related chronic diseases such as heart disease, diabetes, gallbladder disease, osteoarthritis, and some cancers. Obesity-related chronic diseases burden our current healthcare system and government-supported healthcare reimbursement programs with exorbitant costs, which is adding to the national debt and bankrupting our country.

The most cost-efficient and effective method of action to curtail childhood obesity and improve overall health is prevention. A great deal of funding and resources are devoted in an attempt to curtail the childhood obesity epidemic in the United States. Efforts are being focused on the environmental factors, improving the quality of foods available to kids at home, school, and in commercial food service establishments. This unit concentrates on various factors such as the influence of prenatal nutrition, school meals, and restaurant foods.

The Healthy, Hunger-Free Kids Act has prompted the USDA to modify the standards for the National School Lunch and Breakfast programs. Schools that participate in the National School Lunch and Breakfast program are now required to implement the guidelines. The lower calories in school meals that provide more fruits, vegetables, and whole grain are designed to improve the overall health of the nation's children and adolescents.

Another hot topic in childhood nutrition is restaurants that cater to children. Historically, eating out was only for adults. As the food industry began realizing that most parents succumb to the desires of their children, kiddie menus began to surface. To appease the little ones, restaurateurs quickly developed menus filled with chicken nuggets, French fries, and mac-n-cheese, with a free hot fudge sundae for dessert.

Advertisements for the rapidly increasing array of caffeinated energy drinks give children and adolescents the impression that athletic performance is enhanced by drinking beverages with high amounts of caffeine. Many health professionals are concerned about the health effects of caffeine on youth; parents need to be educated about the potential consequences of the stimulant in growing children.

The articles in this unit were compiled to demonstrate different views of nutrition that influence the health of mothers, children, and adolescents, with an emphasis on obesity. Many of the articles provide solutions to the problem; however, solving the obesity epidemic in the United States is a challenging task. The problem is multifactorial and took decades to develop. The solutions, which will essentially be a change in our entire societal culture, will also have to be multifactorial and will take years to see marked results. The articles in this unit can be used as supplemental information for topics on maternal, child, adolescent nutrition, and the obesity epidemic.

Article

Prepared by: Janet Colson, *Middle Tennessee State University*

Childhood Obesity: Is It Being Taken Seriously?

Honor Whiteman

Learning Outcomes

After reading this article, you will be able to:

- Explain why childhood obesity continues to be a problem.
- Discuss the roles that parents have in childhood obesity prevention.
- Describe the role that schools should take to help reduce childhood obesity.

"Childhood obesity is not a cosmetic issue or something the child will just grow out of. Obese children tend to become obese adults, and there are many medical issues associated with obesity. Children are now taking the same type of medications as their parents to manage blood pressure, diabetes, and cholesterol. This is frightening but true," Dr. Rani Whitfield, a spokesperson for the American Heart Association, told *Medical News Today.*

Unfortunately, what Dr. Whitfield says is no exaggeration. Over the past 30 years, the rate of childhood obesity has more than doubled in children and quadrupled in adolescents.

The prevalence of obesity in children aged 6–11 years increased from 7 percent in 1980 to 18 percent in 2012, while the percentage of obese adolescents aged 12–19 years soared from 5 percent to 21 percent in the same period.

These significant increases have led to a rise in obesity-related health conditions among children and adolescents. A 2007 population-based survey of 5–17-year-olds revealed that around 70 percent of obese children and adolescents have at least one risk factor for cardiovascular disease, and it has been well established that the condition can increase the risk of musculoskeletal diseases, diabetes, and cancer.

The effects of childhood obesity can persist well into adulthood, and there is global concern that if rates of childhood obesity continue to rise, so will the prevalence of related medical conditions. This will not only put the health of future generations at risk, but it will also put an enormous strain on the economy. Such concerns have led to the launch of public health campaigns in an attempt to tackle childhood obesity, such as the Let's Move initiative launched by First Lady Michelle Obama in 2010. But how have rates of childhood obesity reached such a high? Is enough being done to tackle the problem? And are we taking childhood obesity as seriously as we should? *Medical News Today* investigates.

Why have we seen such an increase in childhood obesity?

Weight status in children is determined by body mass index (BMI)-for-age percentiles. This calculates a child's weight category based on their age and BMI. A child is deemed overweight if their BMI-for-age percentile is over 85 percent and deemed obese if it is over 95 percent. There is no doubt that the main causes of childhood obesity are an unhealthy diet and lack of physical activity.

Amanda Staiano, PhD, co-chair of the Public Affairs Committee at The Obesity Society—the leading organization dedicated to the study of obesity—told *Medical News Today:* "The availability of liquid calories and empty calories, combined with a deluge of fast food and junk food advertisements, have changed the way children eat. The majority of children fail to meet the recommended 60 minutes of daily physical activity and spend a huge amount of time sitting. The way we've structured our daily lives makes it hard for children to live healthily."

It is clear that lifestyle changes have had a significant impact on childhood obesity over the past 30 years. Children used to consume one snack a day, while 1 in 5 school-age children now eats up to six snacks a day. Food and drink portion sizes are also bigger than they were 30 years ago. In the mid-1970s, a standard sugar-sweetened drink was 13.6 ounces, while it stands at 20 ounces today. Furthermore, the Harvard School of Public Health in Boston, MA, state a child's daily calorie intake from sugary beverages rose by 60 percent between 1989 and 2008.

Although availability of junk food and drink has decreased in schools, the Centers for Disease Control and Prevention (CDC) state that more than half of middle and high schools in the US still offer them for purchase.

And the advertising industry, health care professionals believe, has not helped rates of childhood obesity, with past studies suggesting that children exposed to junk food commercials are more likely to become obese.

Levels of physical activity have also reduced over the past three decades. The CDC state that last year, only 29 percent of high school students participated in the recommended 60 minutes of exercise a day.

Gone are the days when children would run around and play for hours after school. Now, they are more likely to engage in sedentary behaviors, such as watching TV, playing computer games, or using social media. Children now spend an average of 7.5 hours a day using entertainment media.

There are other factors that have been associated with the development of childhood obesity. Genetic disposition is one.

A 2012 study reported by *Medical News Today* discovered two gene variants that researchers claim increase the risk of childhood obesity. A more recent study by researchers from the University of Cambridge in the UK revealed that a gene mutation called KSR2 may cause obesity by causing continued hunger pangs.

But health care experts believe it is primarily unhealthy diets and lack of exercise that have caused rates of childhood obesity to soar. "Although heredity may explain some of the obesity epidemic, it does not justify the explosion we've had over the last 30 years," Dr. Whitfield told us.

Parents not taking childhood obesity seriously.

It seems encouraging children to eat a healthy diet and exercise more is the route to success against childhood obesity. The aforementioned Let's Move initiative is focused on doing just that. But is childhood obesity taken seriously enough for such campaigns to work?

A recent report from the CDC found that 30.2 percent of children and adolescents in the US misperceive their weight status. Around 48 percent of obese boys and 36 percent of obese girls consider their weight to be normal, according to the report.

A 2013 study published in the journal *Maternal & Child Nutrition* found that 62 percent of parents of obese children perceive their child as being of a healthy weight. Dr. Eliana Perrin, associate professor of pediatrics at North Carolina Children's Hospital, told *Medical News Today:* "[Parents] often do not recognize when their children are becoming overweight. Because young children at a healthy weight look skinny and because children who are overweight are becoming the norm, parents often do not realize when their children are not on a healthy track. I think they only start to worry when obesity affects their day-to-day lives."

Dr. Perrin is the lead author of a study we reported on earlier this year that claimed many parents adopt infant and feeding practices that increase a child's risk of obesity later in life.

She told us that parents need support to ensure their children adopt healthier lifestyles—something that is echoed by Staiano: "Parents should be talking with their child's pediatrician about how to attain a healthy weight and make healthier choices with their child—even if the pediatrician doesn't bring it up. Parents are the best advocates for their children," she said, adding:

"Parents can play a role by speaking up at PTA meetings and parent-teacher conferences, advocating for healthier meals in daycares and schools, and demanding that the places children visit, such as schools and parks, are promoting healthy eating and physical activity."

Could schools do more to help tackle childhood obesity?

There is certainly an onus on schools to do more to encourage children to adopt healthy behaviors. In the United States, around 32 million students eat school meals every day, and for many of these children, school meals account for up to 50 percent of their daily energy intake.

Schools have already been subject to new guidelines for school meals, developed by the US Department of Agriculture (USDA) in 2012.

These guidelines require schools to have a higher offering of whole-grain rich foods, offer only fat-free or low-fat milk products, offer fruits and vegetables to all students every day of the week, limit calories based on the age of the student to ensure they receive the correct portion size, and increase focus on lowering the amount of saturated trans fat and salt in foods.

Earlier this year, we reported on a study led by the Harvard School of Public Health, revealing that since these guidelines have been launched, students now eat more fruits and vegetables. But schools need to do more than just offer healthy foods, according to Dr. Whitfield: "Schools play a very critical role in encouraging healthy behaviors in children. Many children spend a significant amount of time at school where both good and bad habits can develop. Physical activity and health education should be mandatory for those in kindergarten through high school."

Staiano noted that schools are under a lot of pressure to teach core subjects but agrees that healthy living is something they should be educated about. "Schools have a responsibility to create a safe, supportive place where the healthy choice is the easy choice," she said.

But she added that encouraging children to adopt healthier lifestyles should not stop at school. Staiano noted that during school breaks, some communities offer structured summer programs that offer physical activity and healthy snacks to children.

"Neighborhood soccer and softball leagues can encourage healthy competition and physical activity as well as positive social interaction," she added. "Attractive parks with equipment catered to a variety of age ranges can provide family-friendly activity to get parents moving, too."

Fight against childhood obesity remains an uphill battle.

Overall, it seems childhood obesity is receiving much more attention, and health care professionals are in agreement that obesity campaigns—such as the Let's Move initiative—have helped raise awareness of the issue.

Some US states have even seen a reduction in rates of childhood obesity. A report from the CDC revealed that between 2008 and 2011, Florida, Georgia, Missouri, New Jersey, South Dakota, and the US Virgin Islands showed a minimum decrease of 1 percent in their childhood obesity rates.

But although such figures show we are heading in the right direction, Staiano told us there is still a lot more work to be done. "Childhood obesity remains at a historical high," she said. "These declines are still within the margin of error, and it is important to continue following trends to see if the trends plateau or continue to go up."

"We are certainly making some progress," added Dr. Perrin, "but given the abundance of marketing to children of unhealthy foods, the lack of easy ways to incorporate healthy activity into children's usual days, and the simultaneous unfairness of obesity stigma, it's an uphill battle."

But it seems Michelle Obama, for one, is not giving up the fight anytime soon: "In the end, as First Lady, this isn't just a policy issue for me. This is a passion. This is my mission. I am determined to work with folks across this country to change the way a generation of kids thinks about food and nutrition."

Critical Thinking

1. Explain why childhood obesity is considered an uphill battle.
2. Describe three things that could be done in your community to reduce childhood obesity.

Create Central

www.mhhe.com/createcentral

Internet References

American Academy of Pediatrics
www.aap.org

Healthy Children
www.healthychildren.org

Let's Move!
www.letsmove.gov

The Obesity Society
www.obesity.org

Honor Whiteman writes for *Medical News Today* and is interested in medical diagnostics, neurology, stem cell research, and cancer research.

Article Prepared by: Janet Colson, *Middle Tennessee State University*

Iodine Deficiency in Pregnancy: A Global Problem

Maia V. Dutta and Janet Colson

Learning Outcomes

After reading this article, you will be able to:

- List the roles that iodine plays in pregnancy.
- Explain how iodine deficiency is diagnosed.
- Describe the practices women should take to prevent iodine deficiency during pregnancy.

Iodine deficiency continues to be a global problem, despite strategies to eliminate the condition, and is the most frequent cause of preventable brain damage in children. Approximately 2 billion people worldwide are iodine deficient, and every year it is estimated that 38 million newborns are affected by the deficiency in developing countries (WHO/UNICEF/ICCIDD, 2007). Iodine is a trace element that is essential for the production of the thyroid hormone; consequently, adequate dietary intake of iodine is especially critical during pregnancy and lactation to prevent maternal and fetal hypothyroidism, which can result in miscarriage, infant mortality, and irreversible cognitive and neurological impairment of the fetus (Stagnaro-Green & Pearce, 2013).

Iodine is a trace element that is essential for the production of the thyroid hormone.

The effects of severe iodine deficiency during pregnancy have been studied extensively. A severe deficiency results in cretinism, the condition characterized by stunted physical and mental growth (Zimmermann, 2012). However, the effects of mild-to-moderate iodine deficiency (MMID) during pregnancy are not fully understood; emerging evidence suggests that MMID can cause gestational hypothyroxinemia, which may also have significant consequences for the fetus, and is often undetected (Suárez Rodríguez, Azcona San Julián, & Alzina de Aguilar, 2013). Many studies have reported that certain populations of pregnant women continue to be at risk for iodine deficiency, even in areas that are considered to be iodine sufficient (Berbel, Obregon, Bernal, Escobar del Rey, & Morreale de Escobar, 2007). Understanding the consequences and prevalence of iodine deficiency during pregnancy can help childbirth educators raise awareness, recommend testing, and provide nutritional guidance to ensure adequate iodine intake.

Iodine and Thyroid Physiology

The hypothalamus releases the thyrotropin-releasing hormone, which stimulates the pituitary gland to secrete thyroid-stimulating hormone (TSH), also called thryrotropin (Ghirri, Lunardi, & Boldrini, 2014). TSH stimulates iodine uptake and the secretion of thyroxine (T_4) and triiodothyronine (T_3), collectively referred to as thyroid hormones (TH). The thyroid gland requires approximately 60 mg of iodine per day for production of TH. T_4 is converted into T_3, which is the more active hormone and plays an important role in metabolism by binding to receptors in target tissues to regulate gene expression (Higdon, 2003).

TH might exist in the bloodstream in both free and bound forms—in the latter case they are bound to the protein thyroxine-binding globulin (TBG). Free (unbound) levels of TH represent the amount of hormone immediately available for use by cells. The concentration levels of TH in the blood are related to the levels of TSH via a negative feedback loop.

When TH levels are high, TSH production is suppressed, and vice versa (Estrada, Soldin, Buckey, Burman, & Soldin, 2014).

Thyroid hormones control numerous metabolic pathways and regulate growth and development of multiple organs, particularly the brain and the central nervous system during development (Ghirri et al., 2014). TH is mandatory for normal neuronal migration and myelination of the fetal brain (Zimmermann, 2012).

Changes in Iodine Needs during Pregnancy

The increased metabolic needs during pregnancy affect the functioning, and hence the iodine needs, of the thyroid. Following conception, circulating total T_4 and TBG concentrations increase by 6–8 weeks and remain high until delivery. Human chorionic gonadotrophin (HCG), produced by the fertilized egg, has a thyrotropic effect (i.e., it can stimulate the secretion of TH) which in turn reduces the serum TSH in the first trimester. Therefore, during pregnancy, women have lower serum TSH concentrations than before pregnancy (Stagnaro-Green et al., 2011).

By weeks 10–12, the fetal thyroid develops the ability to store iodine provided by the placenta. Maternal transfer of iodine to the fetus is estimated at 50–75 micrograms per day toward the end of gestation (Moleti, Trimarchi, & Vermiglio, 2014). During gestation and lactation, the mother is the only source of iodine for the fetus and newborn (Berbel et al., 2007).

Iodine is primarily excreted through the urine. During early pregnancy, renal blood flow and glomerular filtration increases, which causes a significant increase in renal clearance of iodine. This reduces circulating iodine and results in an increased uptake of iodine by the thyroid gland (Moleti et al., 2014). As a result of all these changes, pregnant women need approximately 50 percent more iodine than non-pregnant women.

Recommended Iodine Intake during Pregnancy

In the United States, the Recommended Dietary Allowance (RDA) for iodine for a non-pregnant woman is 150 mcg and increases to 220 mcg during pregnancy and to 290 during lactation (Table 1). The World Health Organization (WHO) and UNICEF recommend 250 mcg of iodine per day for pregnant women ("Iodine Fact Sheet for Health Professionals," 2011). Furthermore, to prevent iodine deficiency during pregnancy and build adequate iodine stores for the fetus, the American Thyroid Association recommends a daily supplement containing 150 mcg of iodine (in the form of potassium iodide) for all United States and Canadian women of childbearing age before conception, as well as throughout pregnancy and lactation (Caldwell et al., 2013). However, these countries are considered iodine-replete, and supplementation may need to be increased in areas that are known to be iodine deficient.

Table 1 Iodine Dietary Reference Intakes for Females

Females ages 14+	Recommended Dietary Allowance for iodine (mcg)	Tolerable upper intake level for iodine (mcg)
Non-Pregnant	150	900
Pregnant	220	900
Lactation	290	1100

Adapted from "Iodine Fact Sheet for Health Professionals," 2011.

Sources of Iodine

Iodine is found in saltwater and in the soil, however, the amount is variable and tends to be lower in areas that experience frequent erosion (Ghirri et al., 2014). As a result, humans are susceptible to iodine deficiency because the amount of iodine in foods varies, depending on the content in the soil in which food is grown (Caldwell et al., 2013). One of the best food sources of iodine is seaweed, but as shown in Table 2, the iodine content can vary from 16–2,984 mcg. Dairy products (from the use of iodine feed supplements and iodophor sanitizing agents), grains, certain fish, and egg yolks are also good food sources. Fruits and vegetables contain variable amounts of iodine, depending on the iodine content in the soil in which it

Table 2 Food Sources of Iodine

Food	Estimated mcg per serving
Seaweed, whole or sheet, 1 gram	16–2,984
Cod, baked, 3 ounces	99
Yogurt, plain, low-fat, 1 cup	75
Iodized salt, 1.5 g (approx. 1/4 teaspoon)	71
Milk, reduced fat, 1 cup	56
Fish sticks, 3 ounces	54
Bread, white, enriched, 2 slices	45
Fruit cocktail in heavy syrup, 1/2 cup	42
Shrimp, 3 ounces	35
Ice cream, chocolate, 1/2 cup	30
Macaroni, enriched, 1 cup	27
Egg yolk, 1 large	24

Adapted from "Iodine Fact Sheet for Health Professionals," 2011.

was grown, fertilizer use, and irrigation practices. This variation also influences the iodine content of animal products because of the iodine content of the foods they consume ("Iodine Fact Sheet for Health Professionals," 2011).

Iodized table salt is also an important source of iodine. One quarter teaspoon (1.5 g) contains approximately 71 mcg of iodine ("Iodine Fact Sheet for Health Professionals," 2011). However, over the last 30 years, health experts recommend reducing salt consumption in an effort to control sodium intake which decreases iodine consumption as a result. Currently, government agencies recommend that adults should limit sodium intake to 1,500 mg which also has the potential to reduce iodine intake. Given that 1/4 teaspoon of iodized salt contains 71 mcg of iodine, and 590 mg of sodium, it is easy to calculate that a person consuming 1,500 mg of sodium from iodized salt will consume less than 200 mcg of iodine per day. This is below the RDA for pregnant and lactating women. Furthermore, according to the 2005–2010 National Health and Nutrition Examination Survey (NHANES), iodized salt is not a major source of iodine in the diets of most Americans (Caldwell et al., 2013). The majority of salt consumed in the United States comes from processed foods (70–80 percent) and food manufacturers usually do not use iodized salt. It is interesting to note that not all vitamin and mineral supplements contain iodine.

Diagnosing Iodine Deficiency

The most common method to diagnose iodine status is by measuring urinary iodine concentration (UIC) from a spot-urine test or, for more accuracy, a median 24-hour urine iodine collection. Approximately 90 percent of iodine consumed is excreted in the urine, thus an individual's iodine intake is reflected by the amount excreted in the urine. The WHO has determined that a UIC of 150–249 mcg/l indicates adequate iodine intake in pregnant women, and values less than 150 mcg/l indicates iodine deficiency ("Iodine Fact Sheet for Health Professionals," 2011). Lactating women are considered iodine deficient if UIC values are below 100 mcg/l (Ghirri et al., 2014) assuming that about 100 mcg will be incorporated into the breast milk (WHO/UNICEF/ICCIDD, 2007). However, UIC only provides an estimate of the iodine status of an individual, especially during pregnancy and lactation because iodine concentrated in the mammary glands and milk excreted lowers the UIC output (Ghirri et al., 2014). To obtain a more accurate determination of iodine deficiency in individuals, at least 10 spot or 24-hour urine samples are recommended (Konig, Andersson, Hotz, Aeberli, & Zimmermann, 2011).

Other methods for measuring iodine status include goiter palpation/ultrasonography, serum TSH or thyroglobulin levels. Goiter assessment reflects a long-term response to iodine deficiency, and hence is not representative of recent iodine intake. TSH is a useful marker in the neonatal period for infants, but it is a relatively insensitive indicator in older children and in adults because concentrations usually remain within normal ranges when iodine deficient. Thyroglobulin (a storage protein in the thyroid gland involved in the production of T_3 and T_4, not to be confused with TBG) can be useful in indicating both low and excess iodine intake. In addition, it is also an early indicator of iodine repletion (Ghirri et al., 2014). These tests are used less frequently because of cost and/or time constraints.

Consequences of Mild-to-Moderate Iodine Deficiency

Recent studies have indicated that MMID during pregnancy may also have significant consequences for the offspring, such as cognitive and psychomotor delays, autism, and increase the oxidative stress of pregnant women. A sample of these studies is discussed below.

Bath, Steer, Golding, Emmett, and Rayman (2013) examined mothers' iodine status and children's cognitive abilities of 1,040 mother-child pairs from the Avon Longitudinal Study of Parents and Children cohort. The mothers were moderately iodine deficient (median UIC of mothers was 91.1 mcg/l). They found that children whose mothers were iodine deficient were more likely to score in the lowest quartile for verbal IQ, reading accuracy, and reading comprehension, compared to those whose mothers were iodine sufficient.

Costeira et al. (2011) conducted a longitudinal study aimed at assessing the relationship between maternal iodine and thyroid status during all three trimesters and the psychomotor development of their offspring. This study was conducted in an iodine deficient area in Portugal on 86 infants and their mothers. The serum of newborns was tested for total thyroxine (TT_4), free T_4 (FT_4), and total triiodothyronine (TT_3) three days after birth and from mothers during each trimester. Infant psychomotor development was assessed at 12, 18, and 24 months using the Bayley Scale of Infant Development. They found that children born to mothers with low serum FT_4 levels during the first trimester of pregnancy had lower psychomotor scores at 18 and 24 months than controls. Their findings demonstrate the importance of adequate iodine status during the early part of pregnancy.

MMID has been shown to cause gestational hypothyroxinemia, which is characterized by normal levels of TSH, but low levels of free T_4. As mentioned earlier, under normal conditions, a low level of T_4 stimulates the production of TSH in an effort to increase T_4 levels. However, during MMID, T_3 levels increase while T_4 levels decrease in an effort to conserve iodine. Kasatkina et al. (2006) investigated the relationship between maternal FT_4 and the cognitive function of offspring, and also examined the thyroid status of pregnant women living in a mildly iodine deficient industrialized city. Two groups of pregnant women were included in this study: those with thyroid-corrected gestational hypothyroxinemia in the first trimester and those with normal levels of FT_4. Serum TSH, FT_3, and FT_4 were measured in all pregnant women. Basic psycho-neurological functions were measured at ages 6, 9, and 12 months using the Gnome mental development scale in 13 children from the thyroid-corrected group and 10 children from the normal group. The results showed that maternal hypothyroxinemia during early pregnancy (5–9 weeks) correlated significantly with delayed cognitive performance of offspring at ages 6, 9, and 12 months. Furthermore, this study found that by correcting gestational hypothyroxinemia before the ninth week of pregnancy with levothyroxine (synthetic TH) the prognosis of the offspring improved and the development of the offspring is similar to children born to mothers with normal T_4 levels.

Henrichs et al. (2010) found that gestational hypothyroxinemia results in cognitive delay of offspring. This study investigated whether low FT_4 levels in pregnant women with normal TSH levels negatively affect the cognitive development of their children. The authors also assessed whether continuous measures of maternal FT_4 and TSH levels during early pregnancy predict verbal cognitive functioning at 18 and 30 months, as well as non-verbal cognitive functioning at 30 months. Their results show that infants born to mothers with mild or severe hypothyroxinemia were more likely to have lower FT_4 levels than those of mothers with normal thyroid function. Both mild and severe hypothyroxinemia was found to be associated with a higher risk of expressive language delay at 18 and 30 months, whereas severe hypothyroxinemia was also associated with an increased risk of non-verbal cognitive delay in offspring. Maternal TSH was not found to be associated with cognitive outcomes in the offspring.

Hamza, Hewedi, and Sallam (2013) explored the relationship between iodine status in autistic children and their mothers and its relationship to the characteristics of autism. The authors hypothesized that because autism may occur as the fetal brain is developing and may have environmental triggers, such as nutrient deficiencies, hypothyroxinemia caused by iodine deficiency may cause autism. This pair-matched case-controlled study was conducted in Egypt, which is considered to be iodine deficient. Fifty autistic children and their mothers were compared to age and sex matched controls and their mothers. It was found that 54 percent of autistic children and 58 percent of their mothers were iodine deficient. However, none of the members of the control group were iodine deficient. As UIC decreased, the severity of autism increased. Positive correlations were also found between the autistic group and their mothers regarding UIC, thyroid function and thyroid volume.

Iodine has also been found to act as an antioxidant or indirectly stimulate antioxidant enzymes. Vidal et al. (2014) assessed the relationship between UIC, oxidative stress, and antioxidant status during pregnancy. They found that pregnant women with optimal iodine levels had low oxidative stress and optimal antioxidant status compared to pregnant women with mild iodine deficiency, indicating that iodine contributes to antioxidant status during pregnancy. The resulting oxidative stress caused by iodine deficiency is also linked to increased risk of preeclampsia (Gulaboglu, Borekci, & Delibas, 2010).

Conclusion

Iodine is a micronutrient required for the manufacture of thyroid hormones, which are mandatory for the proper development of the fetal brain and central nervous system during pregnancy. Recent studies have indicated that even a mild-to-moderate iodine deficiency during pregnancy may have a variety of adverse consequences, such increased oxidative stress in mothers, and autism, lower IQ's, and other cognitive and psychomotor delays in children. Since iodine requirements increase during pregnancy and lactation, it is essential that women consume adequate amounts of iodine before, during and after pregnancy.

Iodine deficiency, especially during pregnancy, appears to be re-emerging, even in countries such as the United States, which were previously considered to be iodine sufficient. To protect women and their infants from the potential adverse effects of iodine deficiency, childbirth educators can implement the following measures:

- Recommend a pre-natal vitamin that contains 150 mcg of iodine to pregnant women or women who are planning to become pregnant.
- Recommend iodized table salt as a source of sodium, rather than processed foods.
- Provide nutritional guidance by encouraging the use of 24-hour dietary recalls to estimate iodine intake and recommend iodine containing foods, such as dairy products and salt water fish.
- If an iodine deficiency is suspected, recommend testing, such as urinary iodine concentration or thyroid function tests.

References

Bath, S. C., Steer, C. D., Golding, J., Emmett, P., & Rayman, M. P. (2013). Effect of inadequate iodine status in UK pregnant women on cognitive outcomes in their children: Results from the Avon Longitudinal Study of Parents and Children (ALSPAC). *The Lancet, 382*(9889), 331–337.

Berbel, P., Obregon, M. J., Bernal, J., Escobar del Rey, F., & Morreale de Escobar, G. (2007). Iodine supplementation during pregnancy: a public health challenge. *Trends in Endocrinology & Metabolism, 18*(9), 338–343. doi: 10.1016/j.tem.2007.08.009

Caldwell, K. L., Pan, Y., Mortensen, M. E., Makhmudov, A., Merrill, L., & Moye, J. (2013). Iodine status in pregnant women in the National Children's Study and in U.S. women (15–44 years), National Health and Nutrition Examination Survey 2005–2010. *Thyroid, 23*(8), 927–937. doi: 10.1089/thy.2013.0012

Costeira, M. J., Oliveira, P., Santos, N. C., Ares, S., Saenz-Rico, B., de Escobar, G. M., & Palha, J. A. (2011). Psychomotor development of children from an iodine-deficient region. *Journal of Pediatrics, 159*(3), 447–453. doi: 10.1016/j.jpeds.2011.02.034

Estrada, J. M., Soldin, D., Buckey, T. M., Burman, K. D., & Soldin, O. P. (2014). Thyrotropin isoforms: implications for thyrotropin analysis and clinical practice. *Thyroid, 24*(3), 411–423. doi: 10.1089/thy.2013.0119

Ghirri, P., Lunardi, S., & Boldrini, A. (2014). Iodine supplementation in the newborn. *Nutrients, 6*(1), 382–390. doi: 10.3390/nu6010382

Gulaboglu, M., Borekci, B., & Delibas, I. (2010). Urine iodine levels in preeclamptic and normal pregnant women. *Biological Trace Element Research, 136*(3), 249–257. doi: 10.1007/s12011-009-8539-y

Hamza, R. T., Hewedi, D. H., & Sallam, M. T. (2013). Iodine deficiency in Egyptian autistic children and their mothers: relation to disease severity. *Archives of Medical Research, 44*(7), 555–561. doi: 10.1016/j.arcmed.2013.09.012

Henrichs, J., Bongers-Schokking, J. J., Schenk, J. J., Ghassabian, A., Schmidt, H. G., Visser, T. J., . . . Tiemeier, H. (2010). Maternal thyroid function during early pregnancy and cognitive functioning in early childhood: the generation R study. *Journal of Clinical Endocrinology and Metabolism, 95*(9), 4227–4234. doi: 10.1210/jc.2010-0415

Higdon, J. (2003, 2010). Linus Pauling Institute: Micronutrient Research for Optimum Health. Retrieved May 11, 2014, from http://lpi.oregonstate.edu/infocenter/minerals/iodine/

Iodine Fact Sheet for Health Professionals. (2011). Retrieved May 11, 2014, from http://ods.od.nih.gov/factsheets/Iodine-HealthProfessional/

Kasatkina, E. P., Samsonova, L. N., Ivakhnenko, V. N., Ibragimova, G. V., Ryabykh, A. V., Naumenko, L. L., & Evdokimova, Y. A. (2006). Gestational hypothyroxinemia and cognitive function in offspring. Neuroscience and *Behavioral Physiology, 36*(6), 619–624. doi: 10.1007/s11055-006-0066-0

Konig, F., Andersson, M., Hotz, K., Aeberli, I., & Zimmermann, M. B. (2011). Ten repeat collections for urinary iodine from spot samples or 24-hour samples are needed to reliably estimate individual iodine status in women. *Journal of Nutrition, 141*(11), 2049–2054. doi: 10.3945/jn.111.144071

Moleti, M., Trimarchi, F., & Vermiglio, F. (2014). Thyroid Physiology in Pregnancy. *Endocrine Practice, 20*(5), 1–26. doi: 10.4158/EP13341.RA

Stagnaro-Green, A., Abalovich, M., Alexander, E., Azizi, F., Mestman, J., Negro, R., . . . Postpartum. (2011). Guidelines of the American Thyroid Association for the diagnosis and management of thyroid disease during pregnancy and postpartum. *Thyroid, 21*(10), 1081–1125. doi: 10.1089/thy.2011.0087

Stagnaro-Green, A., & Pearce, E. N. (2013). Iodine and pregnancy: a call to action. *Lancet, 382*(9889), 292–293. doi: 10.1016/S0140-6736(13)60717-5

Suárez Rodríguez, M., Azcona San Julián, C., & Alzina de Aguilar, V. (2013). Ingesta de yodo durante el embarazo: efectos en la función tiroidea materna y neonatal. *Endocrinología y Nutrición, 60*(7), 352–357. doi: http://dx.doi.org/10.1016/j.endonu.2013.01.010

Unknown. (1897). Sporadic Cretinism Before and After Treatment. *Appleton's Popular Science Monthly, 51.*

Vidal, Z. E., Rufino, S. C., Tlaxcalteco, E. H., Trejo, C. H., Campos, R. M., Meza, M. N., . . . Arroyo-Helguera, O. (2014). Oxidative stress increased in pregnant women with iodine deficiency. *Biological Trace Element Research, 157*(3), 211–217. doi: 10.1007/s12011-014-9898-6

WHO/UNICEF/ICCIDD. (2007). Assessment of iodine deficiency disorders and monitoring their elimination (3 ed.). Geneva.

Zimmermann, M. B. (2012). The effects of iodine deficiency in pregnancy and infancy. Paediatric and Perinatal Epidemiology, 26(Suppl 1), 108–117. doi: 10.1111/j.1365-3016.2012.01275.x

Critical Thinking

1. Compare the effects of severe iodine deficiency to the effects of mild to moderate iodine deficiency on pregnancy outcome.
2. Plan a diet for a woman during the second trimester of pregnancy that will provide adequate iodine without exceeding the upper limit for sodium.

Create Central

www.mhhe.com/createcentral

Internet References

American College of Nurse-Midwives
www.midwife.org

American Congress of Obstetricians and Gynecologists
www.ACOG.org

American Thyroid Association
www.thyroid.org

Mia Dutta and Janet Colson are with the Nutrition and Food Program at Middle Tennessee State University.

Article

Prepared by: Janet Colson, *Middle Tennessee State University*

Ultimate Food Fight Erupts as Feds Recook School Lunch Rules

Nirvi Shah

Learning Outcomes

After reading this article, you will be able to:

- Evaluate the nutrition standards set by the Healthy, Hunger-Free Kids Act for meals served in the National School and Breakfast programs.
- Critique the breakfast and lunch standards of the Act.

Across the country, school cafeteria managers, farm lobbyists, food companies, celebrity chefs, students, and parents have started the ultimate food fight.

The skirmish is over the U.S. Department of Agriculture's efforts, prompted by the recent passage of the Healthy, Hunger-Free Kids Act, to rewrite the rules about meals served through the National School Lunch and Breakfast programs. At stake is what will and won't be offered in the breakfasts and lunches schools serve millions of children every weekday.

"It's not your grandmother's school lunch anymore," Nancy Rice, the head of the School Nutrition Association, said at one of the advocacy group's gatherings last month.

The first rewrite of school-meal rules in 15 years, the proposed standards aim to cut sodium, boost the amount and types of fruits and vegetables students are offered, cut saturated fat, increase whole grains, and for the first time, limit calories. (The new proposed standards don't set limits on or address sugar, in part because sugar wasn't addressed in school meal requirements created by the Institute of Medicine. The USDA based its proposal largely on the Institute's recommendations.) The proposed rules, intended to simultaneously combat childhood obesity and malnutrition, have drawn thousands of emails, letters, and drawings that voice opinions about the proposed nutrition standards for school meals. And some of the interest has been high-profile, including school food activist Jamie Oliver, also known as "The Naked Chef," who has thrown his support behind the changes; the Berkeley, Calif.-based organic and natural foods company Annie's Homegrown, which created a website devoted to sending thank-you notes to the USDA for adding more vegetables to school meals; and the Washington-based National Potato Council, which also has a new website pushing for more potatoes to be allowed in school meals.

The proposed rules were published in January and comments are expected to roll in until the April 13 deadline. It may be next year before the rules are final, giving schools until at least the 2012–13 school year to put the new standards into practice. But stakeholders are asking for many concessions, saying some of the requirements would be impossible or have already proved so in school cafeterias.

"It is difficult to have one-size-fits-all," Agriculture Secretary Tom Vilsack told school nutrition directors in March. "I feel your pain. The trick is doing the balancing act . . . between what is appropriate . . . and fiscally responsible."

One of the biggest concerns is the expected cost to school districts: $6.8 billion over five years on food and labor. Some districts would have to buy new kitchen equipment, too.

The New Menu for Cafeterias

The nutrition standards for school meals would change dramatically under the new Healthy, Hunger-Free Kids Act. Among the proposed changes:

All Meals

- Milk: One-cup servings of unflavored milk must be 1 percent milk-fat or fat-free, and one-cup servings of flavored milk must be fat-free.
- At first, half of bread products served must be made with at least 51 percent whole grains. Two years after the USDA implements the nutrition regulations, all breads served must be at least 51 percent whole grain.

Breakfast

- Students must be offered one full cup of fruit at breakfast. Only half a cup could be juice, and that would have to be 100 percent fruit juice. Fruit could be replaced with vegetables.

- A meat or meat alternative, such as eggs, yogurt, or cheese, would have to be served every day. Tofu is not an approved meat alternative.
- The calorie range is 350 to 500 for elementary students, 400 to 550 for middle schoolers, and 450 to 600 for high schoolers.
- No starchy vegetables—potatoes, corn, peas, or lima beans—are allowed.
- Over the course of 10 years, schools must reduce sodium to 430 milligrams or less per breakfast for elementary students, 470 milligrams or less for middle schoolers, and 500 milligrams or less for high schoolers.

Lunch

- Elementary and middle students must be offered a one-half cup serving of fruit every day. High school students must be offered a cup every day.
- The calorie range is 550 to 650 in elementary school, 600 to 700 in the middle grades, and 750 to 850 in high school.
- Elementary and middle school students must be offered at least one ¾-cup serving of vegetables every day; one cup for high school students.
- Starchy vegetables must be limited to a one-cup serving a week.
- A one-half-cup serving of dark-green vegetables must be offered at least once a week.
- A one-half-cup serving of orange vegetables must be offered at least once a week.
- A one-half-cup serving of legumes—black beans, black-eyed peas, garbanzo beans, green peas, kidney beans, lentils, lima beans, soy beans, split peas, and white beans—must be served once a week.
- Over 10 years, schools must reduce sodium to 430 milligrams or less per lunch in elementary school, 470 milligrams or less in middle school, and 500 milligrams or less in high school.

The price tag was a main reason the American Association of School Administrators, the National School Boards Association, and the Council of the Great City Schools lobbied against the law. Because of the cost, the state of the economy, and the possibility that additional federal money per meal to meet the requirements may not materialize until after they go into effect, the Arlington, Va.-based AASA, in its comments, said districts need more time to put the final regulations into practice. The School Nutrition Association, a group of 55,000 school nutrition directors based in National Harbor, Md., also wants more time, in part because some foods required aren't available in some regions.

Adding more fresh fruits and vegetables this year to school meals in Norfolk, Va., cost about $500,000, said Helen Phillips, the school district's senior director of school nutrition and president-elect of the School Nutrition Association. But at least in her district, changes in anticipation of the federal regulations have been put in over time, allowing her to space out the added costs. For districts with less progressive menus, costs could shoot upward more quickly.

"The cost is big anyway," Ms. Phillips said. But compounding the change, "food costs are at an all time high."

But Margo G. Wootan, the director of nutrition policy at the Center for Science in the Public Interest in Washington, which lobbied for the law, finds neither the timeline nor the costs insurmountable.

"There are lots of school districts that are serving healthy meals under the current reimbursement rate," Ms. Wootan said, referring to how much school districts are paid by the USDA per meal.

The federal agency has suggested districts raise prices, if necessary, to offset costs, although school nutrition directors fear that could turn off some students.

Whole-Grain Everything

Aside from cost, there are concerns about nearly every part of the regulations. One proposed rule requires schools to switch all breads—tortillas, pizza crust, pancakes—to whole grains. At first, half of all bread products must be whole-grain rich, or made with at least 51 percent whole grains. Two years after the rules are final, all grains served would have to be whole-grain rich.

In the Sioux Falls, S.D., schools, Child Nutrition Supervisor Joni Davis said her 21,500-student district is halfway there.

"We've been talking to vendors, and they're listening," Ms. Davis said, although at first, they thought she was "a little bit crazy" for asking for whole-grain breading on chicken patties.

But the Anne Arundel County schools in Maryland abandoned a yearlong effort to switch to whole grains for some lunch items, said Jodi Risse, the supervisor of food and nutrition services in the 75,000-student district. While students didn't seem to notice the change in breakfast breads, they quickly learned to avoid pizza and egg rolls made with whole grains. "We couldn't tell as adults," Ms. Risse said, but for students, "over a few months we saw the consumption of egg rolls just go away. They probably don't eat it that way anywhere else." And there can be a tradeoff when adding whole grains: more sugar. For example, when the Schwan Food Co. of Marshall, Minn., reformulated the pizza it makes for schools to increase whole grains, it added sugar, a comparison of the printed nutrition facts for the two products shows. The USDA said it hopes that calorie requirements will keep sugar levels in check.

'Bok Choy? Watercress?'

In the Burlington, Vt., schools, Food Service Director Doug Davis said his 4,000-student district has easily incorporated orange and dark-green vegetables into menus, in part because of a farm-to-school program that emphasizes local produce.

Lunch Letters

In letters to the Agriculture Department, children thank the federal agency for the proposed nutrition rules:

"Those are the kinds of things that grow best for us," Mr. Davis said, so students are used to eating kale and butternut squash. The proposed rules require at least one half-cup serving each of dark-green and orange vegetables a week. They include bok choy, broccoli, collard greens, dark green leafy lettuce, kale, mustard greens, romaine lettuce, spinach, turnip greens, and watercress, and acorn squash, butternut squash, carrots, pumpkin, and sweet potatoes.

Burlington students eat vegetables, including zucchini and carrots, in breakfast breads, too.

But back in Sioux Falls, Ms. Davis said her district hasn't been big on squash and pumpkin, and including dark-green vegetables, other than broccoli, may be tricky.

"Bok choy? Watercress? That's going to be different. Can you put broccoli on your menu every week as your dark green?" she said. "When we think of kids trying new vegetables, the first time they look at it. The second time they smell it. And the fourth, maybe, they eat it."

Besides the challenge of adding new items is the required serving size, said Bob Bloomer, a regional vice president for Chartwells-Thompson Hospitality of Charlotte, N.C., which provides meals for about 470 Chicago public schools. The proposed regulations would require a minimum of one cup of fruit at breakfast for all students, only half of which may be 100 percent fruit juice. For elementary and middle school students, another half cup of fruit and a ¾-cup serving of vegetables would be offered at lunch, when high schoolers get a full cup each of fruits and vegetables.

"A cup of vegetables? No high school student is going to take a cup of vegetables," Mr. Bloomer said. He and others worry much of the additional produce will end up in the garbage instead of students' stomachs.

Potato Pushback

While children must be served more veggies, the proposal also says cafeterias must reduce starchy items. Potatoes, corn, green peas, and fresh lima beans—those that weren't picked dry off the plant—would be limited to one cup total per week at lunch. Sweet potatoes aren't considered a starchy vegetable in the proposal.

"It doesn't make any sense at a time when you're telling kids to consume more vegetables," said John Keeling, the executive vice president and chief executive officer of the National Potato Council. He said the bad rap on french fries has tainted the popular, cheap tuber, which is high in fiber and potassium and low in calories.

Many schools serve "fries" that are actually baked in the oven, he said. His organization recommends allowing four half-cup servings of spuds a week, plus a serving of another starchy vegetable, and allowing potatoes at breakfast. The School Nutrition Association goes further: They asked for four half-cup servings of potatoes a week in elementary school, and no limits on the number of days those half-cup servings are offered in middle and high school per week—as long as kids can't take seconds and neither potatoes nor any other vegetable could be fried.

The recommendation isn't because cutting back on potatoes isn't impossible, said Ms. Phillips, of the SNA. In her menus in Norfolk, Va., there are weeks when potatoes aren't offered at all. But other districts may rely more heavily on potatoes. "It goes back to where districts are currently," she said, and "a concern . . . that we do have for children. Some of their favorite vegetables are starchy vegetables. To limit them to just that to one cup a week might discourage them from eating vegetables at all."

But Ms. Wootan of the Center for Science in the Public Interest, said the problem with potatoes isn't whether they are fried or roasted.

"It's just the variety," she said. "If kids were eating carrots as their only vegetable at every meal, that wouldn't be a good thing either."

Got (Fat-Free Chocolate) Milk?

The National Dairy Council worries that chocolate milk, long the dairy king among students, may be less inviting in fat-free form. Flavored milks that are anything but fat-free wouldn't be allowed under the new guidelines, although schools could serve unflavored milk with up to 1 percent milk-fat. "We want to make sure there are not unintended consequences," said Ann Marie Krautheim, senior vice president of nutrition affairs of the Council, based in Rosemont, Ill. In other words, if students dislike fat-free flavored milk, they might not drink milk at all.

But in Anne Arundel, students never noticed the switch to skim chocolate and strawberry milk this school year, Ms. Risse said. To make up for the missing fat, the milk has a little more sugar and flavoring, but the district's milk consumption is virtually unchanged. For some districts, however, including Norfolk and Burlington, fat-free flavored milk isn't available from the closest dairies, one reason the School Nutrition Association wants more time before the regulations take effect.

"We need to get the standards out there, let industry meet the standards, and then have time to bid those items," Ms. Phillips said.

Districts do have 10 years to cut back on sodium. While that's enough time for manufacturers to reformulate recipes and for districts to develop spice blends to compensate for the reduced salt, the sodium requirements are unrealistic, said the School Nutrition Association, adding that they are so low they're less than what a hospital might serve a patient on a low-sodium diet.

"School food will taste so dramatically different from what a child would eat at home and at a restaurant that participation will drop," Ms. Phillips said. The association endorses only the first two phases of sodium reduction, but not the final limits. She pointed out that a cup of milk has 120 milligrams of sodium naturally, or about 1/5 of what will be allowed.

In Chicago, the district has already cut sodium to the level required in the first phase of the reductions. Mr. Bloomer said he has been hounding food manufacturers to cut sodium further in processed foods they supply to the district. And district policy doesn't allow added salt on vegetables, to which a blend of spices is now added. Some kids haven't been impressed.

"No matter how good a fresh vegetable is, it needs a little bit of something," he said, which his district adds in the form of spices and herbs.

Whether it's no-salt-added vegetables, roasted butternut squash, or fat-free chocolate milk, by far the biggest challenge for school districts will be to convince kids to eat what will be offered after all the meticulous meal planning and calorie counting.

David Just, a professor at Cornell University in Ithaca, N.Y., and co-director of the school's Center for Behavioral Economics in Child Nutrition Programs, works on ways to get students to eat healthier at lunch through the placement of items, renaming foods, and other subtle measures.

"It isn't nutrition until it's eaten," he said.

Critical Thinking

1. Describe the nutrition standards set by the Healthy, Hunger-Free Kids Act for meals served in the National School and Breakfast programs.
2. Explain why sugar is not addressed in the Healthy, Hunger-Free Kids Act.
3. Critique the breakfast and lunch standards. What do you think will be the most challenging standards to meet?
4. How will these new standards impact food suppliers and food companies?

Create Central

www.mhhe.com/createcentral

Internet References

Food Research and Action Center—National School Lunch Program
http://frac.org/federal-foodnutrition-programs/national-school-lunch-program

Food Science and Human Nutrition Extension
www.fshn.uiuc.edu

Healthy Hunger-Free Kids Act
www.fns.usda.gov/cnd/Governance/Legislation/CNR_2010.htm

School Nutrition Association
www.schoolnutrition.org

Article

Prepared by: Janet Colson, *Middle Tennessee State University*

Feeding the Kiddie

A Brief History of the Children's Menu

MICHELE HUMES

Learning Outcomes

After reading this article, you will be able to:

- Trace the history of children's menus in the United States.
- Describe the changes and recommendations about the foods considered appropriate for children since the late 1800s.

At the age of 4, children of the near-extinct Kawésqar tribe of Chilean Patagonia spear and roast their own shellfish. This is eight years earlier than when kids who vacation in Cape Cod, Mass., come of shellfish age—that is, if the children's menus found in every clam shack in the area are anything to go by. If a child is younger than 12, Arnold's Lobster & Clam Bar will serve them a grilled cheese sandwich or a hot dog. But no clams.

Children tend to rise to the culinary bar we set for them, and children's menus in America set the bar very low indeed. To look at the standard kids' menu, greasy with prefab items like chicken fingers, tater tots, and mac-and-cheese, you might think that industrial food manufacturers have been responsible for setting it. But the delusion that a child even needs a special menu is a lot older than the chicken nuggets that have come to dominate it. In fact, the children's menu dates back to Prohibition, when, remarkably, it was devised with a child's health in mind . . .

Depending on where you stand vis-à-vis childrearing, the golden age of youth dining in America either began or ended with the Volstead Act. In the century leading up to the dry laws, children rarely ate out. A child had to be relatively well-off in order to dine in public, and a guest at a hotel to boot. (Restaurants not attached to hotels didn't tend to serve children, reasoning that they got in the way of boozy grown-up fun.) But the lucky boy or girl who could tick these boxes was assured of a pretty good time. When the English novelist Anthony Trollope toured the United States in 1861 (his two volumes of crotchety travelogue were later published as *North America*), he was astonished to see 5-year-old "embryo senators" who ordered dinner with sublime confidence and displayed "epicurean delight" at the fish course.

Prohibition spelled the end for 5-year-old epicures. Taking effect in January 1920, the dry laws forced the hospitality industry to rethink its policy on children: Could it be that this untapped market could help offset all that lost liquor revenue? The Waldorf-Astoria in New York thought so, and in 1921 it became one of the first establishments to beckon to children with a menu of their very own. But even as restaurants began to invite children in, it was with a new limitation: They could no longer eat what their parents ate.

The earliest children's menus didn't look so different from the playful ones we know today. The Waldorf-Astoria put Little Jack Horner on the cover of their pink-and-cream booklet; as he brandishes his plummy thumb, a dish runs away with a spoon. But then there was the food—the bland, practically monastic food, appearing all the more austere for the teddy bear picnic taking place overleaf. Here was flaked chicken over boiled rice; here were mixed green vegetables in butter; here was a splat of prune whip. And the one dish that appeared without exception—the chicken nugget of the Jazz Age—was a plain broiled lamb chop.

The ubiquitous lamb chop embodied the highest principles of scientific childrearing, the prevailing doctrine of the early-20th-century nursery. Its central text was *The Care and Feeding of Children,* by the pediatrician Emmett Holt. First published in 1894, it stayed in print for nearly half a century, instructing mothers, nurses, and, apparently, chefs that young children were not to be given fresh fruits, nuts, or raisins in their rice pudding. Pies, tarts, and indeed "pastry of every description" were "especially forbidden," and on no account were such items as ham, bacon, corn, cod, tomato soup, or lemonade to pass a child's lips before his 10th birthday.

Emmett Holt didn't tend to explain his rules, so we're forced to guess at his reasoning. Pork was probably out because it was likely to carry parasites, and the prejudice against raw fruit dates back to antiquity, when the physician Galen observed that consuming it often ended in diarrhea (which can be fatal in small children). But guidelines like the one permitting only stale breads for children seem capricious if not punitive, and the closest Holt ever came to explaining them was his assertion that children who are allowed delicious foods soon reject the plain ones. Although he stopped short of saying what it was that was so inherently great about the plain ones, he seems to have believed there was moral danger in sensual pleasure, and damnation in indulgence.

It was this hodgepodge of medicine and morality that informed the first 20 years of children's menus. Restaurants packed them with everything Emmett Holt said to, and they did it proudly. The Biltmore Hotel in Los Angeles was one of several establishments that advertised that their children's fare had been "approved by the American Child Health Association" (of which Holt was the founding vice president). This meant that while parents dined on marrow dumplings in consommé, shirred eggs with asparagus and chicken livers, and barracuda in meunière sauce, their children were steered toward cream of vegetable soup served with a plain omelet. Some restaurants, like the one attached to Chicago's Edgewater Beach Hotel, even boasted a kiddie menu created "Under supervision of house physician."

The idea that a child's meal required the supervision of a Holtean physician was, of course, nonsense. As a boy, even Emmett Holt didn't eat in the style of Emmett Holt. His sister Eliza Cheeseman once wrote him a letter reminding him of the bountiful picnics of their youth, when they had feasted on chicken pie and wild blackberry pie, on biscuits with cheese and pickles, and on as many pieces of cake as they could get away with—all washed down with great quantities of that deadly lemonade. "You ate all this," she deadpanned, "and still live."

By the World War II, the country had come around to Eliza's point of view. With the 1946 publication of *Baby and Child Care,* Benjamin Spock succeeded Emmett Holt as the nation's chief childrearing expert, and the very word "childrearing," which has a whiff of livestock management about it, gave way to the gentler notion of "parenting," which emphasized nurture over discipline. Yet, for all the collective relaxing over children's diets in the postwar years, the children's menu was not abandoned. Restaurants had grown reliant on its marketing benefits; children didn't want to give up booklets that doubled as clown masks or featured punch-out airplanes; and parents, quite understandably, had become attached to the low prices. So the children's menu persisted. Meanwhile, a growing processed-food industry made it irresistibly cost-effective to rewrite it with junked-up, dumbed-down foods. By the 1970s, the children's menu as we know it today was basically in place: The design was as colorful as ever, but the food had been restricted to its present-day palette of browns and yellows.

Today, nutritionists are rightly appalled by the insipid, mostly fried fare designated for children. In response, a growing number of restaurants have tasked themselves with building a healthier children's menu, but the approach taken by casual-dining chains like Red Lobster and Applebee's is superficial: Instead of throwing out the chicken nuggets, they're counting on sides of broccoli to magically counteract them. But even a more thorough revamp would be missing the point—namely, that children never needed a separate bill of fare to begin with. If there is any argument to be made for holding onto the kids' menu, it is that contemporary portion sizes are more than a child can handle. (They're more than most adults can handle, for that matter.) Moving forward, the industry might do well to look backward, to the children's options offered in Parisian restaurants at the turn of the 20th century. This 1900 menu, from the Restaurant Gardes, has the right idea: a child's cut-price prix fixe (*couvert d'enfant*) that doesn't offer different food—just less of it.

Critical Thinking

1. How does the first children's menu used by the Waldorf Astoria in the 1920s compare to children's menus of today?
2. What were pediatrician Emmett Holt's nutrition guidelines for children?
3. Describe the influence of the American Child Health Association in the early 1900s. What current organization or office serves the same purpose today?
4. Design a children's menu for a family-style restaurant that meets the MyPlate guidelines.
5. Compare the food options and nutritional quality of the foods on a children's menu of a fast-food restaurant to the menu of a high-end restaurant.

Create Central

www.mhhe.com/createcentral

Internet References

American Restaurant Association
www.ameribev.org

Nutrition Menu Labeling May Lead to Lower-Calorie Restaurant Meal Choices for Children
http://pediatrics.aappublications.org/content/early/2010/01/25/peds.2009-1117.full.pdf+html

United States Department of Agriculture—MyPlate
www.myplate.gov

***The Care and Feeding of Children* (1902), L. Emmett Holt**
www.gutenberg.org/files/15484/15484-h/15484-h.htm

Article

Prepared by: Janet Colson, *Middle Tennessee State University*

The Use of Caffeine in Energy Drinks

AMELIA M. ARRIA ET AL.

Learning Outcomes

After reading this article, you will be able to:

- Compare the amount of caffeine that the FDA recognizes as Generally Recognized As Safe (GRAS) to the amount of caffeine in various energy drinks.
- Summarize the health effects (including fatalities and injuries) that may result after people consume caffeinated energy drinks.

Dear Commissioner Hamburg:

Recent reports of health complications, emergency department visits, injuries, and deaths related to energy drink consumption have spawned widespread concern among scientists, health professionals, legislators, state and local law enforcement officials, and consumers regarding the safety of highly caffeinated energy drinks. As researchers, scientists, clinicians, and public health professionals who have studied and conducted research on energy drinks, we are writing this letter to summarize the scientific evidence on this issue and encourage action.

Given the evidence summarized below, we conclude that there is neither sufficient evidence of safety nor a consensus of scientific opinion to conclude that the high levels of added caffeine in energy drinks are safe under the conditions of their intended use, as required by the FDA's Generally Recognized as Safe (GRAS) standards for food additives. To the contrary, the best available scientific evidence demonstrates a robust correlation between the caffeine levels in energy drinks and adverse health and safety consequences, particularly among children, adolescents, and young adults.

Description of Energy Drinks and Related Products

Energy drinks are a relative newcomer to the U.S. marketplace and have surged in popularity in recent years, particularly among adolescents. Energy drinks are flavored beverages that contain added amounts of caffeine as well as other additives such as taurine, guarana (a natural source of caffeine), and ginseng.[1–3]

The U.S. energy drink industry has grown rapidly since the drinks were first introduced,[3,4] and is projected to reach $19.7 billion in sales by 2013.[2] Between 2006 and 2012, Monster Energy®, the largest U.S. energy drink manufacturer, tripled its sales.[5] As a result of aggressive marketing, energy drinks are particularly popular among adolescents.[4,6,7] As noted in a 2010 study commissioned by the FDA,[a] "[e]nergy drinks are typically attractive to young people," and 65% of energy drink consumers are 13- to 35-year-olds.[8] More recent reports show that 30 to 50% of adolescents and young adults consume energy drinks.[7,9–11] According to *Monitoring the Future,* the federally funded national annual survey of students in grades eight through twelve, 35% of eighth graders and 29% of both tenth and twelfth graders consumed an energy drink during the past year, and 18% of eighth graders reported using one or more energy drinks every day.[12]

Energy drinks vary with respect to caffeine content and concentration.[1,13] The caffeine content of many energy drinks is not disclosed on the product label,[2] and in these cases, information about caffeine content must be derived from Internet sources of unknown validity. In general, the caffeine concentration of energy drinks is much higher than that of sodas, for which the FDA has recognized 200 parts per million of caffeine (approximately 71 mg per 12 fl oz serving) as GRAS.[14] By contrast, the most popular energy drinks, like Monster Energy®, contain between 160 and 240 milligrams of caffeine per can. Many energy drinks contain as much as 100 mg of caffeine per 8 fl oz serving[2] with some containing as much as 300 mg per 8 fl oz serving.[13] In addition, many energy drink brands are sold in larger containers that hold multiple servings (16 to 24 fl oz/473 to 710 mL).[1] While some energy drink manufacturers properly classify their drinks as beverages, others label their beverages as dietary supplements.[b]

[a]This report discusses the mean per capita daily caffeine intake from energy drinks as calculated by estimates from data provided by the Beverage Marketing Corporation. The mean per capita daily intake tells us nothing about the number of individuals who are ingesting large quantities of these products. The report relied on data that is now out of date and made assumptions based on caffeine levels in 16 oz serving sizes, rather than the new 24 oz sizes. Further, the report also acknowledged that "very limited reliable information is available of the number and age distribution of regular energy drink consumers" and "there may be underreporting for young person[s]".[8]

[b]Energy "shots" are a subset of energy drinks that come in smaller containers (usually 1.4 to 3 oz) and have even higher caffeine concentration than regularlysized energy drinks. Many contain B vitamins, taurine, flavoring, and sweeteners. Other "energy products" available for purchase include gel packs, candies, gum, snacks, energy powders, inhalers, and strips, all containing various amounts of added caffeine.

Although some brands of coffee contain amounts of caffeine that exceed the FDA's established GRAS levels for soda, energy drinks differ from coffee in three important ways. First, the caffeine in coffee is naturally occurring, while the caffeine in energy drinks is added by the manufacturer and is thus subject to regulation by the FDA as a food additive. Second, many energy drinks and related products containing added caffeine exceed the caffeine concentration of even the most highly caffeinated coffee.[13,15] Third, coffee is typically served hot, tastes bitter, and is consumed slowly by sipping. By contrast, energy drinks are typically carbonated, sweetened drinks that are served cold and consumed more rapidly. Indeed, energy drinks are often marketed in a manner that encourages consumers to ingest large quantities quickly (*e.g.,* "pound down," "chug it down"[c]). Unlike coffee, energy drinks are marketed in a manner designed to appeal to youth and are highly popular with youth. A scientific review funded by the National Institutes of Health has concluded that the risk for energy drink overdose is increased by the combination of marketing that specifically targets youth and the developmental risk-taking tendencies of adolescents.[7]

Health Complications Associated with the Consumption of Energy Drinks

We are particularly concerned about the health effects of energy drink consumption by children and adolescents. Younger individuals tend to have greater sensitivity to a given serving of caffeine than adults because they are more likely to have a lower body mass and are less likely have already developed a pharmacological tolerance from regular caffeine consumption. The American Academy of Pediatrics' Committee on Nutrition and the Council on Sports Medicine and Fitness recently concluded that "rigorous review and analysis of the literature reveal that caffeine and other stimulant substances contained in energy drinks have no place in the diet of children and adolescents."[16]

The Institute of Medicine has similarly recommended that any drinks containing caffeine should not be sold to children at school.[17] Pediatric professionals concur and further state that energy drinks "are not appropriate for children and adolescents and should never be consumed."[16] Other experts have concluded that children and adolescents should not consume more than 100 mg of caffeine per day,[7] less than the amount in a single can of most energy drinks.

With respect to adults, the FDA has noted that consumption of 400 mg of caffeine by healthy adults in the course of a day is not associated with adverse health effects.[18] That standard for "healthy adults" does not take into consideration that individuals have varying sensitivities to caffeine.[19–24] Moreover, consumption of 400 mg "in the course of the day" is an important qualification because consumers can ingest 400 mg of caffeine from energy drinks very quickly. Metabolism of caffeine appears to be non-linear at high doses. In one study using caffeine-experienced human subjects, an increase in caffeine dose from 250 to 500 mg was associated with significant increases in the half-life as well as a decrease in the clearance of caffeine from the blood, resulting in higher caffeine levels that were sustained much longer compared with the lower dose.[25] An additional consideration is that the negative effects of caffeine at high blood levels could be compounded by the accumulation of its metabolites (e.g., paraxanthine, theophylline, theobromine), which are active stimulants themselves.[25,26]

Our work as public health professionals has included examination of the surveillance methods used to track adverse health effects associated with energy drink consumption (e.g., emergency department visits for caffeine-related cardiac events). Despite widespread use of energy drinks, there are no systematic data collection methods to ascertain the prevalence of possible adverse health complications related to energy drinks and related products. Therefore, the following information likely underestimates the actual prevalence of adverse health effects associated with these beverages.

Fatalities and Injuries

According to information submitted to the FDA through its voluntary Adverse Event Reporting System, consumption of Monster Energy® was implicated in the deaths of five individuals, and reports of 13 deaths have cited the possible involvement of 5-Hour Energy.®[27] The FDA has not disclosed the ages of the deceased individuals in these cases. However, details reported elsewhere indicate that in one case, a 14-year-old girl reportedly died of a cardiac arrhythmia induced by caffeine after consuming two 24 oz Monster Energy® beverages over two consecutive days.[28] Also reported to the FDA were 21 claims of adverse reactions, some requiring hospitalization, which were reportedly associated with the consumption of Red Bull.®[29] These reports only refer to three of the energy products on the market, and of course do not include injuries and deaths that were not voluntarily reported to the FDA. Also, between October 2010 and September 2011, about half of all calls to the National Poison Data System for energy-drink-related caffeine toxicity concerned children under 6 years old. This incidence is far greater than for accidental ingestion of other forms of caffeine.[30]

Emergency Department Visits

The Drug Abuse Warning Network (DAWN) reports U.S. emergency department (ED) visits using a probability sampling strategy. DAWN conducted a special analysis of the data related to energy drink consumption, which revealed a ten-fold increase in ED visits from 2005 to 2009 (1,128 to 13,114).[31] DAWN recently issued an update to that report which showed that the number of energy-drink-related ED visits doubled between 2007 and 2011, from 10,068 to 20,783.[32]

[c]Labels of Monster Energy® products.

Cardiovascular Complications

Caffeine produces a number of cardiac effects, which appear in a more pronounced manner in caffeine-naïve subjects and in those consuming higher doses of caffeine. The consumption of highly caffeinated energy drinks has been associated with elevated blood pressure, altered heart rates, and severe cardiac events in children and young adults, especially those with underlying cardiovascular diseases. A few studies have examined the effects of caffeine consumption on heart rate and blood pressure in children and adolescents.[33,34]

Higher doses of caffeine have been associated with caffeine intoxication, resulting in tachycardia, elevated blood pressure, vomiting, hypokalemia (from beta-adrenergic stimulation), and cardiac arrhythmias (atrial flutter, atrial fibrillation, atrioventricular nodal reentrant tachycardia, and ventricular fibrillation).[1,3]

A study of young adults found that the consumption of a sugar-free energy drink containing 80 mg of caffeine was associated with changes in platelet and endothelial function great enough to increase the risk for severe cardiac events in susceptible individuals.[35] These findings show how acute effects of caffeine administration on heart rate might result in cardiovascular events requiring hospitalization, especially in at-risk youth. Caffeine's effects on blood pressure have been found to be more pronounced among African American children than White children.[36,37]

The consumption of energy drinks before or during exercise might be linked to an increased risk for myocardial ischemia. In healthy individuals who consume caffeine and then exercise afterwards, significant reductions in myocardial blood flow have been noted by indirect laboratory measures.[38] Several mechanisms have been postulated to explain this effect, including the ability of caffeine to block adenosine receptors that modulate coronary vasomotor tone.[38] This vasoconstrictive effect might be more pronounced among caffeine-naïve individuals or those who acutely ingest higher doses of caffeine, such as are present in energy drinks.

Seizures

In addition to cardiac events, cases have been reported of new-onset seizures attributed to energy drink consumption among 15- to 28-year-olds.[39–42] In all of these cases, seizures ceased after the individuals abstained from consuming energy drinks.

Childhood Obesity

Energy drinks have also been shown to contribute to youth obesity due to their high calorie and sugar content.[7,43] One 24-oz can of Monster Energy® contains 81 grams of sugar, which is equivalent to 6.75 tablespoons.[2] The American Academy of Pediatrics' Committee on Nutrition reports findings that the consumption of excessive carbohydrate calories from energy drinks increases risk for pediatric overweight and that "energy drinks have no place in the diet of children and adolescents."[16] In addition, adolescents are at risk for increased consumption of high-calorie energy beverages due to marketing claims that they enhance physical and mental performance and increase energy.[13]

Other Health Issues

Youth with higher caffeine intake commonly report troubling neurological symptoms, including nervousness, anxiety, jitteriness, and headache.[44–46] In one review, youth consuming 100 to 400 mg of caffeine daily from dietary sources report jitteriness and nervousness.[44] Studies have also linked high caffeine intake to reduced sleep, poor academic performance, daytime sleepiness (falling asleep at school), aggressive behavior, and social and attention problems among youth.[47–53] With regard to energy drinks in particular, studies have shown negative behavioral effects among youth including jitteriness, anxiety, and dizziness, which might undermine students' ability to stay on task, focus, and perform well.[6] Although many energy drink manufacturers assert that additives such as taurine and B-vitamins improve physical or cognitive performance, current evidence does not support these claims.[54] Finally, energy drinks that have higher titratable acidity levels than sports drinks have been associated with comparatively more tooth enamel loss.[55]

Health and Safety Effects of Combining Energy Drinks with Alcohol

Energy drinks also pose unique dangers when combined with alcohol. Although the FDA and CDC have concluded that the combination of alcohol and energy drinks is unsafe and poses serious health risks,[18,56] the latest available national data from *Monitoring the Future* indicated that 26% of high school seniors consumed an alcoholic beverage containing caffeine during the past year.[12] Because individuals who consume energy drinks with alcohol underestimate their true level of alcohol-related impairment (*i.e.,* a "wide-awake drunk"),[57–59] the bulk of scientific evidence suggests that individuals who combine energy drinks with alcohol are more likely to engage in risky behavior than if they were only consuming alcohol.[60–64] Accordingly, consuming energy drinks mixed with alcohol is associated with serious alcohol-related consequences such as sexual assault and driving while intoxicated.[60] One study found that individuals who mix alcohol and energy drinks are more likely to report heavy drinking,[65] while another study documented a link between frequent consumption of energy drinks and increased risk for alcohol dependence among college students.[66]

Conclusion

Based on our own research and our review of the published literature cited herein, we conclude that there is no general consensus among qualified experts that the addition of caffeine in the amounts used in energy drinks is safe under its conditions of intended use as required by the GRAS standard, particularly for vulnerable populations such as children and adolescents. On the contrary, there is evidence in the published scientific literature that the caffeine levels in energy drinks pose serious potential health risks, including increased risk for serious injury or even death. We therefore urge the FDA to take prompt action to protect children and adolescents from the dangers of highly caffeinated energy drinks, including applying the existing GRAS standard for sodas to energy drinks and other beverages that contain caffeine as an additive. We also urge the FDA to require that manufacturers include caffeine content on product labels.

Sincerely,

Amelia M. Arria, Ph.D.
Director
Center on Young Adult Health and Development
University of Maryland School of Public Health
8400 Baltimore Avenue, Suite 100
College Park, MD 20740
aarria@umd.edu

Mary Claire O'Brien, M.D.
Associate Professor
Department of Emergency Medicine
Department of Social Science and Health Policy
Wake Forest School of Medicine
One Medical Center Boulevard
Winston-Salem, NC 27157
mobrien@wakehealth.edu

Roland R. Griffiths, Ph.D.
Professor
Departments of Psychiatry and Neuroscience
Johns Hopkins University School of Medicine
5510 Nathan Shock Drive
Baltimore, MD 21224
rgriff@jhmi.edu

Patricia B. Crawford, Dr.P.H., R.D.
Adjunct Professor and Director
Atkins Center for Weight and Health
CE Nutrition Specialist
119 Morgan Hall
University of California
Berkeley, CA 94720
pbcraw@berkeley.edu

Additional Signatories

Kavita Babu, M.D., FACEP, FACMT
Fellowship Director
Division of Medical Toxicology
Assistant Professor
Department of Emergency Medicine
UMass Memorial Medical Center
55 Lake Avenue North
Worcester, MA 01655
kavitambabu@gmail.com

Bruce A. Goldberger, Ph.D.
Professor and Director of Toxicology
Departments of Pathology and Psychiatry
University of Florida College of Medicine
4800 S.W. 35th Drive
Gainesville, FL 32608
bruce-goldberger@ufl.edu

William C. Griffin III, Ph.D., R.Ph.
Research Assistant Professor
Center for Drug and Alcohol Programs
Department of Psychiatry and Behavioral Sciences
Medical University of South Carolina
MSC 861
67 Presidential Street
Charleston, SC 29425
griffinw@musc.edu

John P. Higgins, M.D., M.B.A. (Hons), M.Phil., FACC, FACP, FAHA, FACSM, FASNC, FSGC
Associate Professor of Medicine, The University of Texas Health Science Center at Houston
Director of Exercise Physiology, Memorial Hermann Ironman Sports Medicine Institute
Chief of Cardiology, Lyndon B. Johnson General Hospital
Principal Investigator HEARTS (Houston Early Age Risk Testing & Screening Study)
Division of Cardiology
6431 Fannin Street, MSB 4.262
Houston, TX 77030
john.p.higgins@uth.tmc.edu

C. Tissa Kappagoda, M.D.
Professor Emeritus
Heart and Vascular Services
Lawrence J. Ellison Ambulatory Care Center
University of California Davis Health System
4860 Y Street, Suite 0200
Sacramento, CA 95817
ctkappagoda@ucdavis.edu

Steven E. Lipshultz, M.D., FAAP, FAHA
George E. Batchelor Professor of Pediatrics and Endowed Chair in Pediatric Cardiology
Professor of Epidemiology and Public Health
Professor of Medicine (Oncology)
Leonard M. Miller School of Medicine, University of Miami
Chief-of-Staff, Holtz Children's Hospital of the University of Miami-Jackson Memorial Medical Center
Director, Batchelor Children's Research Institute
Member, Sylvester Comprehensive Cancer Center, Miami, Florida
Department of Pediatrics (D820)
University of Miami, Leonard M. Miller School of Medicine
P.O. Box 016820
Miami, Florida 33101
slipshultz@med.miami.edu

Kristine Madsen, M.D., M.P.H., FAAP
Fellow, American Academy of Pediatrics
Assistant Professor
School of Public Health, University of California Berkeley
Department of Pediatrics, University of California San Francisco
King Sweesy and Robert Womack Endowed Chair in Medical Research and Public Health
219 University Hall
Berkeley, CA 94720
madsenk@berkeley.edu

Cecile A. Marczinkski, Ph.D.
Assistant Professor
Department of Psychological Science
Northern Kentucky University
349 BEP, 1 Nunn Drive
Highland Heights, KY 41099
marczinskc1@nku.edu

Kathleen E. Miller, Ph.D.
Senior Research Scientist
Research Institute on Addictions
University at Buffalo
1021 Main Street
Buffalo, NY 14203
kmiller@ria.buffalo.edu

Jeffrey Olgin, M.D., FACC
Gallo-Chatterjee Distinguished Professor of Medicine
Professor of Medicine & Chief, Division of Cardiology
University of California San Francisco
505 Parnassus Avenue
Room M-1182A, Box 0124
San Francisco, CA 94143
olgin@medicine.ucsf.edu

Kent A. Sepkowitz, M.D.
PhysicianInfectious Disease Service
Department of Medicine, Infection Control
Memorial Sloan-Kettering Cancer Center
1275 York Avenue
New York, NY 10065
sepkowik@mskcc.org

Jennifer L. Temple, Ph.D.
Assistant Professor
University at Buffalo
Departments of Exercise and Nutrition Sciences and Community Health and Behavior
3435 Main Street
1 Farber Hall
Buffalo, NY 14214
jltemple@buffalo.edu

Dennis L. Thombs, Ph.D., FAAHB
Professor and Chair
Department of Behavioral & Community Health
EAD 709N School of Public Health
3500 Camp Bowie Boulevard
University of North Texas Health Science Center
Fort Worth, TX 76107
dennis.thombs@unthsc.edu

Charles J. Wibbelsman, M.D.
President
California Chapter 1, District IX
American Academy of Pediatrics
Kaiser Permanente
2200 O'Farrell Street, Teen Clinic
San Francisco, California 94115
charles.wibbelsman@kp.org

References

1. Wolk BJ, Ganetsky M, Babu KM. Toxicity of energy drinks. *Curr Opin Pediatr.* 2012; 24(2): 243–251.
2. Heckman MA, Sherry K, Gonzalez de Mejia E. Energy drinks: An assessment of their market size, consumer demographics, ingredient profile, functionality, and regulations in the United States. *Compr Rev Food Sci Food Saf.* 2010;9(3):303–317.
3. Higgins JP, Tuttle TD, Higgins CL. Energy beverages: Content and safety. *Mayo Clin Proc.* 2010;85(11):1033–1041.
4. Blankson KL, Thompson AM, Ahrendt DM, Vijayalakshmy P. Energy drinks: What teenagers (and their doctors) should know. *Pediatr Rev.* 2013;34(2):55–62.
5. Edney A. Monster energy drinks cited in death reports, FDA says. *Bloomberg News: Businessweek.* 2012; http://www.businessweek.com/news/2012–10-22/monster-energy-drinks-cited-in-death-reports-fda-says. Accessed February 12, 2013.
6. Pennington N, Johnson M, Delaney E, Blankenship MB. Energy drinks: A new health hazard for adolescents. *J Sch Nurs.* 2010;26(5):352–359.
7. Seifert SM, Schaechter JL, Hershorin ER, Lipshultz SE. Health effects of energy drinks on children, adolescents, and young adults. *Pediatrics.* 2011;127(3):511–528.
8. Somogyi LP. *Caffeine intake by the US population.* Silver Spring, MD: Food and Drug Administration; 2010.
9. Malinauskas BM, Aeby VG, Overton RF, Carpenter-Aeby T, Barber-Heidal K. A survey of energy drink consumption patterns among college students. *Nutr J.* 2007;6(1):35–41.
10. Simon M, Mosher J. *Alcohol, energy drinks, and youth: A dangerous mix.* San Rafael, CA: Marin Institute; 2007.
11. Miller KE. Wired: Energy drinks, jock identity, masculine norms, and risk taking. *J Am Coll Health.* 2008;56(5): 481–490.
12. Wadley J. *Marijuana use continues to rise among U.S. teens, while alcohol use hits historic lows.* Ann Arbor, MI: University of Michigan; 2011.
13. Reissig CJ, Strain EC, Griffiths RR. Caffeinated energy drinks—A growing problem. *Drug Alcohol Depend.* 2009; 99(1–3):1–10.
14. U.S. Code of Federal Regulations, nr 21CFR-182.1180. Food and Drug Administration. 2012.
15. McCusker RR, Goldberger BA, Cone EJ. Caffeine content of specialty coffees. *J Anal Toxicol.* 2003;27(7):520–522.

16. Committee on Nutrition and the Council on Sports Medicine and Fitness. Sports drinks and energy drinks for children and adolescents: Are they appropriate? *Pediatrics.* 2011;127(6):1182–1189.
17. Institute of Medicine. *Nutrition standards for foods in schools: Leading the way toward healthier youth.* Washington, DC: National Academies Press; 2007.
18. Food and Drug Administration. *Warning letter to Phusion Projects Inc.* College Park, MD: Food and Drug Administration; 2010.
19. Adan A, Prat G, Fabbri M, Sànchez-Turet M. Early effects of caffeinated and decaffeinated coffee on subjective state and gender differences. *Prog Neuropsychopharmacol Biol Psychiatry.* 2008;32(7):1698–1703.
20. Alsene K, Deckert J, Sand P, de Wit H. Association between A2A receptor gene polymorphisms and caffeine-induced anxiety. *Neuropsychopharmacology.* 2003;28(9):1694–1702.
21. Yang A, Palmer A, de Wit H. Genetics of caffeine consumption and responses to caffeine. *Psychopharmacology.* 2010;211(3): 245–257.
22. Temple JL, Ziegler AM. Gender differences in subjective and physiological responses to caffeine and the role of steroid hormones. *J Caffeine Res.* 2011;1(1):41–48.
23. Cornelis MC, El-Sohemy A, Campos H. Genetic polymorphism of the adenosine A2A receptor is associated with habitual caffeine consumption. *Am J Clin Nutr.* 2007;86(1):240–244.
24. Sepkowitz KA. Energy drinks and caffeine-related adverse effects. *JAMA.* 2013;309(3):243–244.
25. Kaplan GB, Greenblatt DJ, Ehrenberg BL, Goddard JE, Cotreau MM, Harmatz JS, Shader RI. Dose-dependent pharmacokinetics and psychomotor effects of caffeine in humans. *J Clin Pharmacol.* 1997;37(8):693–703.
26. Denaro CP, Brown CR, Wilson M, Jacob P, Benowitz NL. Dose-dependency of caffeine metabolism with repeated dosing. *Clin Pharmacol Ther.* 1990;48(3):277–285.
27. Center for Food Safety and Applied Nutrition. *Voluntary and mandatory reports on 5-Hour Energy, Monster Energy, and Rockstar energy drink.* Washington, DC: Food and Drug Administration; 2012.
28. Kilar S, Dance S. Family sues energy drink maker over girl's death. *The Baltimore Sun.* 2012; http://articles.baltimoresun.com/2012–10-19/health/bs-hs-monster-energy-drink-death-20121019_1_energy-drink-monster-energy-monster-beverage-corp. Accessed February 12, 2013.
29. Center for Food Safety and Applied Nutrition. *Voluntary reports on Red Bull energy drink.* Washington, DC: Food and Drug Administration; 2012.
30. Seifert SM, Seifert SA, Schaechter J, Arheart K, Benson BE, Hershorin ER, Bronstein AC, Lipshultz SE. Energy drink exposures in the American Association of Poison Control Centers (AAPCC) National Poison Data System (NPDS) database. Paper presented at: Annual Meeting of the North American Congress of Clinical Toxicology; 2012; Las Vegas, NV.
31. Drug Abuse Warning Network. *Emergency department visits involving energy drinks.* Rockville, MD: Substance Abuse and Mental Health Services Administration, Center for Behavioral Health Statistics and Quality; 2011.
32. Drug Abuse Warning Network. *Update on emergency department visits involving energy drinks: A continuing public health concern.* Rockville, MD: Substance Abuse and Mental Health Services Administration, Center for Behavioral Health Statistics and Quality; 2013.
33. Temple JL, Dewey AM, Briatico LN. Effects of acute caffeine administration on adolescents. *Exp Clin Psychopharmacol.* 2010;18(6):510–520.
34. Turley KR, Gerst JW. Effects of caffeine on physiological responses to exercise in young boys and girls. *Med Sci Sports Exerc.* 2006; 38(3):520–526.
35. Worthley MI, Anisha P, Sciscio Pd, Schultz C, Prashanthan S, Willoughby SR. Detrimental effects of energy drink consumption on platelet and endothelial function. *Am J Med.* 2010;123(2):184–187.
36. Savoca MR, MacKey L, Evans CD, Wilson M, Ludwig DA, Harshfield GA. Association of ambulatory blood pressure and dietary caffeine in adolescents. *Am J Hypertens.* 2005;18(1):116–120.
37. Savoca MR, Evans CD, Wilson ME, Harshfield GA, Ludwig DA. The association of caffeinated beverages with blood pressure in adolescents. *Arch Pediatr Adolesc Med.* 2004;158(5):473–477.
38. Higgins JP, Babu KM. Caffeine reduces myocardial blood flow during exercise. *Am J Med.* in press.
39. Calabrò RS, Italiano D, Gervasi G, Bramanti P. Single tonic–clonic seizure after energy drink abuse. *Epilepsy Behav.* 2012;23(3):384–385.
40. Iyadurai SJP, Chung SS. New-onset seizures in adults: Possible association with consumption of popular energy drinks. *Epilepsy Behav.* 2007;10(3):504–508.
41. Babu KM, Zuckerman MD, Cherkes JK, Hack JB. First-onset seizure after use of an energy drink. *Pediatr Emerg Care.* 2011;27(6):539–540.
42. Trabulo D, Marques S, Pedroso E. Caffeinated energy drink intoxication. *BMJ Case Rep.* 2011;28(8):712–714.
43. Clauson KA, Shields KM, McQueen CE, Persad N. Safety issues associated with commercially available energy drinks. *J Am Pharm Assoc.* 2008;48(3):e55–e63.
44. Temple JL. Caffeine use in children: What we know, what we have left to learn, and why we should worry. *Neurosci Biobehav Rev.* 2009;33(6):793–806.
45. Bernstein GA, Carroll ME, Crosby RD, Perwien AR, Go FS, Benowitz NL. Caffeine effects on learning, performance, and anxiety in normal school-age children. *J Am Acad Child Adolesc Psychiatry.* 1994;33(3):407–415.
46. Heatherley SV, Hancock KMF, Rogers PJ. Psychostimulant and other effects of caffeine in 9- to 11-year-old children. *J Child Psychol Psychiatry.* 2006;47(2):135–142.
47. Calamaro CJ, Mason TBA, Ratcliffe SJ. Adolescents living the 24/7 lifestyle: Effects of caffeine and technology on sleep duration and daytime functioning. *Pediatrics.* 2009;123(6):e1005–e1010.
48. James JE, Kristjansson AL, Sigfusdottir ID. Adolescent substance use, sleep, and academic achievement: Evidence of harm due to caffeine. *J Adolesc.* 2011;34(4):665–673.
49. Pettit ML, DeBarr KA. Perceived stress, energy drink consumption, and academic performance among college students. *J Am Coll Health.* 2011;59(5):335–341.
50. Martin CA, Cook C, Woodring JH, Burkhardt G, Guenthner G, Omar HA, Kelly TH. Caffeine use: Association with nicotine use, aggression, and other psychopathology in psychiatric and pediatric outpatient adolescents. *Scientific World Journal.* 2008;8:512–516.
51. Warzak WJ, Evans S, Floress MT, Gross AC, Stoolman S. Caffeine consumption in young children. *J Pediatr.* 2011;158(3):508–509.
52. Anderson BL, Juliano LM. Behavior, sleep, and problematic caffeine consumption in a college-aged sample. *J Caffeine Res.* 2012;2(1):38–44.
53. Drescher AA, Goodwin JL, Silva GE, Quan SF. Caffeine and screen time in adolescence: Associations with short sleep and obesity. *J Clin Sleep Med.* 2011;7(4):337–342.

54. McLellan TM, Lieberman HR. Do energy drinks contain active components other than caffeine? *Nutr Rev.* 2012;70(12): 730–744.
55. Jain P, Hall-May E, Golabek K, Zenia Agustin M. A comparison of sports and energy drinks—Physiochemical properties and enamel dissolution. *Gen Dent.* 2012;60(3): 190–199.
56. Centers for Disease Control and Prevention. *Fact sheets: Caffeinated alcoholic beverages.* Atlanta, GA: Centers for Disease Control and Prevention; 2010.
57. Ferreira SE, de Mello MT, Pompeia S, de Souza-Formigoni ML. Effects of energy drink ingestion on alcohol intoxication. *Alcohol Clin Exp Res.* 2006;30(4):598–605.
58. Marczinski CA, Fillmore MT, Henges AL, Ramsey MA, Young CR. Effects of energy drinks mixed with alcohol on information processing, motor coordination and subjective reports of intoxication. *Exp Clin Psychopharmacol.* 2012;20(2):129–138.
59. Arria AM, O'Brien MC. The "high" risk of energy drinks. *JAMA.* 2011;305(6):600–601.
60. O'Brien MC, McCoy TP, Rhodes SD, Wagoner A, Wolfson M. Caffeinated cocktails: Energy drink consumption, high-risk drinking, and alcohol-related consequences among college students. *Acad Emerg Med.* 2008;15(5):453–460.
61. Arria AM, Caldeira KM, Kasperski SJ, O'Grady KE, Vincent KB, Griffiths RR, Wish ED. Increased alcohol consumption, nonmedical prescription drug use, and illicit drug use are associated with energy drink consumption among college students. *J Addict Med.* 2010;4(2):74–80.
62. Miller KE. Alcohol mixed with energy drink use and sexual risk-taking: Casual, intoxicated, and unprotected sex. *J Caffeine Res.* 2012;2(2):62–69.
63. Thombs DL, O'Mara RJ, Tsukamoto M, Rossheim ME, Weiler RM, Merves ML, Goldberger BA. Event-level analyses of energy drink consumption and alcohol intoxication in bar patrons. *Addict Behav.* 2010;35(4):325–330.
64. Howland J, Rohsenow DJ. Risks of energy drinks mixed with alcohol. *JAMA.* 2013;309(3):245–246.
65. Berger LK, Fendrich M, Chen H-Y, Arria AM, Cisler RA. Sociodemographic correlates of energy drink consumption with and without alcohol: Results of a community survey. *Addict Behav.* 2011;36(5):516–519.
66. Arria AM, Caldeira KM, Kasperski SJ, Vincent KB, Griffiths RR, O'Grady KE. Energy drink consumption and increased risk for alcohol dependence. *Alcohol Clin Exp Res.* 2011;35(2):365–375.

Critical Thinking

1. What level of caffeine is generally recognized as safe by the FDA in beverages?
2. Why are the manufacturers of energy drinks not required to include the amount of caffeine on the label?
3. Compare the effect that caffeine has on an adult who has been drinking two cups of coffee each morning plus a 20 oz. cola every afternoon for many years to a 12-year-old who has never consumed caffeine, yet drinks three 16-ounce cans of Monster Energy Drink at a friend's party.
4. Which of the health problems associated with consumption of caffeinated energy drinks poses the most severe problems to children and adolescents? Explain your answer.
5. The co-authors of this letter to FDA include 18 medical experts from research hospitals and universities from throughout the United States. What other groups could send a letter to FDA with their opinions about energy drinks?

Create Central

www.mhhe.com/createcentral

Internet References

American Beverage Association
www.ameribev.org

Caffeinated Energy Drinks—A Growing Problem
www.ncbi.nlm.nih.gov/pmc/articles/PMC2735818

Caffeinated energy drinks in children
www.ncbi.nlm.nih.gov/pmc/articles/PMC3771720/013

Energy Drinks: Exploring Concerns about Marketing to Youth
www.aap.org/en-us/advocacy-and-policy/federal-advocacy/Documents/SchneiderSenateCommerceCommitteeEnergyDrinksTestimony_7_31_13.pdf

Acknowledgments: Special thanks are extended to Brittany A. Bugbee, Kimberly M. Caldeira, Kaitlin A. Hippen, and Kathryn B. Vincent.

Unit 3

UNIT

Prepared by: Janet Colson, *Middle Tennessee State University*

Nutrients

Nutrition is a relatively new, yet rapidly evolving science. Early research dealing with nutrition began in the mid-18th century with investigations related to how the body requires and uses calories from carbohydrates, protein, and fats. In the early 20th century, scientists began to discover, investigate, and identify vitamins and minerals and their effects on human health. Although the fundamentals of nutrition were discovered 100 years ago, breakthroughs of their relationships to health are reported daily. More recently, research is expanding beyond the nutrients with investigations of phytochemicals—substances found in plant foods that promote health but are not technically classified as nutrients.

A vast amount of knowledge about nutrients has been discovered, and scientists continue to investigate the best way for these nutrients and phytochemicals to be provided safely and in proper amounts to facilitate optimal functioning of the human body. In 2013, more than 22,000 scientific articles were published in peer-reviewed journals on some aspect of nutrition and food. In addition to the science-based, peer-reviewed articles, a quick search of the Internet reveals almost 350 million nutrition-related sites or articles available—with much of the information based on unsubstantiated claims.

The articles of this unit have been selected to present current knowledge about nutrients, with particular emphasis on the nutrients of concern outlined in the *Dietary Guidelines for Americans (DGA), 2010.* The *DGA* stress decreasing "solid" fats, added sugar, and sodium, while increasing fruits, vegetables, and whole grains. A challenge of understanding nutrition is being able to interpret scientific nutrition studies and translate the results into nutrient-specific recommendations. Articles in this unit were chosen to help students gain a better understanding of current research and limitations of some published research.

Too often the resounding message about nutrition and our diets is that we eat too much of the "bad stuff" and not enough of the "good." But most people are confused on which nutrients fit into each of the categories. One of the best examples of confusion is the ever-changing advice about fats. Early Americans ate real butter, lard, and whole fat milk; in the 1960s, people were told to stay away from the animal fats they had eaten for centuries and were encouraged to use commercially prepared shortening and margarine made from vegetable oils. Nutritionists taught that saturated (animal) fat is bad while unsaturated (vegetable) fat is good. But was this advice based on sound research? Students of nutrition are encouraged to trace the ever-changing recommendations about dietary fat and decide which type is best for health.

The USDA and HHS currently recommend that all American adults strive to limit sodium intake to 1,500 mg rather than the previously recommended 2,300 mg. The reason for lowering the recommended amount across the board is that over 70% of the population fit into groups that are at high risk for developing hypertension, stroke, and heart disease. The challenge of meeting this guideline is that it will be difficult to consume processed foods or dine out in restaurants in the United States. A proposed next step of the USDA is to address the amount of sodium in the processed foods, which is the main source of sodium in the U.S. diet

An important message that is often overlooked is that our diets commonly lack certain vitamins and minerals that are beneficial. Many people think that Vitamin K's only role is to aid in coagulation. Students should recognize that the vitamin has two forms; vitamin K-1 (phylloquinone) is derived from plants, whereas vitamin K-2 (menaquinon) is the form produced by bacteria in the gut. Recent research focuses on vitamin K-2 and its roles in bone and heart health.

Antioxidants are powerful substances that can work for or against you, depending on the amount you consume. Do we need to eat pomegranates, blueberries, and kale to get our daily dose of antioxidants or are supplements just as good? Are all antioxidants vitamins—or are all vitamins antioxidants? And what about the phytochemicals, are they all beneficial or can we consume too much of them? These and other questions are addressed in articles in this unit.

Sports nutrition and foods to improve physical performance are popular topics among the general population and within the profession of nutrition and dietetics. A growing number of Americans are increasing their levels of physical activity in an effort to meet or exceed the exercise recommendations published in the *DGA, 2010.* As a result, more people are exercising at the level of "athlete" rather than occasional exerciser, and they need to know how to properly fuel and hydrate for optimal athletic conditioning.

The articles selected for this unit will provide additional information to the macronutrient and micronutrient sections of a general nutrition course. Several of the articles also address the challenges of interpreting and evaluating scientific nutrition research.

Article

Prepared by: Janet Colson, *Middle Tennessee State University*

Vitamin K2: A Little-Known Nutrient Can Make a Big Difference in Heart and Bone Health

AGLAÉE JACOB

Learning Outcomes

After reading this article, you will be able to:

- Compare food sources and functions of vitamin K1 and K2.
- Explain the influence that a diet low in saturated fats may have on vitamin K2 status.

Ever since vitamin K was discovered in the early 1930s, all the attention has been directed toward its role in coagulation. Although both the K1 (phylloquinone) and K2 (menaquinone) forms of the vitamin were identified at that time, they were thought to be simple structural variations. It's only in the 21st century that the distinct nature of vitamin K2 was finally recognized.

Vitamin K1 deficiency is rare and almost nonexistent, unlike vitamin K2 deficiency.[1] Because of the possibility of vitamin K2 deficiency, it's important for RDs to be aware of this little-known nutrient and the beneficial impact it can have on their clients' and patients' heart and bone health.

Bone Health

Optimizing bone health isn't as simple as getting enough dietary calcium. Beyond the obvious importance of this mineral, other factors, such as vitamin D and magnesium intake, low-grade systemic inflammation, weight-bearing exercise, and intestinal health, also impact bone mineral density, and vitamin K2 should be added to the list.

This fat-soluble vitamin is required to activate osteocalcin, an important protein secreted by osteoblasts, the body's bone-building cells. When vitamin K2 is activated, osteocalcin can draw calcium into the bones where osteoblasts then incorporate it into the bone matrix.[2] In addition, vitamin K2, when combined with vitamin D3, helps inhibit osteoclasts, the cells responsible for bone resorption.[3]

According to a recent study, the incidence of hip fractures in Japanese women seemed to be strongly influenced by their vitamin K2 intake. In Tokyo, the regular consumption of natto, a fermented soy food high in vitamin K2, is associated with a significantly lower risk of hip fractures compared with western Japan where natto isn't frequently eaten.[1] Studies examining the influence of vitamin D and vitamin K (including K1 and K2) intake in institutionalized elderly patients compared with home-dwellers also showed that a higher intake of these nutrients reduced bone fractures.[1]

Since 1995, high doses of vitamin K2 supplements have become an approved treatment for osteoporosis in Japan where studies support its benefit in the prevention of further decline in bone mineral density. Some women have experienced an increase in bone mass as a result of this intervention.[1] Although these results are promising, more studies are needed to confirm their applicability to other populations.

Heart Health

The same osteocalcin protein that vitamin K2 activates also triggers the activation of another protein called matrix gla protein (MGP), which is responsible for removing excess calcium that can accumulate in soft tissues such as arteries and veins.[2] This role takes on significant importance considering that about 20% of atherosclerotic plaques are comprised of calcium, from the early to the more advanced stages of heart disease development.[2]

Vitamin K2-activated MGP is considered the strongest factor in preventing, and possibly even reversing, tissue calcification involved in atherosclerosis, as described in the October 2008 issue of *Thrombosis and Haemostasis.* Patients with diabetes have been shown to have lower MGP levels in their arteries, possibly contributing, at least partly, to the higher risk of arterial calcification and cardiovascular disease seen in this population.

Data from the Rotterdam Study, which followed more than 4,800 subjects aged 55 and older for up to 10 years, showed associations between vitamin K2 intake and aortic calcification. Subjects diagnosed with severe aortic calcification had a lower intake of vitamin K2 compared with subjects with mild to moderate aortic calcification.[4]

Calcium Supplementation with K2 Deficiency

Many physicians recommend calcium supplements to postmenopausal women to help prevent or treat osteoporosis. The question is whether they should, especially if postmenopausal women are deficient in vitamin K2, which may put them at risk of developing cardiovascular diseases. Calcium is the main mineral present in the bone matrix, but supplementing with it doesn't necessarily result in stronger bones if it accumulates in veins and arteries instead of in bones.

Further study is needed to answer this question about the efficacy and safety of calcium supplementation if a postmenopausal woman is deficient in vitamin K2. But based on the current literature, calcium supplements probably shouldn't be recommended. A large-scale meta-analysis published in the December 2007 issue of the *American Journal of Clinical Nutrition* found that calcium supplementation doesn't lower the risk of hip fracture in men or women—in fact, it may increase it.

Results from a 2011 meta-analysis published in *BMJ,* which other researchers have replicated, showed that calcium supplementation with or without vitamin D significantly increased the risk of myocardial infarction or stroke in postmenopausal women. The data were taken from the Women's Health Initiative that included a cohort of 36,282 women. The dietary calcium intake of the women averaged around 800 mg/day, while those supplementing with calcium obtained an additional 585 mg/day.[5] Could their higher risk of cardiovascular diseases be caused by a deficient intake of vitamin K2? Additional study is needed to determine this and whether supplementing with vitamin K2 alone or in combination with calcium can produce better outcomes for bone and heart health.

Food Sources of Vitamin K2

In the meantime, it wouldn't hurt to suggest that clients and patients eat foods rich in vitamins K1 and K2 for optimal health. While vitamin K1 mostly is found in leafy greens, animal products are the best food source of vitamin K2. The ideal way to obtain dietary vitamin K2 is to eat meat, especially organ meat (mainly liver), chicken, beef, bacon, and ham, according to data published in the January 2006 issue of the *Journal of Agricultural and Food Chemistry.* Egg yolks, but not egg whites, also provide valuable amounts of this fat-soluble nutrient as do high-fat dairy products, particularly hard cheeses made with whole milk.

Natto is the only vegetarian source of vitamin K2 because of a specific strain of bacteria used in its fermentation process. It should be noted that although intestinal bacterial synthesis is possible, it doesn't appear to be sufficient in preventing vitamin K2 deficiency in most people.[2]

The reason we can get vitamin K2 from animal-derived foods is because animals have a unique ability to synthesize vitamin K2 from the vitamin K1 they obtain from grass. For this reason, meat, eggs, and dairy from pastured and grass-fed animals contain higher levels of vitamin K2 compared with their grain-fed counterparts.[2]

Many of the best food sources of vitamin K2 also are high in saturated fat, which has been accused of contributing to heart disease without adequate evidence to support this claim. A rigorous meta-analysis, including 347,747 subjects followed for up to 23 years, published in the January 2010 issue of the *American Journal of Clinical Nutrition* clearly showed that there's a lack of significant evidence for blaming saturated fats for the development of coronary heart disease and cardiovascular diseases. Accordingly, subjects in the Rotterdam Study with the highest vitamin K2 intake consumed more total and saturated fats and also had lower total cholesterol values and higher levels of heart-protective HDL cholesterol.[4] Therefore, RDs shouldn't be afraid to recommend foods high in vitamin K2 despite their higher saturated fat content while monitoring their clients' cardiovascular risk profile, especially if they emphasize high-quality, grass-fed and pastured animal sources.

Dietitian's Perspective

Although serum vitamin K2 levels aren't reliable, undercarboxylated osteocalcin represents an indirect marker for vitamin K2 status that should become more available in the future, providing a useful assessment tool for RDs and their clients and patients. Vitamin K2 supplementation also is available in the form of MK-4, a synthetic version produced from an extract of the plant Nicotiana tabacum, and MK-7, a more natural form sourced from natto, as alternatives to help clients meet their vitamin K2 requirements.

The current Dietary Reference Intake for vitamin K doesn't differentiate between the types of this fat-soluble vitamin, but this hopefully will change with future revisions. In the meantime, knowing that food sources of vitamins K1 and K2 are different and that vitamin K2 deficiency is prevalent, RDs should look for ways to help their clients incorporate good sources of vitamin K2 into their diet to ensure proper calcium utilization in the body.

Comparison of Vitamins K1 and K2

	Vitamin K1	**Vitamin K2**
Other name	Phylloquinone	Menaquinone
Role	Coagulation	Proper calcium utilization
Food sources	Leafy greens and green vegetables	Liver, meat, egg yolks, high-fat dairy, and natto
DRI	90 to 120 mcg/day	Not yet determined
Deficiency	Rare	Prevalent

References

1. Vermeer C, Shearer MJ, Zittermann A, et al. Beyond deficiency: potential benefits of increased intakes of vitamin K for bone and vascular health. ***Eur J Nutr.*** 2004;43(6):325–335.
2. Rheaume-Bleue K. ***Vitamin K2 and the Calcium Paradox: How a Little-Known Vitamin Could Save Your Life.*** 1st ed. Ontario, Canada; Wiley: 2011.
3. Plaza SM, Lamson DW. Vitamin K2 in bone metabolism and osteoporosis. ***Altern Med Rev.*** 2005;10(1):24–35.
4. Geleijnse JM, Vermeer C, Grobbee DE, et al. Dietary intake of menaquinone is associated with a reduced risk of coronary heart disease: the Rotterdam Study. ***J Nutr.*** 2004;134(11):3100–3105.
5. Bolland MJ, Grey A, Avenell A, Gamble GD, Reid IR. Calcium supplements with or without vitamin D and risk of cardiovascular events: reanalysis of the Women's Health Initiative limited access dataset and meta-analysis. ***BMJ.*** 2011;342:d2040.

Critical Thinking

1. Which form of vitamin K is involved in coagulation and which form may help reduce the risk of chronic diseases such as atherosclerosis and osteoporosis?
2. What is natto and why is it a good source of vitamin K2?
3. Locate and summarize a peer-reviewed article that describes the role of vitamin K2 and cancer.
4. Explain why many Americans who are concerned about cardiovascular health may have low dietary intake of vitamin K2.
5. Visit the supplement section in your local pharmacy. What form of vitamin K is provided in multivitamin supplements? Which form is found in vitamin K supplements?

Create Central

www.mhhe.com/createcentral

Internet References

Academy of Nutrition and Dietetics
www.eatright.org

Linus Pauling Institute—Vitamin K
http://lpi.oregonstate.edu/infocenter/vitamins/vitaminK

USDA Nutrient Database
ars.usda.gov/Services/docs.htm?docid=17477

Aglaée Jacob, MS, RD, CDE, is a freelance writer who specializes in diabetes education and digestive health, and currently is studying naturopathic medicine in Toronto.

Article

Prepared by: Janet Colson, *Middle Tennessee State University*

Paranoia about Fats Is Driven by Junk Science

When it comes to fats such as omega-3s and omega-6s, it's not just a matter of the right fats, but the right ratio.

JILL RICHARDSON

Learning Outcomes

After reading this article, you will be able to:

- Trace the history of dietary fat recommendations—saturated vs. unsaturated and omega-3 vs. omega-6.
- Describe the contributions that Ralph Holman and Artemis Simopoulos have made about the roles that various fatty acids have on health.

You've heard about omega-3s. You probably know you need to eat them. You've likely heard that they're found in fish. But odds are, there's a lot more you need to know about this family of healthy fats.

Over the last century, Americans have become increasingly confused about fats. Travel back to the Little House on the Prairie, and you'd find Americans happily adding lard, cream and butter to their food. In the 20th century, these saturated animal fats went out of vogue, and "healthier" products like margarine graced American tables instead. Today, no healthy eater would touch the trans-fats in margarine—although they might opt for a trans-fat-free margarine made with palm oil instead.

What's the right answer? And where do omega-3s fit in? As you'll see, while we need omega-3 rich foods in our diet, the bottom line is that we must eat less of another kind of fat, omega-6s, to get the benefit of the omega-3s.

We Don't Need Fat . . . Do We?

To understand Americans' troubled relationship with fat, one must begin when scientists first identified that food was made from protein, carbohydrates and fat. Our bodies can turn carbs into fat, they figured, so we don't actually need fat to survive. Wrong! But it wasn't easy to prove this, at least until modern medicine perfected intravenous feeding (total parenteral nutrition, in hospital-speak).

In a strange twist of fate, scientist Ralph Holman's mother fell ill and ultimately died after a long period receiving fat-free intravenous nutrition. Holman researched the role of fat in human nutrition and he was convinced that certain fats—essential fatty acids—are needed for humans to survive. But he had not been able to prove it.

"Holman watched helplessly as [his mother] died of the very deficiency that he was working to prevent," wrote Susan Allport in *The Queen of Fats: Why Omega-3s Were Removed from the Western Diet and What We Can Do to Replace Them.* Holman lost his mother, but with her death, he proved humans must eat certain fats to survive.

Bad Science Gets Popularized

Careful scientists often assume that there is still plenty we do not know, refraining from making public recommendations until all of the facts are in. (For an example of this, see the recent Michael Pollan article about microbes' role in human health; he emphasizes that the science is so new there aren't many concrete recommendations yet.) But every now and again, a charismatic and arrogant scientist will popularize a current working theory, right or wrong.

Such was the case with Ancel Keys, nicknamed "Monsieur Cholesterol" for popularizing the term and pontificating against it. President Eisenhower had a heart attack in 1955, and suddenly the entire nation was interested in cardiovascular health. Keys had the answer: don't eat fat. He later amended this to an also overly simplified mantra of "saturated fat, bad; unsaturated fat, good."

An obedient nation swapped out butter and lard for unsaturated vegetable oils, especially soybean oil. (Soybean oil is often labeled "vegetable oil" at the store.) But unsaturated vegetable oils are not all equal. They might be monounsaturated or polyunsaturated. Within the polyunsaturated fats, there are omega-6s and omega-3s. And even within those categories, there are different fats with different properties. (You may have heard of the highly sought-after omega-3s EPA and DHA.)

Fat Chemistry 101

Fats are easier to understand once you have a very basic idea of their chemical structure. To grossly oversimplify, fats are basically long chains of carbons connected mostly by single bonds. Scientists classify fats by the number of carbons in the chain, the number of double bonds between the carbons, and the placement of these double bonds.

With the exception of palmitic acid, a saturated fat with 16 carbons, most fats we eat have 18 carbons. With no double bonds, an 18-carbon fat molecule is called stearic acid, a saturated fatty acid. Add one double bond and you've got oleic acid. With two double bonds, it becomes linoleic acid (LA), and with three double bonds, it's alpha-linolenic acid (ALA). (Allport recommends remembering these two similarly named fats by remembering that the molecule with the extra double bond—linolenic—has the name with an extra letter in it.)

Omega-6 vs. Omega-3: It's the Ratio, Stupid

What makes a fat classified as an omega-3, omega-6 or even omega-9? The placement of the double bond closest to the end of the molecule. LA, with its last double bond six spots from the end, is an omega-6. ALA, with its last bond three spots from the end, is an omega-3. And oleic acid, with its last and only bond nine spots from the end, is an omega-9. Omega is the last letter of the Greek alphabet, so the name "omega-3" denotes the double bond is three away from the omega end, the tail end, of the molecule.

Our bodies can make fat, we can add carbons to fat molecules, and we can even add double bonds to fat molecules. However, we cannot add double bonds any closer than nine spots from the end. If you eat an omega-3, it remains an omega-3. If you eat an omega-6, it remains an omega-6.

Here's the catch: we usually eat fat molecules with 18 carbons, but we need longer chain fatty acids for important purposes in our bodies. After we eat LA (an omega-6) and ALA (an omega-3), the two compete for the same set of enzymes to elongate and desaturate them into arachadonic acid (ARA, an omega-6), eicosapentaenoic acid (EPA, an omega-3), and docosahexaenoic acid (DHA, an omega-3).

Omega-3s are stronger competitors to gain use of these enzymes, but they can't compete if we flood our bodies with omega-6s. And that's what we do.

A healthy omega-6 to omega-3 ratio is somewhere around 4:1, and some scientists think it could be even closer to 2:1. Americans average something more like 10:1.

The Systematic Flooding of Our Food System with Omega-6s

How did we get where we are today? Consider our food system: lots of shelf-stable packaged foods, plenty of cheap, grain-fed animal products, and a consumer base convinced that saturated fats are bad and polyunsaturated fats are good. Each of these factors adds up to more omega-6s and less omega-3s.

Omega-3s are often found in leafy greens. You might not think of spinach as a fatty food—and it isn't—but within the tiny bit of fat in raw spinach, you'll find five times more omega-3s than omega-6s. Seeds, on the other hand, tend to have more omega-6s than omega-3s. Out of the world's most popular vegetable seed oils (soy, sunflower, rapeseed, peanut, cottonseed, olive, sesame, corn, and safflower), only rapeseed (canola) has a favorable ratio of omega-6s to omega-3s.

Consider your average supermarket. How much space is devoted to seeds and their oils compared to leafy greens? Check out any packaged food on the market. Odds are you'll find corn and soy . . . both seeds. What did the animals that produced the meat, milk, and eggs eat? Probably a lot of corn and soy. Even factory farmed cattle, which still eat some grass, eat more seeds (again, mostly corn and soy) than their ancestors did a century ago.

Omega-6s are more shelf-stable than omega-3s. Flax oil, high in omega-3s, must be stored in dark bottles in the fridge, and even still it must be consumed quickly before it goes rancid. And seeds, full of omega-6s, are higher in calories than leafy greens, so factory farms prefer them as a quick way to fatten livestock. And, as Americans learned from "experts" that saturated fat is bad and polyunsaturated fat is good, the food industry gave us what we asked for—but usually in the form of shelf-stable omega-6s.

Another factor comes from our ability to produce vegetable seed oils. Using a simple mechanical process one can extract olive oil and avocado oil. To extract other oils, like soybean oil, chemical solvents are used. Until about a century ago, all soybean oil extraction was done mechanically (and not very efficiently), but soybean oil was hardly the major food source it is today.

Extracting soybean oil with hexane, a toxic chemical that can cause nerve damage, was just one innovation that made soybean oil ubiquitous in our food supply. As factory farming increased—and with it the demand for soybean meal—the result was an increase of its byproduct, soybean oil. Also important: making soybean oil more palatable to consumers. That requires the oil to be degummed, refined, bleached, and deodorized. Partial hydrogenation also allowed vegetable oils to stand in where we previously used saturated fats (i.e., margarine instead of butter).

The advent of these technologies made an unprecedented amount of vegetable seed oils—and omega-6s—available in our food supply. By 1986, a whopping 81.7 percent of the vegetable oil Americans ate came from soybeans. The tide turned a bit over the next decade, as canola oil gained a reputation as a healthy oil—but more than three-quarters of the vegetable oil in the U.S. still came from soybeans.

A study found that the single largest source of omega-6s (58 percent) in the U.S. food was soybean oil—more than meat, fish, eggs, milk, cheese, lard, and other vegetable oils combined. Soybean oil does not have the worst ratio of omega-6 to omega-3—other oils like cottonseed, sunflower, safflower, and corn are all far worse. But since it is so prevalent in our food, it's the biggest culprit all the same.

The Science Revisited

The title of a recent piece by omega-3 pioneer Ralph Holman is telling: "The Slow Discovery of the Importance of Omega-3 Essential Fatty Acids in Human Health." While we were tripping over ourselves to rid our diets of all fats, or saturated fats, or animal fats, or trans-fats, as one trend gave way to the next, scientists like Holman were carefully piecing together the importance of omega-3s in reducing inflammation and heart disease. Sadly, as they were figuring out the importance of the ratio of omega-6 to omega-3s, the nation's ratio kept tipping in the wrong direction.

Artemis Simopoulos, author of *The Omega Diet,* is one of the scientists who made great contributions to understanding the importance of omega-3s. A physician and the president of the Center for Genetics, Nutrition, and Health, she went back and looked at the raw data from Ancel Keys' famous Seven Countries Study.

Undertaken in the late 1950s, the study examined diet and heart disease in Yugoslavia, Finland, Italy, the Netherlands, Greece, Japan, and the U.S. It "clearly showed that the people who had the lowest rate of heart disease and cancer and who lived the longest were the people who lived on the island of Crete, in Greece," she explains. Simopoulos recognized Keys' mistakes in interpreting the data. He neglected to distinguish between omega-6s and omega-3s.

As a Greek, Simopoulos certainly knew something about the traditional Greek diet. "When I was looking at the traditional diet of Crete," she recalls, "I became very much aware that the people in Greece at the time—and I'm talking prior to 1960—they ate a lot of wild plants. And so I studied the wild plants and the composition of the wild plants and I found that wild plants have more antioxidants, more vitamin C, more vitamin E, and more omega-3s" in the form of ALA. "And purslane," a common edible weed in the Mediterranean, "has more omega-3s than any other plant."

One day she was visiting her parents in Greece and she saw the chickens eating purslane. "I questioned whether that egg would be different in composition than the egg you buy in the supermarket where the chickens are fed corn and other grains." Analyzing the eggs, she found they contained equal amounts of omega-6 and omega-3s, whereas a typical egg in U.S. supermarkets has a ratio of 20:1.

The difference was not just the purslane that the Greek chickens ate. "They eat grass, they eat bugs, and they eat worms," notes Simopoulos—adding that bugs and worms are high in ALA, EPA and DHA. "What's fascinating is that the amount of DHA in egg yolk [from her chickens] is equivalent to mother's milk at one month of age."

Other top sources of omega-3s are fish, particularly wild-caught fish, and seaweed. Like the bugs, worms and wild plants eaten by the Greek chickens, wild-caught fish and seaweed are not cultivated by humans.

The Bottom Line: Eat Less Omega-6s

While we usually consume omega-3s as ALA, our bodies require EPA and DHA. EPA is commonly used in our membranes, whereas DHA is important in our brains and eyes. And with a few exceptions (for example, premature babies and people with hypertension), humans can turn ALA into EPA and DHA. But, remember, that only happens if you do not consume so much omega-6s that they monopolize the enzymes needed.

According to Simopoulos, traditionally only 2% of energy came from omega-6 and 1% came from omega-3s. "The ratio was either balanced or it was 2:1," she says. And we won't achieve that ratio unless we dramatically bring down the amount of omega-6s we eat.

How do we do this? The people of Greece have a good idea: use olive oil. A healthy, monounsaturated fat, it does not play into the omega-6 vs. omega-3 ratio. Eat your fish and eat your greens (even seaweed) to get omega-3s, but boot the omega-6s from your diet.

Critical Thinking

1. How did Ralph Holman determine that humans must consume essential fatty acids to survive?
2. What criticism does Artemis Simopoulos have about Ancyl Keys' recommendations that "saturated fat, bad; unsaturated fat, good"?
3. Describe foods consumed in the traditional Mediterranean diet and the effect they have on health.
4. What is ratio of omega-3 to omega-6 fatty acids in the typical American diet? What is the desirable ratio?
5. Using MyPlate.gov, evaluate the fatty acid content of your diet. What is the ratio of omega-3 to omega-6? What steps can you take to improve this ratio?

Create Central

www.mhhe.com/createcentral

Internet References

Dietary Guidelines for Americans 2010
www.health.gov/dietaryguidelines/2010.asp

Essential Fatty Acids—Linus Pauling Institute Micronutrient Research for Optimum Health
http://lpi.oregonstate.edu/infocenter/othernuts/omega3fa

Omega-6 Me: One Woman's Journey to the Dark Side of the American Food supply
www.susanallport.com/files/Omega-6_Me.doc

The Slow Discovery of the Importance of ω3 Essential Fatty Acids in Human Health
http://nutrition.highwire.org/content/128/2/427S.full

Jill Richardson is the founder of the blog *La Vida Locavore* and a member of the Organic Consumers Association policy advisory board. She is the author of *Recipe for America: Why Our Food System Is Broken and What We Can Do to Fix It.*

Article

Prepared by: Janet Colson, *Middle Tennessee State University*

Antioxidants: More Is Not Always Better

These powerful nutrients can work for or against you, depending on how you consume them.

CONSUMER REPORTS

Learning Outcomes

After reading this article, you will be able to:

- Describe the health benefits of antioxidants.
- List possible adverse effects that taking high amounts of a single antioxidant can cause.

Grocery-store shelves are full of products with labels bragging that they contain antioxidants, and implying that you're just a few bites—and bucks—away from better health:

- "The #1 antioxidant fruit," boasts a can of Wyman's wild blueberries.
- "Antioxidant Advantage," promises a banner on Tropicana Pure Premium Orange Juice.
- "The antioxidant power of 6 servings of fruits and vegetables," claims the website for the food supplement Go Greens Super Fruits & Veggies drink mix.

But it's not that simple. More is not necessarily better when it comes to antioxidants. And research has found that how you consume them can make a big difference in your health. In fact, two recent lawsuits have challenged manufacturer claims about antioxidants, alleging that product labels are misleading consumers. To help you distinguish the myths from the truth, here's a close look at the latest on antioxidants.

MYTH: Antioxidants are all vitamins

There are thousands of antioxidants, but relatively few of them are vitamins. Some are minerals and others are enzymes, which are protein molecules that facilitate chemical reactions necessary for cells to function properly. Vitamins C and E, the minerals selenium and zinc, and pigments such as carotenoids are all promoted for their antioxidant abilities. Polyphenols (or flavonoids), the most plentiful and common form of antioxidants, are found in fruit, vegetables, whole grains, tea, chocolate, and red wine.

What antioxidants have in common is their ability to block the action of free radicals: unstable chemical fragments that can wreak havoc on healthy components in your body's cells. This damage can cause cells to grow and reproduce abnormally, part of a dangerous chain reaction. In time, that process is thought to play a role in chronic conditions including cancer, cardiovascular disease, Alzheimer's, Parkinson's, and eye diseases such as cataracts and age-related macular degeneration.

Your body produces free radicals during exercise and when converting food into energy. And your body generates antioxidants to help stabilize them. Other factors—cigarette smoke, alcohol consumption, and exposure to sunlight and environmental contaminants like pesticides—trigger the production of more free radicals, which can potentially overwhelm your body's natural defenses. Antioxidants in the food you eat, such as fruit, vegetables, and whole grains, can come to the rescue.

Substances known as antioxidants also have other beneficial effects, including combatting inflammation.

MYTH: All antioxidants are created equal

"Different antioxidants fight different free radicals," says Jeffrey Blumberg, Ph.D., director of the Antioxidant Research Lab at Tufts University. "There is an antioxidant defense network. It's like an army; you have generals and colonels and lieutenants. Each one has a different job."

And they work well together. For example, vitamin C recycles vitamin E. Once a molecule of vitamin E neutralizes a free radical, vitamin C converts that molecule of E back to its antioxidant form, allowing it to combat more free radicals. "So if you take a lot of vitamin E but your vitamin C intake is low, you won't see much antioxidant benefit," Blumberg says.

The synergistic effect among thousands of antioxidants is a major reason doctors, dietitians, and others advise people to eat a wide range of fruit, vegetables, whole grains, and legumes. Even though scientists have yet to pinpoint all the ways those healthy compounds protect against disease, many observational studies suggest that people who consume a greater amount of antioxidant-rich foods have a lower risk of certain diseases than people who don't.

For example, a study published in the October 2012 *American Journal of Medicine* that followed more than 32,000 Swedish women for 10 years concluded that those whose diets contained the most antioxidants had a 20 percent lower risk of a heart attack compared with women who consumed the least.

MYTH: It's important to eat pomegranates, berries, and other "super fruits"

"All fruits are 'super,' " Blumberg says. "There's no scientific or regulatory definition of 'super fruit.' It can mean anything—therefore, it's meaningless." Each fruit or vegetable has a unique combination of healthy compounds, including antioxidants. By eating only those billed as "super," you shortchange your health by skipping those combinations of nutrients in other produce.

And what if you dislike a particular fruit or vegetable? "Nature tends to group similar nutrients in foods that have the same color, so find foods you like in as many colors as you can," says Tricia Psota, Ph.D., a clinical research dietitian at the National Institutes of Health's Clinical Center. If you don't like kale or spinach, opt for broccoli or green pepper. Instead of oranges, consider mangoes or papaya.

MYTH: You should amp up your intake with supplements

Focus on food instead. Overall, clinical trials that have examined the disease-fighting capability of specific antioxidant nutrients in supplement form haven't shown very promising results. One of the exceptions is the Age-Related Eye Disease Study led by the National Eye Institute. It found that a combination of antioxidants and zinc supplements reduced the risk of developing advanced age-related macular degeneration in people who already had an intermediate stage of the disease.

Talk with your physician about supplement use, however, because some studies have suggested that some can cause harm. Selenium supplements of 200 micrograms a day have been linked to a higher incidence of recurrence of nonmelanoma skin cancers in people who previously suffered such a cancer. And despite earlier findings that men who took vitamin E or selenium had a lower risk of prostate cancer, a large study of about 35,000 men, published in 2011, found that those who had taken 400 international units of vitamin E a day were 17 percent more likely to develop prostate cancer over seven years.

Scientists don't know why the studies have been disappointing, but they have some theories."Some people would argue that the trials have focused too much on high doses of single or limited combinations of nutrients," says Howard Sesso, Sc.D., an epidemiologist at Brigham and Women's Hospital in Boston and associate professor at the Harvard Medical School. He says another explanation might be that supplements can't replicate the complex, beneficial effects of a healthy diet.

MYTH: If some antioxidants are good, more are better

"Too much of a good thing can be problematic," especially when it comes from dietary supplements, says Susan Mayne, Ph.D., an epidemiologist at the Yale School of Public Health. So beware of multi- and single-antioxidant capsules labeled "megadoses," which contain more than the recommended daily values for antioxidants. Some evidence suggests that when taken in megadoses, antioxidants can become pro-oxidants, which increase the production of free radicals, especially in people who smoke or drink alcohol. "Supplements can have unpredictable interactions in these cases," Mayne says. "They can flip from potentially healthful to being harmful." In one study, heavy smokers who took high-dose beta-carotene, alone or with vitamin E, were more likely to get lung cancer.

It's much less likely that you'll consume too many antioxidants from food. But eating one type of fruit or vegetable in excessive amounts can result in some odd, if harmless, effects. For example, consuming extremely large amounts of carrots or other beta-carotene-rich vegetables can result in orange-tinted skin. And eating an excessive amount of tomatoes can cause yellow-orange skin discoloration.

But most Americans eat too little, not too much, fruit and vegetables. If you want to boost your intake, stick to normal serving sizes and choose a wide variety of produce.

MYTH: Packaged food with labels touting antioxidants will boost your health

Antioxidant claims on packaged food don't always mean a health benefit. "Unfortunately, 'antioxidant' is a very loosely used term," says Joy Dubost, Ph.D., a nutritionist and spokeswoman for the Academy of Nutrition and Dietetics. "Outside the lab, it has become more of a marketing term than a scientific term."

Some food manufacturers add an antioxidant, such as vitamin C or E, and then label the product as containing antioxidants, presumably in hopes of boosting sales. Kellogg's Fiber-Plus Antioxidants Dark Chocolate Almond bars, for example, have 20 percent of the daily value of vitamin E and zinc. But they also contain 7 grams of sugar and 5 grams of fat. You can avoid processed food and eat an ounce of dry-roasted almonds, which provides more vitamin E, and 3 ounces of lean beef, which has more zinc.

Some food manufacturers even advertise antioxidant "power," represented by ORAC, or oxygen radical absorbance capacity values. But ORAC measures antioxidant activity in a test tube, not in the human body. So if you're tempted by Mystic Harvest Purple Corn Tortilla Chips, which are supposed to have an ORAC score of 6,000, don't be. "We don't know what these values mean biologically," Dubost says, but they don't guarantee better health.

A class-action lawsuit filed in November 2012 against the makers of 7Up Cherry Antioxidant Soda claimed that the packaging and marketing could lead consumers to think that the antioxidants in the soft drink come from fruit, when they really come from added vitamin E, and a 12-ounce can provides only 15 percent of the daily value.

Another class-action lawsuit, filed in April 2012 against Hershey, alleges that the chocolate giant makes "misleading" and "unlawful" claims regarding antioxidants. For example, certain packages of Hershey Special Dark Kisses state that "Cocoa is a natural source of flavanol antioxidants." While cocoa is a reasonable source of antioxidants, the suit alleges that many—if not all—of Hershey's cocoa or chocolate products undergo alkalization, a process that reduces or virtually eliminates the flavanol content.

Both companies have publicly denied any wrongdoing. The maker of 7Up Cherry Antioxidant said that in a decision unrelated to the lawsuit it has produced a new version of 7Up Cherry without antioxidants.

As scientists continue to explore how antioxidants work in the body, the best health advice remains the simplest: Make sure your diet contains plenty of varieties of fruit, vegetables, whole grains, and legumes.

Critical Thinking

1. How do antioxidants function within the body?
2. Explain why Susan Mayne does not consider that pomegranates and blueberries are "super fruits."
3. What happens when a person take vitamin E supplements every day while eating a diet that consists of French fries, bananas, and hot dogs?
4. What is a pro-oxidant and what effect does it have on the body?
5. What does ORAC measure? What is Joy Dubost's opinion regarding the ORAC level in a food?

Create Central

www.mhhe.com/createcentral

Internet References

Antioxidants and Cancer Prevention. National Cancer Institute
www.cancer.gov/cancertopics/factsheet/prevention/antioxidants

Antioxidants and Health: An Introduction. National Center for Complementary and Alternative Medicine
http://nccam.nih.gov/health/antioxidants/introduction.htm

Dietary Supplement Labeling Guide: Chapter VI. Claims—Antioxidants. Food and Drug Administration
www.fda.gov/Food/GuidanceRegulation/GuidanceDocumentsRegulatoryInformation/DietarySupplements/ucm070613.htm

Article

Prepared by: Janet Colson, *Middle Tennessee State University*

Athletes *and* Protein Intake

Experts weigh in on whether the Recommended Dietary Allowance for highly physically active people is adequate.

DENSIE WEBB

Learning Outcomes

After reading this article, you will be able to:

- Compare the protein needs of a trained athlete to the needs of someone who is just beginning a program of strength training.
- Which amino acid appears to be the most critical for an athlete? What role does this amino acid play in muscle protein synthesis?
- Discuss the health consequences of a diet that provides 25–35 percent of total calories from protein.

Controversy exists among medical experts regarding the role protein plays in maintaining optimal health. They debate about when to consume it, how much to consume, and what type is best, especially for athletes and highly active people.

The Recommended Dietary Allowance (RDA) for protein, 0.8 g/kg of body weight per day, is designed to maintain nitrogen balance in the body for the average adult; a negative nitrogen balance indicates that muscle is being broken down and used for energy. (RDAs for protein in children are higher on a gram-per-body-weight basis than for adults. RDAs also are greater for women who are pregnant [1.1 g/kg/day] or lactating [1.3 g/kg/day]).

While maintaining nitrogen balance is critical for health, studies now suggest that the RDA may not be the amount of protein needed to promote optimal health. To achieve that, they say, more protein is needed, and studies now suggest that athletes, active people, and older individuals require even more.

Dietary proteins are in a constant state of flux in the body, being broken down into amino acids, transformed into other compounds, and sometimes reassembled into other proteins. They also are used for energy, a mechanism that increases when energy intake is low or when protein intake is inadequate. Muscle protein then becomes a source of energy, resulting in a negative nitrogen balance. This is a critical concern for athletes, who are regularly involved in energy-demanding activities.

It stands to reason then that athletes and active individuals would require more protein, and high-quality proteins, on a daily basis than those who spend their days sitting at a desk in front of a computer screen. (High-quality proteins contain all nine essential amino acids in amounts similar to amino acid requirements; animal proteins are higher quality than plant proteins.) While adequate high-quality protein is critical for good health and optimal athletic performance, the amount needed isn't the one-size-fits-all recommendation the RDA suggests.

Today's Dietitian spoke with experts to determine the latest protein requirements for athletes and highly active people.

How Much Is Enough?

While it's generally accepted that athletes need more protein than sedentary people, recommendations vary significantly depending on the type of athlete, current body weight, total energy intake, whether weight loss or weight gain is the goal, exercise intensity and duration, training status, the quality of the dietary protein, and the individual's age. The general rule of thumb is 1.2–1.4 g/kg of body weight for endurance athletes and 1.2–1.7 g/kg of body weight for strength and power athletes, says Christopher Mohr, PhD, RD, a nutrition consultant and writer and the co-owner of Mohr Results, a weight-loss company in Louisville, Kentucky. The greater the number of hours in training and the higher the intensity, the more protein is required. Other research has recommended as much as 2 g/kg of body weight to prevent muscle loss in athletes who have reduced their energy intake.

While physical activity increases protein needs, it also increases the efficiency with which muscles use dietary protein, even in older individuals. One study found that a moderate increase in physical activity among a group of older subjects enhanced the response to protein intake, suggesting that increased exercise may help prevent and treat muscle loss that occurs with aging.

What about the recreational athlete, otherwise known as the weekend warrior? "The research shows that most people would benefit from added protein, from increased satiety to increased muscle synthesis," Mohr says. "People generally consume only around 15–16 percent of total calories as protein, so there's certainly room to increase protein intake." Some have suggested that recreational athletes should aim for daily intakes closer to 1.1–1.4 g/kg of body weight per day, 38–75 percent greater than the current RDA. Endurance athletes, such as marathon runners, should be in the range of 1.2–2 g/kg of body weight, and strength athletes, such as weight lifters, should be in the range of 1.4–2 g/kg of body weight.

According to Nancy Clark, MS, RD, CSSD, a sports nutrition counselor and the author of *Nancy Clark's Sports Nutrition Guidebook,* different protein recommendations aren't needed for men vs. women. "[They're] based on grams per kilogram of body weight," she says. In addition, active people shouldn't focus on protein alone. "Have protein/carbohydrate combinations, protein to build and repair muscle tissue and carbs to fuel." The ratio of protein to carbohydrate can vary greatly, depending on protein intake.

Unlike endurance training, single sessions of resistance exercise, regardless of workout length or intensity, don't appear to increase protein use during the workout itself. However, amino acid uptake after a resistance training session does increase, indicating that the amino acids are being used for muscle repair and construction. Protein utilization appears to be higher for individuals who are less fit.

When beginning endurance training, nitrogen balance may be negative for the first two weeks, and protein requirements may be higher in the first week of strength training to support new muscle growth. After one to two weeks of training, however, typically the body adapts and the protein utilization decreases. In general, adequate calorie and carbohydrate intake reduces the need for amino acid oxidation for energy and spares dietary protein and muscle tissue. Protein sparing is based on the concept that if adequate energy is consumed from carbohydrate and fat then dietary protein is available for protein-unique functions (i.e., protein synthesis [tissue, hormones, neurotransmitters, enzymes, etc.]). To protect muscle protein, consider counseling athletes to temporarily increase protein intake when starting a new training program or entering a new training phase.

Protein-Rich Foods and Supplements

- Beef tenderloin steak, lean only (3.5 oz): 29 g
- Salmon (4 oz): 29 g
- NOW Pea Protein Powder (33-g scoop): 24 g
- Swanson Whey Protein Powder (23-g scoop): 20 g
- Solgar Whey to Go Powder (25-g scoop): 20 g
- Lentils (1 cup): 18 g
- BOOST High Protein Drink (8 oz): 15 g
- Greek yogurt (5 oz): 14 g
- Kashi GOLEAN cereal (1 cup): 13 g
- Skim milk (8 oz): 8 g
- Tofu, firm (3.5 oz): 7 g
- Egg, large (1 large): 6 g
- Beneprotein Instant Protein Powder (7 g scoop): 6 g

Sources: Reference and Company Websites.

Type of Protein to Consider

The International Society of Sports Nutrition recommends that high-quality proteins be consumed. It highlights milk-derived whey protein isolate and casein and egg white and soy protein isolate as proteins that provide essential amino acids that are readily taken up by muscle to optimize nitrogen balance and muscle protein synthesis.

Research suggests that of all the essential amino acids, leucine may be the limiting factor in initiating muscle protein synthesis, and that leucine-rich proteins may be the best way to boost muscle protein synthesis after intense physical activity. Some researchers suggest that protein quality based on leucine content is important when consuming small meals or when the total amount of protein consumed is less than optimal.

The mixture of proteins in the American diet averages about 8 percent leucine. The range of protein thought to stimulate muscle protein synthesis after a meal is about 2.5–3.5 g. Dairy products, beef, poultry, seafood, pork, peanuts, beans, lentils, and soybeans are among the foods richest in leucine.

What about protein powder supplements? "They're not necessary," Mohr says. "[But] are they convenient for those on the go looking for a quick, quality meal? Absolutely. Blend with a little milk, veggies, and nuts or nut butter and you have a great meal to go."

When to Eat Protein

Just as important as the amount and type of protein athletes should eat is when they should eat it. As a result of physical activity, muscle breaks down. If protein intake is low, that muscle isn't replaced. Those who are acclimated to regular exercise experience less muscle protein breakdown. However, protein needs are greater during intense bouts of training. The general consensus is that protein ingestion after exercise, when muscle is most sensitive to nutrient intake, will boost muscle protein synthesis and recovery.

Athletes aside, "Most people eat only about 10–15 percent of total protein in the morning, about 20 percent or so in the afternoon, and the remainder at dinner. Since our bodies don't store protein, spreading that intake more evenly throughout the day would be beneficial," Mohr says.

"Research has shown that adults need at least 30 g of protein at two or more meals to maintain healthy muscles," says Donald Layman, PhD, professor emeritus in the department of food science and human nutrition at the University of Illinois at Urbana-Champaign. "Small meals, such as breakfast or lunch, often contain less than 15 g of protein and provide no benefit to muscle health."

A study recently published in the *Journal of Nutrition* found that muscle protein synthesis was 25 percent higher when protein was evenly distributed across breakfast, lunch, and dinner compared with a more typical pattern, when most protein was consumed at the evening meal, even when total protein intake was the same. Protein that's evenly distributed throughout the day may be especially important for older, physically active adults, as older individuals experience a resistance to muscle protein synthesis in response to meals containing less protein; in other words, the protein threshold to trigger muscle protein synthesis is higher in older individuals.

According to Douglas Paddon-Jones, PhD, an associate professor at the University of Texas Medical Branch at Galveston and a protein researcher, "The same basic model of consuming a moderate amount of high-quality protein three times a day applies to different aged athletes. But moderate for different sized people might range from 15 g to 40-plus grams per meal."

Protein Specific Guidelines

- Develop a meal plan that will supply adequate calories, carbohydrate, and protein each day.
- Distribute the protein equally across meals.
- Emphasize high-quality protein.
- Base protein intake on weight, not on percentage of calories.
- Base protein intake on the individual's sport and intensity level.
- Recommend that active, older individuals boost protein intake, as some may require more to help preserve muscle mass.
- Suggest protein powders to individuals who need added protein on the go and whose calorie intake is low.

— DW

High-Protein Diets

Since added protein intake is critical for athletes and physically active people, should they consume a high-protein diet? Instead of recommending protein as grams per kilogram of body weight, the Institute of Medicine established an acceptable macronutrient distribution range for protein at 10–35 percent of total calories for adults older than 18. The Institute of Medicine defines the acceptable macronutrient distribution range as a range of intake associated with reduced risk of chronic diseases while providing adequate intakes of essential nutrients. The average protein intake in the United States of 15 percent of total calories is well within the acceptable macronutrient distribution range but well below recommended intakes for most athletes. Even the 95th percentile of protein intake for US adults doesn't come close to the highest acceptable macronutrient distribution range for protein at 35 percent of total calories. Higher intakes of high-quality protein recommended for athletes would still be well within the acceptable macronutrient distribution range.

Frequently, concerns are expressed about the possible negative health effects of high-protein intakes; however, an upper limit for protein intake hasn't been established, though the Dietary Reference Intakes warn against exceeding the acceptable macronutrient distribution range. It's important to bear in mind that if calories are limited, high protein intake may displace other important nutrients.

Probably the most common concern expressed is that high-protein intakes may impair renal function. It's true that protein intake, beyond that which supports nitrogen balance, promotes urea formation, and can increase glomerular filtration rate and kidney nitrogen load. There's little evidence that the change in glomerular filtration rate can cause problems in healthy people, as the clearance of urea becomes more efficient with higher protein intakes. However, lower protein intakes, based on an individual's weight and the severity of their condition, are recommended for those with impaired renal function.

For healthy people, a recent study suggested a maximum intake of 2–2.5 g/kg of body weight per day, totaling 176 g of protein per day for an 80-kg (176-lb) individual consuming approximately 2,900 kcal daily. This translates to about 25 percent of calories from protein within the range of 10–35 percent recommended by the 2010 Dietary Guidelines for Americans and the maximum of 35 percent by the acceptable macronutrient distribution range.

A recent study of overweight and obese individuals with type 2 diabetes consuming a diet containing 90–120 g of protein per day found no effect on renal function compared with those consuming 55–70 g/day, suggesting that higher intakes aren't harmful.

However, increased dietary protein can result in elevated urinary calcium, which may contribute to bone loss and the subsequent development of osteopenia and osteoporosis. Yet the role protein plays in bone health is complex. A recent systematic review found that the evidence was inconclusive regarding a significant relationship (either positive or negative) between protein intake and bone health, but that protein likely provided a small benefit to bone health. Moreover, evidence shows an association between dietary protein and increased peak bone mass in both young and older adults.

An interaction exists between calcium and protein intakes; when calcium intakes are low, a high-protein diet could be detrimental to bone. When calcium intakes are higher, protein appears to be beneficial. It has been suggested that protein intakes of greater than 2 g/kg of body weight per day should be avoided if calcium intake is below 600 mg/day.

High-protein diets that consist of excessive intakes of 200–400 g/day can exceed the liver's ability to convert excess nitrogen to urea and lead to nausea, diarrhea, and even death. "I think the biggest message is to avoid the absurd—30-oz steak dinners or carrying around a gallon container of a protein drink all day," Paddon-Jones says.

Recommendations

Developing an individualized nutrition plan for athletes should take into account the individual's health history, the sport he or she plays, weekly training regimens, time of competition, access to food, and travel schedules. When working with athletes, dietitians must gauge a person's readiness for change before offering guidance. Moreover, sports nutrition professionals should discuss the athletes' goals and concerns, answer questions, and ask for the athletes' participation in their meal planning.

Critical Thinking

1. Explain why the recommendations regarding protein needs for athletes are controversial.
2. Design a 24-hour meal plan for a college-age male who has just started a body-building program. Include the serving sizes, the grams of protein provided in each food, and the total grams of protein provided for the entire day.
3. What advice would you give a friend who consistently consumes 35 percent of his calories from protein?

Create Central

www.mhhe.com/createcentral

Internet References

Academy of Nutrition and Dietetics
www.eatright.org

American College of Sports Medicine
www.acsm.org

Densie Webb, PhD, RD, is a freelance writer and industry consultant based in Austin, Texas.

Article

Prepared by: Janet Colson, *Middle Tennessee State University*

Virtual Nutrition Counseling

More dietitians are offering telehealth services for convenience and to meet their clients' changing needs.

LORI ZANTESON

Learning Outcomes

After reading this article, you will be able to:

- Explain what telehealth is and how it may be used to counsel patients.
- Describe how virtual nutrition counseling is beneficial for dietitians and clients.

Counseling clients and patients in a private practice, classroom, hospital, or other clinical setting is the most common way in which nutrition professionals provide nutrition counseling services. But due to the rapid advances in technology, more and more dietitians are branching out of the traditional office and clinical setting and are offering virtual nutrition counseling services remotely. They're counseling clients via cell phone and the Internet, meeting them in local coffee shops and other public venues, and even making house calls.

In this fast-paced digital age, almost everyone stays connected through handheld devices that allow for immediate communication in real time. So it makes sense that cell phones, smartphones, tablets, and other wireless technologies are expanding the ways in which RDs perform their jobs. Technology has made the provision of nutrition counseling more convenient and accessible for both the provider and the client.

Virtual Health Care

Offering virtual health care services, also known as telemedicine or telehealth, isn't new, as other medical professions already are doing it. Physicians provide remote health care via e-mail, smartphones, and two-way video conferencing. Psychologists and psychiatrists offer virtual mental health services, known as e-therapy, e-counseling, or cyber counseling, over the Internet, through e-mail or video conferencing, or by phone. Patients also have access to telenursing, telepharmacy, and telerehabilitation services.

The growing demand for virtual health care services in these and other professions has prompted many telecommunications companies to begin offering video conferencing services. Vsee.com and Securevideo.com are just a few of the well-established services available, which many health care practitioners use to meet with and counsel clients and patients.

In the context of dietetics, nutrition professionals practice telehealth and telenutrition, which, according to Heather R. Mangieri, MS, RDN, CSSD, LDN, owner and nutrition consultant at Nutrition CheckUp and a spokesperson for the Academy of Nutrition and Dietetics (the Academy), is defined by the Academy Definition of Terms List as follows:

> Telehealth is the use of electronic information and telecommunications technologies to support long-distance clinical health care, patient and professional health-related education, public health, and health administration. Telehealth will include both the use of interactive, specialized equipment, for such purposes as health promotion, disease prevention, diagnosis, consultation, therapy, and/or nutrition intervention/plan of care, and non-interactive (or passive) communications, over the Internet, videoconferencing, e-mail or fax lines, and other methods of distance communications for communication of broad-based nutrition information.
>
> Telenutrition involves the interactive use, by a RD or RDN, of electronic information and telecommunications technologies to implement the Nutrition Care

Process (nutrition assessment, nutrition diagnosis, nutrition intervention/plan of care, and nutrition monitoring and evaluation) with patients or clients at a remote location, within the provisions of their state licensure as applicable.

Before delving into telenutrition, Mangieri says "Registered dietitians should do their homework before determining if this is an area they want to explore. The Academy of Nutrition and Dietetics offers extensive information on this area of practice, including practice tips."

Meeting Clients' Needs

According to Ruth Frechman, MA, RDN, CPT, owner of On the Weigh, a nutrition consulting service in Burbank, California, and a national spokesperson for the Academy, "The best way to counsel clients is the way that best suits their needs to receive information. If a client prefers to stay home and is willing to chat by phone or computer, it makes sense to accommodate them."

However, beyond a client's personal preferences, they may have other limitations that prevent them from leaving home, such as a broken-down car or no one available to pick them up after their appointment—both of which can lead to canceled appointments. "[In many cases], using a virtual service can be a win-win for everyone," Frechman says.

The option to eliminate a face-to-face appointment is a convenience many people prefer, she says. Virtual nutrition counseling can allow for a quick session between activities or during a lunch break, and it requires fewer adjustments to daily schedules and eliminates commuting time.

Moreover, virtual nutrition counseling enables dietitians to see clients who travel frequently for work or who live in remote areas and wouldn't be able to commute to a dietitian's office. Amanda Austin, RDN, CLT, a Michigan-based certified LEAP therapist and food sensitivity specialist, recently counseled a patient who worked out of the country. The patient suffered from migraines, digestive problems, fatigue, heartburn, and other symptoms for more than 10 years. She needed to see a dietitian right away but couldn't do so in a traditional setting. "She found me, and within 10 days of implementing the dietary recommendations that I provided her, her symptoms were reduced by 66 percent," Austin says. "By six weeks, all of her symptoms were gone. If she hadn't been able to work with me over the phone, there's no question in my mind that she would still be suffering."

Susan Linke, MBA, MS, RD, LD, CLT, a certified LEAP therapist and certified LEAP therapist mentor, has an office in Dallas but does most of her counseling virtually. Because Dallas is such a large city, teleconsulting has enabled her to expand her practice by reaching clients who otherwise may spend too much time trying to reach her office. "It can save someone an hour commute if they can schedule a phone consult," she says. "If they don't have to dress up to come see me, it saves them even more time."

The clients Linke counsels in her office often prefer follow-up visits by phone, which usually don't last 1 hour like a typical in-person office visit does. Phone calls enable Linke to see more clients and charge less per session. "Clients benefit from that, and I can fit more clients in, so I benefit as well," she says.

However, the nonverbal physical cues and the absence of eye contact during counseling sessions by phone or audio-only video conferencing isn't ideal for all clients. Jan Patenaude, RD, CLT, director of medical nutrition at Oxford Biomedical Technologies in the Grand Junction, Colorado, area, says she doesn't conduct long-distance consults for problems such as eating disorders because making eye contact with the patient and observing the patient are essential.

Clients must be considered on an individual basis to determine whether virtual counseling will be effective. "[Virtual nutrition counseling] isn't appropriate for every counselor or client, and we need to be good judges of when to refer out to somebody for a face-to-face consult," she says.

Making House Calls

Lisa Raum, RD, owner of RD To Go, a mobile version of an office-based private practice, makes house calls and provides on-site services in the Richmond, Virginia, area. She says her clients feel more comfortable in their homes than in a clinical setting. "Clinical settings have a clinical feel. The home is a soothing, warm environment that's more conducive to receiving information," she says.

And counseling sessions at home are more convenient for clients. Often, they're scheduled at the end of the day or in the evening when clients are relaxed and not preoccupied with the day's activities, Raum adds. Also, she invites and encourages family members to join in the conversation at no additional cost. "Nutrition is not specific to the individual," she says. "There's an improved likelihood of buy-in when the whole family is involved."

When Raum is allowed to see her clients' pantries, she helps them identify healthful foods and shows them how to read food labels. Sometimes she takes clients grocery shopping and helps them choose healthful foods for the week. This positive reinforcement gives them the support they need to make healthful dietary changes.

RD Perks

Virtual and nontraditional nutrition counseling have as many benefits for RDs as for clients. After moving to the rural mountains of Colorado, 30 miles from the nearest small town,

Patenaude searched online for work she could do from home. Serendipitously, she found a company looking to help their clients find nutrition services in remote parts of the country. She began working with them and has been providing nutrition counseling by phone for 12 years now.

The ability to work remotely is a huge plus for Patenaude, who often travels between two homes and accompanies her husband on his business trips. "My laptop essentially is my office," she says. "If I have [my laptop] and a cell phone, I'm in business."

Counseling by phone enables Patenaude to make her sessions as long or as short as necessary to meet her clients' needs. When clients meet in a traditional office setting, sessions typically run for a set amount of time, regardless of what clients may need. "It's easy to do 5–10 quick Q & A consults when a client just has a quick question," she says. These quick sessions give her time to garden or hike during the day and schedule longer appointments as early as 6 A.M. or as late as 11 P.M. if a client lives in a different time zone.

The flexibility of working remotely is a major reason Raum chooses to counsel clients in their homes. "I'm interested in having time to pursue multiple interests and having variety in my day," she says. Raum also teaches community college courses and is in graduate school pursuing two master's degrees.

Because of all these activities, she chooses to practice nutrition counseling part-time but says she makes "what many may make full-time." She believes there's enough demand for these services that she could increase her client base tremendously if she chose to aggressively market her business.

Money Matters and Legal Issues

For all the advantages virtual and nontraditional nutrition counseling provide, it doesn't come without challenges. Nutrition counseling, whether virtual or not, is a business, and it requires a business-minded professional to run it effectively. For example, cancellations can be an issue. A house call can take up to 4 hours of Raum's day because of the time it takes to drive to the client. If the client cancels while Raum is standing on the doorstep, she suffers a financial loss. Experience has taught her to require all payments in advance. She sends out an electronic invoice, which gives clients 24 hours to cancel their appointment. The client signs it and pays online using PayPal, which is a free payment service.

In addition, many insurance plans don't cover virtual counseling services, so clients may have to pay out of pocket. If this is the case, not everyone will be able to work with you. Rather than view this as a deterrent, Austin and Raum have found virtual nutrition counseling to be a positive experience. Raum works with clients who want and value her services, so payment isn't an issue. Austin's clients can pay for bundled services in advance, which makes them more committed to her program. "Commitment means better outcomes," she says.

Then there are the legal issues surrounding virtual nutrition counseling. Because telehealth is a relatively new field, it's critical that RDs become familiar with HIPAA and its privacy and security rules. The HIPAA Privacy Rule protects the privacy of individually identifiable health information, and the HIPAA Security Rule sets national standards for the security of electronic protected health information.

Nutrition professionals must take special care when counseling clients via e-mail and the Internet and in public settings such as coffee shops or other eateries, where conversations may be overheard, potentially compromising a client's privacy. When it comes to cell phone and Internet use, dietitians must ensure they have a secure Internet connection when speaking with clients and practice security measures, such as using passwords and installing firewalls on devices.

While there are health care practitioners who use Skype, it isn't considered HIPAA compliant, so nutrition professionals shouldn't use it to counsel clients. There's been much concern about using Skype to provide health care services due to the implementation of the HIPAA Final Rule in March 2013, which enhances a patient's privacy protections, provides individuals new rights to their health information, and strengthens the government's ability to enforce the law. Those who don't abide by the HIPAA Final Rule can be fined up to $1.5 million per violation.

The good news is that there are many HIPAA-compliant services available that health care practitioners can use, such as VSee, which offers video conferencing. It also enables practitioners to use documents to assist the counseling process while ensuring a secure connection. Subscribers to this service can connect from a desktop computer, laptop, or 3G/4G cellular phone. SecureVideo, Vidyo, and Talk to an Expert are similar HIPAA-compliant services.

In addition to being HIPAA compliant, Frechman advises dietitians interested in telehealth to follow the rules in their individual states, which may differ from state to state. For example, in California, Frechman says RDs are required to get a referral from a medical doctor to provide medical nutrition therapy, although it isn't necessary when offering weight-loss and wellness services.

When general nutrition education becomes medical nutrition therapy, it's important for dietitians to know and follow their state's licensure laws. Counseling outside state boundaries for a house call or even by phone or videoconference may violate state licensure laws, though some states will allow RDs to apply for reciprocity to practice in another state.

An Emerging Trend

"Telehealth is an emerging area of practice for many health care professionals," Mangieri says. "Regulations, policies, and standards are in flux until a gold standard becomes consensus, but that hasn't stopped technology from entering into mainstream practice." Dietitians who are considering adding a telehealth or telenutrition service to their practice should use the Scope of Practice Decision Tool offered online by the Academy, Manigieri says.

Virtual nutrition counseling is ripe with potential, but it's a relatively new field and there's room for improvement, Mangieri adds. It would be easier if there were "more online documents and communications that allowed the RD to remain HIPAA compliant," Patenaude says.

Frechman says she'd like to see more insurance reimbursement in this area. "Thinking outside the box with creative ways of doing business will ultimately benefit clients," she says. "In order for new ideas to take place, insurance reimbursement has to be in agreement with innovation."

Despite some of the challenges and legal issues concerning virtual nutrition counseling, it continues to be a growing trend. Dietitians say the advantages far outweigh the disadvantages, and they plan to continue counseling clients and patients by phone and over the Internet or in an otherwise nontraditional manner. They embrace the potential for increasing the accessibility of their services to meet their needs and ultimately the needs of their clients.

Critical Thinking

1. Explain why using Skype to counsel patients is not HIPPA compliant.
2. Investigate your state's rules and regulations regarding the qualifications a person must have to provide virtual nutrition counseling for a patient with type I diabetes. Write an essay discussing your findings.

Create Central

www.mhhe.com/createcentral

Internet References

Academy of Nutrition and Dietetics
www.eatright.org

U.S. Department of Health and Human Services
www.hhs.gov

Lori Zanteson is a food, nutrition, and health writer based in southern California.

Zanteson Lori, "Virtual Nutrition Counseling," *Today's Dietitian*, vol. 16, 4, April 2014, pp. 43.

Article

Prepared by: Janet Colson, *Middle Tennessee State University*

The Quest for a Natural Sugar Substitute

DANIEL ENGBER

Learning Outcomes

After reading this article, you will be able to:

- Explain what stevia is and the source of it.
- Outline the steps involved in testing a new ingredient used to flavor a food.
- In addition to stevia, state the names of two other natural, noncaloric sweeteners and describe their potential as sweeteners.

On a Sunday evening last September, stevia became famous. In the final episode of *Breaking Bad,* an image of the sweetener filled the TV screen. Lydia emptied the packet into her mug of camomile tea, not knowing that Walt, her former partner, had poisoned it. "How are you feeling?" he later asked. "Kind of under the weather, like you've got the flu? That would be the ricin I gave you. I slipped it into that stevia crap that you're always putting in your tea."

In an interview with *The Guardian,* published the next day, the actress who played Lydia laughed about the product anti-placement: "Sorry, stevia," she said. "Oh, I suppose it feels a bit rubbish. Do you think anyone actually bought it anyway?"

Actually, yes. The natural, noncaloric sweetener, made from the leaves of a Paraguayan shrub, now sits in second place in the $400 million market for sugar-bowl sachets. (Sucralose hangs on at No. 1.) When Cargill introduced the leading brand of stevia, called Truvia, in 2008, the company heralded it as "a new category of sweet." Sure enough, imitators followed. A few weeks later, Merisant put out PureVia—made from the same ingredient—and then the manufacturer of Sweet'N Low started filling light green packets with what it called Stevia in the Raw.

That was five years ago, yet most of us have few associations with the product. Splenda, Equal, Sweet'N Low: These are household names. Stevia's still an arriviste, the oddball at the coffee bar.

But the battle for the sugar-substitute market is not about packets on the table; the real money is in being the go-to additive for diet foods, especially diet drinks. When the FDA approved a chemical called cyclamate in 1951, a brand-new industry emerged: No-Cal soda, Diet Rite, and all the other sugar-free refreshments. Cyclamate was banned in 1969 for promoting bladder cancer in rats, but aspartame later took its place. In 1983, Coca-Cola put aspartame-based NutraSweet in Diet Coke, and sales soared. "The rule of thumb is that 60 percent of all high-potency sweetener sales is in beverages," says John Fry, a food scientist and 40-year industry veteran who consults on sweeteners for Cargill. "You have to be in soft drinks, one way or another."

As badly as stevia needs the soft-drink companies, the soft-drink companies may need stevia even more. While sweetened carbonated beverages still make up around one-fifth of all the liquids we consume, the volume sold has dropped, per capita, every year since 1998. We're more afraid of sugar than we've ever been. What yesterday were seen as "empty calories" have today been designated "toxic." Doctors warn that cans of soda put fat into your liver, weaken your response to insulin, and increase your risk of heart disease and diabetes. The panic over sugar has grown so pervasive that other dietary boogeymen—salt and fat and gluten—seem like harmless flunkies in comparison. (In 2012, when the market-research firm Mintel asked consumers which ingredients or foods they were trying to avoid, sugar and added sugar topped the list, by a wide margin.)

The soda companies have tried to tack into the headwind: In 2010, PepsiCo promised to reduce the sugar in its products by 25 percent, and the following year Coca-Cola told the British government that it would cut the calories in soda. But consumers are not content to switch to artificial sweeteners. Sales volume of diet soda fell by 12 percent in the last six years. Far from serving as a life raft for the industry, that business is leaking dollars, too.

The problem is that for all the fear of fructose, consumers have grown just as wary of its beaker-born alternatives. To health fanatics, they seem noxious on their face: Sweet'N Low comes from a derivative of coal; Equal is made from methanol and converts to formaldehyde when digested; Splenda is a chlorinated sugar. Others worry over well-worn rumors of their ill effects—tumors, headaches, and depression. More recent studies hint that diet drinks can cause the very problem they're meant to solve and make us fat instead of thin. (Lab rats fed with noncaloric sweeteners sometimes start to overeat, as if the ersatz sugar primed their rodent tongues for other sweets.)

The science on these questions is inconclusive at best. There's no clear evidence that artificial sweeteners cause cancer or obesity, at least in human beings. But the fear of artificial sweeteners was never quite a function of the scientific evidence—or never of just that. It stems as much from a sense that every pleasure has its consequences: that when we try to hack our taste buds in the lab—to wrench the thrill of sugar from its ill effects—we're cheating at a game we'll never win.

Because it came from a plant, stevia seemed to offer a way to sneak around the rules. "We've been consuming sweetened products for 8,000 years," says Jim Kempland, a former sales manager for NutraSweet and later vice-president of marketing for Sweet Green Fields, a U.S.-based stevia producer. "The enormous rates of obesity both here and globally are not going to curtail our human cravings for sweet things. The alternative, or possibly the solution, would be to ask, How do we create those things naturally, so that they can fit into a lifestyle that allows us to have things we like?"

The beverage companies knew that sales growth in the natural category had almost tripled that of other foods and beverages, driven by the intuition that they're better for our health. What if Diet Coke or Diet Pepsi could be made into a "natural" product—a sweet-tasting drink with zero calories and nothing artificial? Would a more wholesome substitute for sugar—one that comes from plants instead of factories—let us have our sweets and eat them too?

But the industry soon discovered that its salvation would have to be postponed. For all the hype, stevia had a fatal flaw: Its taste.

Deep inside Cargill's corporate headquarters in Wayzata, Minn., where it runs its $136 billion business, a technician in a hairnet put out a bowl of strawberries. Melanie Goulson, a food scientist in the company's corn-milling unit, had taken me to a laboratory kitchen outfitted with frying pans and cleavers and stir-plates spinning fluids with Teflon-coated bars. She waited as I dipped a berry in a sample of white granules and popped it in my mouth.

Truvia felt a lot like sugar on my tongue—much more so than the rival brands—but there was something strange about its sweetness. The flavor dawdled and digressed, until it seemed as if I'd chewed a nub of licorice or soaked my gums in watered-down Campari. This has been stevia's problem from the start: It has a bitter taste that lingers. The defect may be unobtrusive in small doses—the amount you sprinkle in your cappuccino—but it's ruinous at the quantities it takes to make a diet soda. "Anybody who tasted stevia in 2008, when it was just about to be permitted in the United States," Fry says, "would have been painfully aware that this was not an aspartame or a sucralose in terms of sweetness quality."

Goulson and her team have tried to bolster stevia by blending it with other additives. "We're trying to understand how sweet this product should be," she said. "What features do people like? What don't they like? How can we get the recipe just right?" In a perfect world, they'd find a way to sand down the jagged edges of its flavor, so stevia could match the taste of table sugar. (Sugar is "widely accepted as the gold standard for sweet taste," Goulson told me.) At the very least they're hoping to make stevia as appetizing as the chemicals in Diet Coke and Diet Pepsi. "Taste is king," Goulson said. "I mean, the healthiest product in the world really isn't relevant if people don't enjoy the taste."

A member of her team poured out several cups of orange liquid for me to try. It wasn't orange juice but orange drink: The beverages had been watered down by more than half to cut the sugar content, then spiked with stevia and other natural flavors. I knew the first one they handed me would be the taste-test patsy, but even so, its awful flavor caught me by surprise: a hit of sour that slowly faded to a bitter, sticky sweet. Then I tried the second cup. Goulson had tweaked the recipe so that its sweet and sour flavors came and went in harmony. The drink contained the same amount of stevia but tasted more like orange juice. "It's a science and an art," she said. "Depending on the flavor, if you're dealing with an apple-based or orange-based or berry-based system, we may change the ratio of the acids to help that flavor pop out more."

Her artistry has limits, though. It's possible to minimize the aftertaste of stevia, but only when there's still some sugar to go with it. "Generally you've seen 30 percent, 35 percent, 50 percent [sugar] reductions on the market," says Wade Schmelzer, one of Goulson's lab lieutenants. The biggest soft-drink companies have shunted off the product to a little-known and little-loved class of carbonated drinks: the midcalorie soda. In parts of Europe, Coca-Cola now makes Sprite with a mix of stevia and sugar, to cut the calories by 30 percent; last June, it started selling Coca-Cola Life, another stevia-and-sugar drink, in Argentina. PepsiCo has also tried a stevia-sweetened, mid-calorie version of its cola at markets in Australia. For now, their dreams of making fully natural, fully diet soda—the beverage market's killer app—are on hold. "We know that in the end—in an ideal world," Schmelzer said, "the customers would like to be at zero sugar."

Later in the day I met with Mark Brooks, Truvia's business director. "There are those people who love artificial sweeteners," he told me, "and there are those people for whom sugar is it; but the growing segment, and now the biggest segment (and we see this worldwide), is a group that we call the naturally splendids—those people who are really looking for that natural source." Brooks's department guessed that in 2010, 39 percent of household shoppers fit into this latter group, but that number may be rising.

Still, all the splendids in the world won't help the bottom line if Truvia can't appeal on flavor. It's not enough to tell consumers that a product comes from farms in Paraguay. It's not enough to let them think it's better for their health. "At the end of the day," Brooks said, "the consumer will buy you again because you taste great."

Not every natural, noncaloric sweetener comes from stevia. As Cargill tries to grapple with its gremlins, other firms have done their best to find alternatives. In the summer of 2012, McNeil Nutritionals—the maker of Splenda—put out Nectresse, a product made from the Chinese mountain-orchard melon known as *luo han guo,* or monk fruit. Sold in tangerine-colored packets, Nectresse was supposed to be a more natural-seeming natural product. While few of us think of leafy plants as being sweet, monk fruit brings to mind a cantaloupe or a honeydew. "A fruit ingredient in your food or in your beverage is very intuitive for the customer," says David Thorrold, the CEO of BioVittoria, which now controls a major portion of the world's monk-fruit supply.

Even Cargill is developing stevia alternatives. As Nectresse hit the market, the company received a bioprospecting permit from the South African government, giving it the right to exploit the molomo monate plants that grow on rocky slopes in northeast South Africa. At her lab in Minnesota, Goulson tested a sweet-tasting amino acid drawn from those plants and concluded that it would be enough to flavor diet beverages. John Fry called it one of the finest zero-calorie sweeteners he had ever tried.

Yet these ingredients have problems even worse than stevia's. While monk-fruit extract isn't quite as bitter, its flavor can be very slow to build, and it, too, lacks the oomph to sweeten diet soda. (It's also more expensive.) The molomo extract tastes a lot like sugar, but when exposed to UV light, it undergoes a horrid transformation. In the early 2000s, scientists at Coca-Cola added the sweetener to bottles of Sprite, then left them on the roof over the weekend; by Monday morning, the soda had turned urine yellow and developed the smell of feces.

So the beverage-makers have returned to where they started. Coca-Cola set out to find what is often called the holy grail of diet beverages—a natural alternative to aspartame—about 10 years ago. If today we're stuck with stevia, a curly-haired chemist named Grant DuBois may be as much to blame as anyone.

DuBois left Coca-Cola in 2011, after two decades of working for the company's global research and development team. "I was feeding my ideas into this supersecret group responsible for flavor chemistry," he said when we met for breakfast in the suburbs of Atlanta. Now 67, DuBois runs a sweetener consultancy from his Georgia home, and he seemed most at ease while making presentations. The one he'd prepped for me described how hard it is to find a sweetener that works and why the best natural product that we have is a compromise.

A new product should be considered for development, he explained, only if it meets nine specific requirements. It's not enough to find a chemical that's sweet; it also has to sweeten foods in the ways that matter most, to the right degree, without an aftertaste, without a linger and without diminishing effect. And even one that has the taste of granulated sugar would be deficient if it weren't also stable in solution, resilient to hot and cold, safe to drink, cheap to make, and amenable to patenting. An "all-natural" sweetener must meet these nine metrics for success, and then a 10th: It must be taken from a living thing.

That last requirement left DuBois with little room to work. In all, there are about a hundred natural, noncaloric chemicals that, by pure coincidence or some unlikely quirk of evolution, have found a way to hijack the mouth's machinery for sensing sugar. One category comes from animals. Lysozyme, a chemical found in tears and spit, and also in the whites of eggs, can be very sweet. (In hens and turkeys, it's sugary but pungent; in soft-shelled turtle eggs, it tastes more like licorice.) The rest derive from vegetation, including: one compound drawn from crushed hydrangea leaves, used in Japan for sweet tea; another from a Malaysian plant called lemba, with tiny yellow flowers and fruits that look like cloves of garlic; the seeds of a swollen caper berry in Yunnan, China, which locals chew as candy; and monk fruit, a cousin to the cucumber and the bitter melon, which grows in Guangxi.

Most of these, DuBois knew, would never stand a chance. He pushed aside his knife and fork and tilted the laptop's screen to show me why. For the natural-sweetener project, he started with the first and most important of his tests, shown on his display as "Taste Quality Metric 1: Maximal Response." Were any of the natural compounds strong enough to sweeten Diet Coke? At first this seemed an easy obstacle to overcome: Lysozymes are at least 10 times as sweet as sugar; monk-fruit extract is

20 times as strong as lysozyme; and the sweetener drawn from the lemba plant is 10 times more intense than monk fruit. But those numbers correspond only to tiny doses of the chemicals, enough to match the strength of, say, a teaspoon of sugar mixed into a cup of water—a 2 percent solution. To make a cup of Coca-Cola, you'd need much more: about six teaspoons' worth of sugar, for a 10.4 percent solution. (Pepsi is a little sweeter, at 11 percent. Root beers and some fruit-flavored sodas can be 12 percent or more.) That's where many substitutes fall short.

DuBois had a set of graphs tracking how the power of a sweetener changes with its concentration. He included curves for six different compounds, from saccharin to stevia, but they all looked very much the same. Each curve rose steeply, gaining sweetness with every increment in milligrams per liter, then appeared to hit a ceiling, a point at which the sweetness flattened out. Once you reach that threshold concentration, a compound loses its effect: No matter how much more of it you pump into a beverage, you'll never get a sweeter taste. The ceilings for some chemicals are high enough to flavor carbonated drinks. Aspartame, for example, can match the taste of sugar in a 16 percent solution. But others reach their limit much too soon. That's why today you'll never find a Diet Coke that's made with saccharin. At best it would match the sweetness of a sugar drink at 10.1 percent.

He gestured at the curve for stevia, which didn't seem much better than the one for saccharin. "That looks like a death sentence," he said. But when I asked him to name his favorite noncaloric sweetener, DuBois demurred and cleared his throat. "None of them," he said, "tastes like sugar."

We clicked ahead to Metric 2—"Flavor Profile." Most products have at least a hint of bitterness or licorice; some have a metallic note or even menthol cooling. Metric 3 considers how the compound's taste develops on the tongue. Sip a soda made with sugar, and the taste should reach its peak of sweetness in 4 seconds, then fall off 10 seconds later. Zero-calorie substitutes tend to lag behind: They come on too slowly, and then—much worse—they stay too long, clinging to your mouth in a disconcerting glaze. Even aspartame takes an extra second to hit its sweetness high and hangs around an extra four before it goes away.

It's hard enough to handle these requirements, DuBois said, when you're making chemicals from scratch. Never mind if you have to meet them using something natural. As he searched for a plant-based substitute to put in diet beverages, DuBois remembered that he played around with a compound drawn from stevia while working for a start-up in the 1970s. At the time, he figured out a way to make it work about as well as aspartame. "It still had a lingering sweetness, but no bitterness," he said. But his lab work changed the compound's shape. It wasn't natural anymore.

Could the chemical in stevia—called rebaudioside-A—work in an unaltered state? It seemed more promising than any other option on his list. Stevia was commercialized in Japan more than 30 years ago and then bred to make as much Reb-A as possible. While the sweetener has some bitterness and licorice, its warts are modest next to those of monk fruit or lemba or any of the other plant derivatives. Also a company in Kuala Lumpur called Stevian Biotechnology (later renamed PureCircle) said it could produce Reb-A on the cheap. In 2003, DuBois passed along his findings: Coca-Cola should try to make a sweetener from stevia. Others at the company agreed and made a deal with Cargill to get the plant-based ingredient approved. Coke would do the basic scientific work on stevia; Cargill would work on the supply chain. "There was no alternative," DuBois told me, looking very serious. "I decided that of all these 100 or so compounds—all the natural, noncaloric sweeteners that are known—the one that meets the metrics best—and it's not perfect—is Reb-A."

At a greenhouse in East Lansing, Mich., a scientist named Ryan Warner plucked a pair of shriveled-looking leaves from a specimen of stevia. They looked like wrinkled basil, but when I put one in my mouth, it had the taste of Sen-Sen and the feel of leaded paint. Warner laughed as I did my best to gulp it down. "Did you see me spit mine out?" he said.

Since 2010, Warner, an associate professor of horticulture at Michigan State University, has led a team of scientists funded by PureCircle, the top stevia producer, to engineer a better version of the crop. Rather than alter the chemical, scientists are trying to alter the plant. They'd like to find a novel strain that makes sweet-tasting compounds with less bitterness and aftertaste—a kind of superstevia. Every year, he breeds a set of cultivars and tests the composition of their leaves. It's a funny job for someone who has so little interest in sweet taste: "I'm a fat, oil and beer kind of person," Warner told me. "The best dessert is a cheese plate."

What I tasted in his greenhouse might be called Stevia 1.0: It's not so far off from the crude leaf extract that has been sold in health-food stores in the United States since the early 1980s. The composition of these extracts—and thus their taste—varies with the plants from which they're made, which may be one reason that they've never been cleared as a food additive by the FDA (It's possible that chewing on raw stevia is dangerous.)

It's Warner's task to tweak the makeup of the organism, using only natural means. Every stevia plant carries a certain mix of metabolites, called steviol glycosides, that define its sweetness signature. The most abundant glycoside in wild stevia has an overly bitter taste that wouldn't fly in foods or beverages. Enzymes in the plant convert that glycoside into several dozen others, including rebaudioside-A—the substance that DuBois recommended as a natural sweetener. But for any given plant, it's hard to know how much of each you'll get. "There's still not a great understanding of why there's so much variability," Warner said.

Until recently, PureCircle wanted plants that make as much Reb-A as possible. (That was Stevia 2.0.) Now PureCircle hopes that Warner and his team can start this process over and optimize the plant for a different set of glycosides with still fewer imperfections in their flavor. The project could take many years of crossing plants. In the wild, the shrub grows at the borders of grasslands and marsh. When cultivated by farmers—in Paraguay, Kenya, China, and California's Central Valley—the shrub demands enormous care: Crops are often raised from cuttings, dug into the ground by hand. The work seemed just as hard in Michigan. A few miles from the greenhouse, Warner's team had planted rows along a highway and left them under strips of plastic for weed control. When I visited last spring, Warner's seedlings had just gone in that morning. He told me that his team would harvest the foliage and grind it to a powder in the Red Devil—a souped-up paint-shaker on which a member of the lab had drawn a demon-horned Bart Simpson spearing a leaf of stevia with a pitchfork.

Warner tests the light green powders for their glycosides and then selects the ones with better profiles for another round of breeding. The details of his work are secret, but it seems as if he's searching for a pair of chemicals—rebaudioside-D and rebaudioside-X—that tend to show up in very small amounts. If the lab can find a way to make these more abundant, the rewards would be enormous. "These next-generation stevia sweeteners hold a lot of potential for unlocking new growth within the stevia industry," says Robert Brooke, CEO of Stevia First, an agricultural and biotech firm. "Reb-A has done quite well. . . . Reb-D and Reb-X can take it to a whole new level."

The beverage giants feel the same. In a patent filed last September, PepsiCo scientists put out a set of spider plots to show that Reb-D is sweeter than Reb-A, with far less bitterness and licorice. The new ingredient would allow for the creation of a "natural carbonated cola beverage product" sweetened entirely with stevia and without the need for "taste-masking agents." Coca-Cola's researchers followed with a similar patent at the end of May, this one with graphs to show that Reb-X tastes even better than Reb-D and would make an even more delicious can of diet cola.

All these efforts raise a basic question, though. As Grant DuBois discovered in the 1970s, stevia can taste as good as NutraSweet, if you're willing to apply the tools of synthetic chemistry. But even if you avoid these sorts of interventions, what about the science in between—from crossbred crops to lab-grown glycosides and fancy formulations? At what point in the process of refinement does a natural product lose its link to nature?

At the kitchen lab in Minnesota, Goulson offered a taste of what might be next. Her team set out a Sprite-type drink, fizzy lemon-lime, in which the sugar had been cut by 75 percent—more than has been feasible with natural sweeteners so far. "This is outside of the space where anybody has been operating," Goulson said. She'd used an experimental extract that might soon be on the market, and while the soda had a bitter aftertaste, its defects were subdued. Goulson wouldn't tell me much about the mystery ingredient, only that it's "in the world of stevia."

Other signs suggest that Cargill is about to make the jump to next-gen natural sweeteners. On March 6, a multimillion-dollar deal with the Swiss biotech firm Evolva was announced; with Cargill they would develop a yeast-fermented version of stevia. Instead of raising stevia from cuttings of the plant, then steeping the leaves and sucking out the glycosides, Evolva makes them by using microbes to perform the needed feats of biochemistry.

When Evolva gets its system going—which should happen in the next few years—the cost of stevia-based sweeteners could plummet. Cargill wouldn't be beholden to rain and sun and weeds, nor to the natural limits of plant biology. Fermentation would allow the company to make whichever glycoside it wanted, at whatever quantity and purity it needed.

The Evolva process, like another that's in development at Stevia First, makes use of homemade microorganisms, with foreign genes stuffed into their nuclei. That's one way to pump out Reb-D or Reb-X, but what about the consumers who are drawn to "natural" claims—will they still go for stevia when it flows from a vat of GMOs? And will regulators object?

Later that afternoon, I put these questions to David Henstrom, Cargill's global business director for health ingredients and the man now in charge of selling Truvia. "Country by country they have different ways that they describe what you can say is natural and what you can't," he told me. In the United States, food-and-beverage companies get to make the judgment for themselves. "There might be some products that aren't trying to make that hard 'all-natural' claim," he continued. "Some people are claiming naturally sourced. Some people are claiming nature-identical. It comes down to the product and what the product is trying to say and deliver to the customer."

Natural zero-calorie sweeteners have so far been caught between two imperatives: What they want to say and what they can deliver. It used to be that natural sweeteners weren't sweet enough; now they have an added problem: They aren't fully natural.

"'Natural' would mean that I picked it from the ground," said Donna LiVolsi, the director of operations at Cumberland Packing Corporation, which invented Sweet'N Low, the first artificial sweetener sachet, in 1957. I met her near the Navy Yards of Brooklyn, where Cumberland still makes Sweet'N Low, along with value brands of aspartame and sucralose and a couple of natural-sugar substitutes—Stevia in the Raw and Monk Fruit in the Raw. When I asked LiVolsi if she thought these latter two were "natural," she said she couldn't answer, because each consumer has a sense of what the word means to them.

It's a question that has bedeviled beverage-makers, too. In the fall of 2012, a German food company surveyed 4,000 people in eight European countries, to find out how they understood the "natural" claim. Almost three-quarters said they thought that natural products were more healthful and that they'd pay a premium to get them. More than half argued that natural products have a better taste. But the respondents weren't sure what degree or form of processing would be enough to strip a product of its natural status. Some drew a line between sea salt (natural) and table salt (artificial). Others did the same for dried pasta and powdered milk, though both are made by dehydration.

My visit to the Navy Yards showed how confusing this can get. LiVolsi took me through the loading bays, where drums of ingredients arrive in giant bags from overseas, and then into a noisy room where mostly women sit in front of large machines, sweeping packets into pink boxes. A set of tubes suspended from the ceiling ferried blends of saccharin or stevia from an upper floor, and wayward dust dissolved into the atmosphere. With every breath, I could feel a sweetness tingling my tongue like tiny snowflakes.

Every sweetener at Cumberland goes through the same routine, from a blending tub upstairs into a giant hopper and then down across the belts and wheels below. LiVolsi pointed to what looked like a whipping Catherine wheel, with spikes that spurted powder into paper packets, 50 blurring past in every second. It doesn't matter if it's made from Chinese orchard fruit or a derivative of coal, the stuff ends up in this contraption, strobing pink for saccharin, blue for aspartame, gold for sucralose, pale green for stevia. "We get the ingredient, we get the bulking agent, we blend it together, we make the batch, we test the batch, we put it in the packets and life moves on," LiVolsi said. They're different flavors to us, she said, "that's how we look at it."

Some consumers also wonder if the natural sweeteners aren't simply different flavors of the products they've been trying to avoid. At the beginning of July, just as PepsiCo got approval for Reb-D and Coca-Cola said it would be working on Reb-X, a 58-year-old woman living in Hawaii filed suit against Big Stevia. In March she bought a box of Truvia at Walmart because she thought it was a natural product. Now she's convinced it's no such thing. Her complaint declared that "Reb-A is not the natural crude preparation of stevia," and that its manufacture is not "similar to making tea," as Cargill's packaging suggests. Rather, it's "a highly chemically processed and purified form of stevia-leaf extract."

Hers was not the only attack on Cargill's natural sweetener. In ongoing negotiations to settle a similar suit, Cargill has offered to remove the phrase "similar to making tea" from the packaging and/or add an asterisk to the product's tagline, "Nature's Calorie-Free Sweetener," directing people to a website FAQ That page would explain that Truvia contains very little stevia, by weight, and that its main ingredient—erythritol—comes from yeast that may be fed with genetically modified corn sugar. "As with almost all finished food products," the FAQ would say, "the journey from field to table involves some processing."

"Five years ago, these lawsuits were unusual," says Rebecca Cross, an attorney with BraunHagey & Borden in San Francisco who has helped a dozen food-product companies defend themselves against charges of health-claim mischief and natural-product fraud. "Now in California, you have four or five every week. Before 2008, I don't know if you'd get four or five every year."

So far, none of the natural-product cases have gone to trial. They have either been settled out of court or dismissed by a judge. But many more are in the pipeline, and the FDA has done little to clear up the regulations. The agency began to draft a formal definition of the term "natural" in the early 1990s but never finished. It fell back instead on an advisory opinion, hinting only that a natural food is one without artificial or synthetic additives. Judge William Orrick of the U.S. District Court, meanwhile, ruled in October that natural-products lawsuits can't be put off until the feds produce a more specific rule. "The court is skeptical that the FDA will develop a policy regarding the term 'natural' anytime soon," he wrote, "especially since it has considered the matter for over two decades but still has not provided further guidance."

In the face of this uncertainty, manufacturers have chosen to be pragmatic: They won't say that stevia is more healthful than aspartame or sucralose just because of how it's made. Nor will they acknowledge that one form of stevia might be more or less natural than another. "I think the important thing is that there's a choice for everyone, and you can pick what's right for you and what you need," Goulson told me on our tour of tasting labs at Cargill. "What's good for one person may not be good for another."

Earlier, she showed me where her colleague Nese Yurttas feeds Truvia to employees from the Cargill campus or kids from local schools, in order to study their responses. Yurttas earned her masters at the University of Minnesota, working on cheddar-cheese aromas. Now she runs panel tests to see if average consumers like the taste of stevia. In 2011, Yurttas asked a group of children to test diet chocolate milk, with the sugar reduced by 30 percent. They gave it some mixed reviews. "Tasted so good it blowed my head off," one kid told Yurttas. "I think it should be sweeter," another said. On the whole, however, when asked to rate its flavor on a "nine-point hedonic scale," the children gave the drink an average score of 7.9, the same as standard chocolate milk. They liked the taste, all right, but would their parents say it's natural? There is no nine-point scale to measure that.

Critical Thinking

1. Using PubMed available at http://www.ncbi.nlm.nih.gov/pubmed, select one peer-reviewed article that investigates a health aspect related to stevia; summarize the study and its findings.
2. Based on the study selected from the previous question, do you believe stevia will be used widely as a natural sweetener? Explain your answer.
3. Prepare a beverage (such as tea, coffee, or Kool-Aid) that generally has sugar added using a commercially prepared version of stevia (such as Truvia) and a second sample of the beverage using table sugar. Compare the taste of the two beverages and describe the differences.

Create Central

www.mhhe.com/createcentral

Internet References

American Beverage Association
www.ameribev.org

Institute of Food Technologists
www.ift.org/

Stevia.Net
www.stevia.net/

DANIEL ENGBER writes and edits science coverage for *Slate* magazine. He has also written for *Discover, SEED, Popular Science,* and the *Washington Post,* among other publications. His proposal for a scientific approach to professional basketball was featured in the *New York Times Magazine*'s "Year in Ideas."

Unit 4

UNIT

Prepared by: Janet Colson, *Middle Tennessee State University*

Diet and Disease

Research that focuses on the connection between diet and disease has unraveled the role of many nutrients in delaying the onset of certain diseases, preventing diseases, and in some instances reversing disease. The challenging aspect of releasing results from nutrition research is communicating this information in a manner that is not controversial or contradictory to previously released messages. With the increasing interest in health and disease prevention among Americans, media outlets publish scientific findings prematurely and without the physiological context in which the message should be conveyed. Scientific research takes time to answer the questions about health, nutrition, disease, and medicine, whereas consumers want answers to these questions much quicker than scientifically possible.

Medical and nutrition research has changed since the mapping of the human genome. We have come to better understand the role of genetics in the expression of disease and its role in how we respond to dietary change. In addition, research about diet and disease has enabled us to understand the importance and uniqueness of the individual (age, gender, ethnicity, and genetics) and his or her particular response to dietary interventions. Individualizing one's diet to prevent disease and promote health is a concept that we will see developing in the future.

The prevalence of diet- and lifestyle-related diseases in the United States is astronomical. Heart disease, type 2 diabetes, obesity, stroke, high blood pressure, osteoporosis, and certain cancers are diet- and lifestyle-related conditions that affect millions of Americans. Proper nutrition plays a vital role in these diseases. Components of foods such as saturated fats, trans fats, sodium, and added sugars continue to be highlighted as the premier culprits of these diseases.

A recent area of nutrition research focus is the degree of added sugars that are consumed by Americans. The average American consumes 350 to 475 grams of added sugars each day. The most commonly consumed form of added sugars is high-fructose corn syrup, but other forms of sugar such as table sugar, honey, and cane juice are considered to be "added sugar" too. As newer research explores the effects of high-fructose corn syrup on human health, food companies are developing products using other forms of sugar. These "natural sugars" still provide empty calories in the diet that may lead to weight gain if consumed in excess and not balanced by physical activity. Discretionary calories (calories consumed after nutrient needs are met from healthy food and beverage sources) are an effective way to think about the calories that are consumed in relation to the calories needed to provide adequate nutrient intakes. The USDA recommends that empty calories (from solid fats, added sugars, and alcohol) not exceed 260 kcal. for college-age women and 330 kcal. for men. Individual recommendations for empty caloric allowances can be calculated using myplate.gov.

High-fructose sweeteners have been linked to greater risk for heart disease, metabolic syndrome, type 2 diabetes, gout, and accumulation of visceral fat. The link may be caused by increased triglycerides and uric acid in the bloodstream secondary to the way fructose is metabolized.

Research supports the link between consumption of sugar-sweetened beverages and risk of type 2 diabetes, heart disease, hypertension, hypertriglyceridemia, gout, and weight gain. Added fructose has been tied to increased levels of triglycerides in the blood, decreased fat oxidation, increased LDL cholesterol, increased uric acid in the blood, and increased visceral fat. Epidemiological data supports a relationship between fructose sweeteners and heart attacks. Liquid calories from sugar-sweetened beverages are not only empty calories, but they also promote increased calorie intake at meals, possibly through suppression of leptin, a hormone that triggers you to stop eating.

The number one concern of the health of the United States is the prevalence of overweight and obesity. Although much of the attention is centered on childhood obesity and tactics to prevent or curtail it, there is also an ongoing problem with overweight or obesity as our population ages. On average, Americans in their 60s are 10 pounds heavier than they were just a decade ago. A typical woman in her 40s weighs 168 pounds, compared to 143 pounds in the 1960s. People used to start midlife at a lower weight and lose weight when they reached their 50s. Humans need fewer calories as they age because of slower metabolism and the tendency to lose muscle mass and gain fat, especially abdominal fat. Because muscle burns more calories than fat, it is challenging to lose weight in older years and maintain weight while eating the usual intake. Staying lean and eating right can delay onset or prevent certain diseases that plague older Americans, such as osteoporosis, heart disease, hypertension, insulin resistance, memory loss, arthritis, and some cancers.

Approximately 25 million people in the United States have type 2 diabetes and 1 million have type 1 diabetes. The incidence of type 1 diabetes has been increasing at rates of 3–5% per year. The reason for the increase in incidence of type 1 diabetes is unclear. Some speculate the rise in type 1 diabetes may be explained by the hygiene hypothesis while others lean toward the overload hypothesis.

The immune system is commonly taken for granted; however, it is a fascinating system of defense that is essential to our existence and optimal health. Proper nutrition and balanced nutrient intake is required for our immune system to function optimally whereas nutrient deficiencies impair immunity.

The articles in this unit will be useful as a supplement to diet and chronic disease sections of general nutrition courses. The article topics add a slightly different view of the commonly known diet-related diseases and other diseases that are not publicized as often.

Article

Prepared by: Janet Colson, *Middle Tennessee State University*

The Eating Disorder You've Never Heard of

Tempted by potential weight loss, diabetic adolescent girls are tampering with their insulin doses and putting themselves at risk for blindness, kidney failure, and amputated limbs.

KAREN LINDELL

Learning Outcomes

After reading this article, you will be able to:

- Explain what diabulimia is and why people develop the condition.
- List the possible long-term consequences of untreated diabulimia.

Clinicians call it "ED-DMT1," the dual diagnosis of an eating disorder and diabetes ("diabetes mellitus type 1"). Most people call it "diabulimia." But before it even had a name, Maryjeanne Hunt called it her "quirky little weight-management strategy."

In 1971, when she was 10, Hunt found out she had type 1 diabetes. She had to take insulin shots every day and follow a special "diet" for the rest of her life. Her mom was dieting all the time anyway, so it didn't seem like a big deal. But at age 14, while trying on a dress, she noticed her curves in the mirror. She told her mother, "This dress makes me look fat." "Yes," her mom replied, "You look kind of chunky."

Hunt suddenly felt very self-conscious about her body. She then made a connection that hadn't occurred to her when she was diagnosed with diabetes: *I have a tool I can use to get rid of this fat.* Or rather, a tool she could stop using. Before Hunt started taking insulin, her body couldn't absorb glucose, the body's energy source. Diabetics who don't use insulin lose the excess sugar (and calories) in their urine. So to lose weight, Hunt stopped taking insulin, or took just enough to keep herself from going into a diabetic coma. "I played with that, and found what I thought was great success, dropping pounds dramatically," Hunt says. She also found herself in the emergency room, over and over, for the next 22 years, because her body's cells were dropping all the energy they needed to survive. Hunt had no name for it, and neither did doctors in the 1970s. The term *diabulimia* has emerged only in the last 15 or so years.

People with diabulimia are type 1 diabetics who also have an eating disorder. Most deliberately stop taking their insulin, or manipulate the dose, as a way to lose weight. "Diabulimia," a combination of "diabetes" and "bulimia," is a bit of a misnomer. Bulimia is an eating disorder in which a person uses behaviors such as vomiting, laxatives, diuretics, exercise, or other purging behaviors to prevent weight gain. Those with diabulimia are said to "purge" their calories via excess glucose in their urine.

The term "implies that there's one thing women with diabetes struggle with—bulimia—when they have an eating disorder," says Ann Goebel-Fabbri, PhD, a psychologist at the Joslin Diabetes Center in Boston and an assistant professor in psychiatry at Harvard Medical School. Some patients with diabulimia, however, continue to take insulin but still suffer from such eating disorders as anorexia, bulimia, and binge eating.

No one has studied exactly how many people suffer from diabulimia. But according to a study published in *BJM* (formerly the *British Medical Journal*), adolescent females with type 1 diabetes are 2.4 times more likely to develop eating disorders than peers of the same age without diabetes. Other studies show that about 30 percent of females with type 1 diabetes intentionally omit insulin. Because diabulimia is not yet officially recognized as a medical or psychiatric diagnosis, it is often misunderstood or left untreated.

Short and long-term consequences of insulin restriction include eye problems (from blurred vision to blindness), kidney failure, nerve damage, osteoporosis, vascular disease, amputated limbs, and death. People with diabulimia develop these conditions far sooner, and with more severity, than those with diabetes alone. Females, especially adolescents, appear to be at higher risk than males. Goebel-Fabbri says she sees patients in their 20s who've already had treatments for eye disease, or are awaiting kidney transplants. "This should not be happening in 2014," she says. "There's so much hope in diabetes treatment, which can reduce these complications massively. This is a tragedy."

Castlewood Treatment Centers, an eating disorder program with facilities in Missouri, California, and Alabama, sees five to 10 cases each year of patients with diabetes who manipulate insulin, says Deanna James, director of marketing. "It's a huge increase," she says. Five years ago, the centers "did not even ask about that on the assessment, and now it is standard."

To understand why insulin reduction causes weight loss, it helps to understand type 1 diabetes. Food we eat is broken down into glucose, a sugar that circulates in the blood. For non-diabetics, the pancreas pumps out insulin, which allows cells to let glucose in for energy. In people with type 1 diabetes, the immune system attacks cells in the pancreas that make insulin. Type 1 diabetics must check their glucose levels manually; based on their blood sugar levels, and what they plan to eat, they must give themselves insulin. If they don't, or underdose, their bodies can't absorb glucose. The body makes drastic attempts to compensate. It goes into starvation mode and starts to break down muscle and fat, releasing acids called ketones. The ketones build up, leading to diabetic ketoacidosis (DKA), which can be fatal.

According to Ovidio Bermudez, M.D., chief medical director at the Eating Recovery Center in Denver, Colorado, diabulimia, or ED-DMT1, as he prefers to call it, "is a relatively new phenomenon. People have not been diligent about insulin use for a long time; they forget, or are less careful, but it's not intentional. What's new is this manipulation, with the specific purpose of weight loss."

Many of the warning signs of diabulimia apply to other eating disorders, such as negative body image; obsession with weight and nutrition; skipping or restricting meals; eliminating carbohydrates or fats; eating in secret; feelings of guilt and shame about eating; significant weight loss or gain; compulsive exercising; menstrual irregularities; and depression and anxiety. Other warning signs apply to diabetics who restrict insulin, such as symptoms of hyperglycemia, or high blood sugar, including increased thirst and urination, irritability and extreme fatigue. Those with diabulimia might avoid going to see their endocrinologist or doctor. They often test their blood sugar in secret, or not at all, and keep the results from loved ones and doctors. Some add other substances to their insulin to obtain a more "normal" blood sugar reading.

Why might someone with type 1 diabetes be at increased risk for developing an eating disorder? Diabetics, to manage their disease, must closely monitor what they eat, which can lead to an unhealthy focus on calories, carbohydrates, and weight control. Also, type 1 diabetes is a chronic condition that requires daily attention for a lifetime, which can be a physical and emotional struggle.

Erin Williams, co-founder of We Are Diabetes, a support organization for type 1 diabetics who suffer from eating disorders, says when she turned to diabulimia at age 11, "weight wasn't an issue. I was just incredibly embarrassed I was diabetic, a person with a disease. I thought no one would want to be my friend. I wanted to be like everyone else. Why couldn't I go out and have a piece of pizza with my friends? . . . People started taking food away from me, asking why I was eating a Skittle. I had no control over anything in my life." She could, however, control the amount of insulin she put in her body.

Eventually, Williams lost control and turned to binging, because she was constantly hungry without any food being absorbed by her body. "When I binged, the amount of insulin I needed was so high, it did become a weight thing. I thought if I gave myself insulin, I was going to gain weight," she says.

Diabetics often hear that taking insulin will lead to weight gain, but according to Bermudez, "insulin is not a weight-gain hormone; it regulates energy production. The only way to gain weight with insulin is to overeat." The increase in weight that some diabetics experience, he says, is often just the body normalizing itself after being starved.

"If I introduce insulin in a person starved at a cellular level, and they eat at the same time, glucose enters the cell and feeds the cell, so the patient regains weight that was lost," he says. "The body plays a little bit of catch-up, and gains weight back that it should." Goebel-Fabbri says the "weight" gain is often water retention as the body soaks up insulin and water due to dehydration, "but it doesn't last forever."

Some patients with diabulimia need hospitalization or inpatient treatment to become medically stable. Whether treatment is inpatient or outpatient, a team of doctors working closely together is recommended: an endocrinologist, psychotherapist, diabetes educator, registered dietitian and, in many cases, a psychiatrist. The Diabulimia Helpline includes links to treatment centers known to help patients with diabetes and eating disorders.

Dawn M. Holemon, a psychiatrist and medical director at Castlewood Treatment Centers, says patients with diabulimia often require closer monitoring. "You have to be more careful, making sure the person is doing blood-sugar checks, and watching them, because the tests are easy to manipulate," she says. "But you're still dealing with an eating disorder mentality, so you have to start there."

One goal at eating disorder treatment centers is to get patients away from a hyperfocus on food and counting calories and carbs. But diabetics still have to pay attention to those dietary concerns. A less rigid approach to diabetes and eating is usually recommended. "The philosophy at Castlewood is, a balanced meal plan is the way to treat an eating disorder, whether you're a diabetic or not," Holemon says. "It includes everything in moderation." Scare tactics, guilt trips, belittling and shaming are not helpful.

Williams, 30, who is earning a degree in nursing and diabetes education, was treated for diabulimia at age 16 and now suffers from diabetic retinopathy, kidney damage, osteoporosis, ulcers, and neuropathy. She says patients should be careful when checking out eating disorder treatment centers to make sure the staff understand diabetes. "We have different lifestyle needs," she says. "Somebody needs to meet those needs or we're not getting help."

Hunt, now 53, is the author of *Eating to Lose: Healing from a Life of Diabulimia* (Demos Health Publishing). The Boston resident, a financial adviser and mother of 21-year-old twins, believes she would have developed an eating disorder with or without diabetes. "My mother has always had an unhealthy relationship with food," Hunt says. "But I don't just blame her. I also think it's perpetuated in our culture, and it's not just body image. We're a culture of 'not enoughness.' We're never good as we are." Hunt says she didn't get help for her diabulimia until she gave birth, because "I couldn't pass this pathological way of looking at yourself to my kids." She says long-term recovery comes from self-acceptance. "I stopped engaging in the behavior, but I don't think that defines healing from diabulimia," she says. "True healing lies in deep acceptance of yourself, and that is a work in progress."

Critical Thinking

1. Compare the behaviors of a teenage girl who has diabulimia to one who has bulimia. Which do you think is easier to treat? Explain your answer.
2. Design a treatment program for a college-age student who has diabulimia.

Create Central

www.mhhe.com/createcentral

Internet References

American Diabetes Association
www.diabetes.org

American Psychological Association
www.apa.org/

Anorexia Nervosa and Related Eating Disorders
www.anred.com

Karen Lindell is a freelance reporter based in Pasadena, California.

Article

Prepared by: Janet Colson, *Middle Tennessee State University*

We Will Be What We Eat

When it comes to staving off the problems of aging, from bone and muscle loss to high blood pressure and heart disease, your diet is your friend—or enemy.

MERYL DAVIDS LANDAU

Learning Outcomes

After reading this article, you will be able to:

- Discuss why it is more challenging for older adults to lose or maintain their body weight than younger adults.
- Summarize how dietary choices during young adulthood influence the risk for osteoporosis, heart disease, hypertension, diabetes, memory problems, and certain cancers in later life.

If your mental image of an older person is someone frail and thin, it may be time for an update. For the generation currently moving through middle age and beyond, a new concern is, well, growing: obesity. "We're already seeing a large number of obese elderly, and if we don't do something, that figure is sure to rise," laments David Kessler, former commissioner of the Food and Drug Administration and author of *The End of Overeating*. Government figures show that Americans in their 60s today are about 10 pounds heavier than their counterparts of just a decade ago. And an even more worrisome bulge is coming: A typical woman in her 40s now weighs 168 pounds, versus 143 pounds in the 1960s. "People used to start midlife [at a lower weight] and then lose weight when they got into their 50s, but that doesn't happen as much anymore," Kessler says.

People used to start midlife at a lower weight than they do now and then lose weight in their 50s, but not anymore.

If you're entering that danger zone now, be aware that it's not going to get any easier to lose weight, because people need fewer calories as they age. Blame slowing metabolism and the body's tendency starting in midlife to lose muscle mass—a process known as sarcopenia—and gain fat, especially around the abdomen. (Fat burns fewer calories than does muscle.) "All that conspires to make it harder for people to maintain the same body weight when they eat their usual diets," says Alice Lichtenstein, director of the Cardiovascular Nutrition Laboratory at Tufts University. "People have fewer discretionary calories to play with, so they need to make better food choices."

Why do those choices matter? First, carrying an extra 20 or 30 pounds with you into old age doesn't bode well for attempts to head off the myriad diseases that strike in midlife and later and are linked to weight—including diabetes, arthritis, heart disease, and some forms of cancer. (It's probably not a coincidence that one recent study finds that people in their 60s have more disabilities than in years past.)

But paying attention to what you eat isn't only about controlling weight; the need for certain vitamins and minerals increases with age. One is calcium, necessary to protect bones. Another is B_{12}, since some older adults make less of the stomach acid required to absorb the vitamin. More vitamin D also is required. "The skin gets less efficient at converting sunlight into this vitamin, so more is needed from other sources," Lichtenstein says. Fewer than 7 percent of Americans between 50 and 70 get enough vitamin D from the foods they eat, and fewer than 26 percent get enough calcium.

Staying lean and eating right are both crucial for maintaining health through the years. (Kessler recalls a fellow researcher at Yale who, upon realizing the panoply of diseases linked to body weight, promptly lost 30 pounds.) If weight is a problem, it is especially important to cut back on the processed foods that combine sugar and fat. Studies with rats indicate that when the two are added to chow, animals can't easily stop eating, says Kessler. This happens in humans, too, he says, and food manufacturers have taken note and added sugar and fat to many products.

So what should people eat? A healthful diet at midlife is the same as for younger adults—it's just that the stakes may be higher. The focus should be on fruit, vegetables, whole grains, low- and nonfat dairy, legumes, lean meats, and fish. For someone whose current diet is far from this ideal, Lichtenstein suggests starting small: Swap dark-green lettuce for iceberg, load more veggies on the dinner plate, eat more skinless chicken or beans in place of hamburger. And exercise. Walking briskly for at least 30 minutes every day makes it easier to get away with the occasional cookie. With some further fine-tuning of that basic healthful eating plan, you can greatly improve your odds of staving off the major barriers to a vital old age.

Bone Loss

No nutrient can stop bones from losing mass over time, but consuming sufficient calcium and vitamin D can slow the deterioration, says Felicia Cosman, an osteoporosis specialist at Helen Hayes Hospital in West Haverstraw, N.Y., and clinical director of the National Osteoporosis Foundation. Once a person reaches age 50, calcium requirements jump from 1,000 mg to 1,200 mg per day. Cosman recommends adding up the number of servings consumed in a typical day of dairy products and foods that are highly calcium-fortified, such as orange juice and cereal, and multiplying that by the 300 mg each most likely supplies. Add 200 to 300 mg for the combined trace amounts in leafy green vegetables, nuts, and other sources. Then get the remainder in a supplement. By midlife, adults also need at least 800 to 1,000 IU of vitamin D to help the body absorb calcium and, possibly, prevent other diseases, according to the NOF. Sources include fatty fish such as salmon (also important for heart health), egg yolks, and fortified foods, but most people need to supplement.

Heart Disease

By now, every American surely knows the roll call of foods that affect your heart, for better and for worse. Good for the ticker: monounsaturated fats like olive oil and the omega-3 fatty acids found in such cold-water fish as salmon and herring and in flaxseed and walnuts. Harmful: too much red meat and full-fat dairy, because of their saturated fat content, and margarine and baked goods, because of the trans fats they contain.

But expunging troublesome foods from your daily fare can be surprisingly difficult. "Although many supermarket products have removed the trans fats, they're hardly history. Restaurants, especially, continue to use them," cautions Robert Eckel, former president of the American Heart Association and a professor at the University of Colorado-Denver. Some food manufacturers, moreover, have simply swapped out their trans fats for saturated fat, which is equally problematic, Eckel says. Saturated fat should total no more than 7 percent of daily energy intake—about 16 grams for the average 2,000-calorie diet.

Recent research points to another potential heart danger. It's not fat; it's high-fructose corn syrup, commonly found in soda. The decades-long, 88,000-woman Nurses' Health Study found that, even controlling for weight and other unhealthful habits, drinking one 12-ounce can of regular soda daily boosts a woman's risk of later having a heart attack by 24 percent; two or more servings raise the risk by 35 percent. "We don't know exactly why this is, but fructose does increase uric acid and triglycerides in the blood, which are known contributors to hypertension and heart disease," says study coauthor Teresa Fung, associate professor of nutrition at Simmons College in Boston.

Hypertension

Lowering high blood pressure before it contributes to the development of heart disease is vital for people in midlife. It can be accomplished with an eating plan known as the DASH (Dietary Approaches to Stop Hypertension) diet. "The DASH diet has the same effect as taking a blood-pressure-lowering medication," Eckel says. The DASH-Sodium version, which subtracts salt, works as well as up to two medications. The plan is rich in fruits and vegetables (eight to 10 servings a day for someone on a 2,000-calorie diet), grains (six to eight servings daily, with most being whole grains), and low-fat protein sources. And it's low in saturated fats and added sugars. The biggest difference from standard healthful eating advice is DASH's focus on lowering sodium, which can damage artery walls in people sensitive to the nutrient. The diet limits sodium to 2,300 mg a day, while DASH-Sodium slashes it to 1,500 mg—just two thirds of a teaspoon. It's not enough to go easier on the salt shaker; the National Institutes of Health recommends looking for low- or no-salt labels, limiting high-sodium foods like bacon and sauerkraut, and rinsing canned foods. (A one-day sample menu of a DASH eating plan is available on the *U.S. News* website at www.usnews.com/dash.)

Insulin Resistance

Research has repeatedly demonstrated that type 2 diabetes and insulin resistance (a precursor to the disease in which the body begins to respond less well to the hormone that clears glucose from the blood stream) can often be prevented or postponed with a healthful diet, exercise, and weight loss. That three-part combination, in fact, actually has been shown to be more effective than medication. An eating plan aimed at minimizing the risk of insulin resistance does not have to be complex. "I coach people to mentally divide their lunch and dinner plate into thirds, with one third protein, one third nonstarchy vegetables, and the final third a starch like brown rice, whole-wheat pasta, potatoes, or corn," says Nora Saul, a dietitian and diabetes educator at Harvard's Joslin Diabetes Center in Boston. It's also a good idea to get serious about cutting back on sugar and white flour, both of which have a high glycemic index and can spike blood glucose levels.

Memory Problems

Alas, there's no magic bullet that will guarantee protection from dementia. But researchers are finding that a Mediterranean diet—similar to a conventional healthful diet but with an emphasis on fish and olive oil—seems to lower the odds of developing cognitive problems. Scientists at Columbia University followed more than 1,300 people for up to 16 years; those most closely adhering to this diet developed Alzheimer's at half the rate of those who didn't. One caveat: Alcohol (particularly in the form of wine), one element of the Mediterranean Diet that has been suggested to enhance memory function, has not been proved to do so, says Gary Kennedy, director of geriatric psychiatry at Montefiore Medical Center in New York.

Joint Disease

Although age is a risk factor for arthritis, the breakdown of cartilage in the joints is not inevitable. Minimizing weight gain goes a long way toward avoiding this problem, because every extra pound translates to 3 pounds of pressure on the knees while walking. It is also a good idea to limit foods that encourage inflammation in the body, particularly omega-6 fatty acids (found in corn and soybean oils and many snack and fried foods), the Arthritis Foundation says.

Cancer

Some 45 percent of colon cancers, 38 percent of breast cancers, and 69 percent of esophageal cancers would never occur if Americans ate better, weighed less, and exercised more, estimates the American Institute for Cancer Research. "It's not just cancers of the digestive tract. What you eat and what you weigh affect certain other cancer types as well," says Alice Bender, AICR's nutrition communications manager. The organization recommends limiting red meat to 18 (cooked) ounces per week and loading up on plant-based foods, which are high in the phytochemicals and antioxidants known to inhibit cancer cell growth in lab animals. Those with the deepest colors—like purple grapes, blueberries, and leafy green vegetables—tend to have the most beneficial compounds. One recent study, for example, showed that eating foods such as broccoli and kale that have lots of sulforaphane, an antioxidant, suppresses a bacterium linked to stomach cancer.

It looks as if food is the best source of healthful nutrients. "Numerous studies on supplements—of vitamin C, lycopene, beta carotene, and even fiber—have all proved disappointing," Bender says. Yet another reason to swap that cookie for a carrot.

Critical Thinking

1. Why is it more difficult for people over the age of 50 to lose or maintain their weight?
2. Which nutrients are needed in higher quantities by older adults?
3. What is the DASH diet? How many servings of fruits and vegetables and how much sodium is recommended per day on the DASH diet?

Create Central

www.mhhe.com/createcentral

Internet References

Diet and Physical Activity: What's the Cancer Connection?
www.cancer.org/cancer/cancercauses/dietandphysicalactivity/diet-and-physical-activity

Food—American Association for Retired Persons
www.aarp.org/food/healthy-eating

Food and Nutrition for Older Adults: Promoting Health and Wellness
www.eatright.org/About/Content.aspx?id=8374

Food and Your Bones—National Osteoporosis Foundation
http://nof.org/foods

Article

Prepared by: Janet Colson, *Middle Tennessee State University*

Insulin Resistance

Research suggests a nutrient-rich diet plus exercise may prevent and even reverse it.

RITA CAREY RUBIN

Learning Outcomes

After reading this article, you will be able to:

- Identify the major risk factors for developing insulin resistance.
- Discuss the role insulin resistance may play in the development of type 2 diabetes and cardiovascular disease.

Insulin resistance is a state of reduced cellular responsiveness to normal circulating concentrations of insulin in the blood. Much is unknown about the condition's etiology, but research has shown insulin resistance appears to play a role in the pathophysiology of prediabetes, type 2 diabetes, and cardiovascular disease (CVD). While much remains to be discovered about the exact causes of the condition, research has investigated and pinpointed several likely risk factors, including a sedentary lifestyle, central obesity, genetics and, most likely, diet.

To support dietitians in helping clients and patients address and possibly even reverse insulin resistance, this continuing education article reviews the current theory and research regarding the condition's etiology and major risk factors as well as the role it may play in the development of type 2 diabetes and CVD.

History

Research leading to the discovery of what's known today as insulin resistance dates back to the late 1950s, when research scientists Solomon Berson and Rosalyn Yalow developed the radioimmunoassay, a technique used to measure circulating levels of hormones and other substances in the blood. In later research using this technique, Berson and Yalow found that people with type 2 diabetes exhibited higher-than-average levels of circulating insulin than did individuals with normal glucose tolerance.[1]

This finding led to the first speculation that patients with type 2 diabetes may not adequately respond to insulin and thus require more insulin than normal to maintain healthy blood glucose levels. Later studies corroborated these findings, and researchers eventually coined the term "insulin resistance" to describe this condition.[2–4]

In the book *How Fat Works,* author Philip A. Wood defines insulin resistance as a condition in which the body's cells require more and more insulin to achieve normal levels of glucose uptake.[5] According to Wood, a professor of genetics, nutrition science, physiology, and biophysics as well as an experimental pathologist and director of genomics at the University of Alabama at Birmingham, insulin resistance typically develops over many years and eventually can lead to overt diabetes when the pancreas no longer can keep up with a chronically excessive insulin demand.

Pathophysiology

The development of insulin resistance and reduced glucose tolerance may be linked to altered fatty acid metabolism. In normal metabolism, liver and muscle tissue take in circulating plasma fatty acids derived from dietary fats and/or adipose tissue and convert them to fatty acid metabolites such as acyl coenzyme A (acyl-CoA). Molecules of acyl-CoA are then either oxidized in the mitochondria for energy or converted to triglycerides and stored in adipose tissue for later use.[5]

Excess quantities of circulating fatty acids commonly are associated with obesity, insulin resistance, and type 2 diabetes.[6] According to Wood, an overabundance of fatty acids also may result in the abnormal deposition of fat in both liver and muscle tissues.[5] Indeed, studies have shown a strong positive relationship between the accumulation of fat in muscle tissue and insulin resistance.[7] In addition, a positive relationship has been observed between fasting plasma fatty acid concentrations and insulin resistance in muscle.[8] In other words, insulin resistance in muscle diminishes as circulating fatty acids are reduced.

According to Gerald Shulman, MD, PhD, a professor of medicine and cellular and molecular physiology at Yale University School of Medicine, excess fatty acids appear to interfere with a very early step in insulin stimulation of glucose transport across cell membranes. Moreover, Shulman's research suggests that fatty acid metabolites, including acyl-CoA, may be some of the most important biochemical triggers of insulin resistance.[9–11]

Both Shulman and Wood describe the normal biochemical pathway for the transfer of glucose across a cell membrane as follows:[5,9]

- Insulin binds with an insulin receptor on the cell membrane, which activates a protein known as insulin receptor substrate molecule 1 (IRS-1).
- IRS-1 activates the enzyme phosphatidylinositol-3 (PI-3) kinase.
- PI-3 activates a cascade of reactions that ultimately stimulate the translocation of glucose transporter 4 (GLUT4) to the cellular membrane.
- GLUT 4 allows the movement of glucose across the membrane and into the cell.

In an insulin-resistant individual, excess acyl-CoA and other fatty acid metabolites may inhibit IRS-1 activation of PI-3 and the subsequent transfer of glucose into the cell by GLUT 4. Thus, glucose's transfer into the cell is diminished and glucose levels in the blood rise.[9]

In a research review published in 2004 in *Physiology,* Shulman speculated that defects in mitochondrial function that reduce the ability of liver and muscle tissue to adequately oxidize fatty acids may contribute to the intracellular accumulation of metabolites that trigger insulin resistance.[11] A recent review by Pagel-Langenickel and colleagues, published in *Endocrine Reviews,* also provides evidence that dysfunctional mitochondria play an important role in the development of both insulin resistance and type 2 diabetes.[12]

In this substantial research review, the authors cited evidence suggesting that lean insulin-resistant offspring of parents with type 2 diabetes and individuals with severe obesity commonly exhibit a reduction in skeletal muscle cell mitochondrial number and density; genes responsible for turning on mitochondrial metabolic functions are downregulated in patients with diabetes; and decreased levels of fatty acid and glucose oxidation are observed in patients who are obese and/or present with a strong family history of diabetes. According to the review, researchers also are debating whether mitochondrial dysfunction actually may be a cause or just a symptom of insulin resistance.[12]

Vicious Cycle

Once insulin resistance begins, it appears to stimulate a series of events that continue to increase levels of both glucose and insulin in the blood. Under normal circumstances, circulating levels of insulin rise after a meal and reduce gluconeogenesis (the production of glucose from noncarbohydrate substrates) in the liver.

Insulin-resistant liver cells, however, don't respond to this normal cue to stop creating new sources of energy. Thus, the liver continues to produce glucose from substrates such as glycerol (obtained from abundant circulating triglycerides). This continual release of glucose from the liver then stimulates the additional release of insulin from the pancreas and contributes to rising insulin levels in the blood.[5]

In addition, research shows insulin-resistant adipose tissue may not react to rising plasma insulin levels. Normally, insulin reduces the breakdown of adipose tissue (lipolysis) and promotes fat storage after a meal. In people with insulin resistance, lipolysis continues despite elevated levels of insulin. Adipose tissue therefore releases more fatty acids into circulation which, in turn, may aggravate and promote insulin resistance.[5]

Risk Factors

The risk factors for insulin resistance include central obesity, physical inactivity, and genetics.

Central Obesity

The location of fat stores in the body appears to be a strong determinant of insulin resistance. Research indicates that adipose tissue in the hips, buttocks, and thighs is less of a risk factor than is fat deposited centrally, or in the gut.[5,13–15] The specific location of central fat also may be important, as visceral abdominal fat (located deep and around organs) may be more likely to cause insulin resistance than subcutaneous abdominal fat.[15]

Several theories address the role abdominal fat plays in the pathogenesis of insulin resistance, but the exact mechanisms remain undefined. According to Wood, fat that's stored lower in the body is less likely to undergo lipolysis than centrally deposited, visceral fat. Thus, abdominal fat is more likely to contribute to elevated levels of fatty acids circulating in the blood, which, in turn, may promote insulin resistance.[5]

Researchers also have proposed that the endocrine function of adipose tissue influences the development of insulin resistance.[16] For example, adipose tissue contributes to circulating levels of the proinflammatory cytokine interleukin-6 (IL-6), and elevated levels of IL-6 have been positively associated with obesity, impaired glucose tolerance, and insulin resistance.[17] However, the role IL-6 and other mediators of inflammation play in the development of both insulin resistance and type 2 diabetes hasn't been adequately determined, and researchers recommend further investigation.[17]

Sedentary Lifestyle

Many people who are insulin resistant are obese (though some who are lean also can suffer from insulin resistance), but not all obese individuals are insulin resistant.[18] Gerald Reaven, MD, an endocrinologist and professor emeritus of medicine at Stanford University who's considered an expert on insulin resistance, maintains that insulin's ability to stimulate cellular glucose uptake may vary more than sixfold among individuals.[19] In fact, Reaven and his colleagues estimate that only 25% to 35% of this variability in insulin action is related to being overweight.[20] Therefore, obesity is likely only one of several factors that modulate insulin action.

A sedentary lifestyle may be a strong risk factor for developing insulin resistance. In a study of volunteers of both Pima Indian and European ancestry who didn't have diabetes, Bogardus and colleagues found that differences in physical fitness were as powerful as variations in adiposity in the modulation of insulin action.[21] The results of a large observational study by Risérus and colleagues (n = 770) indicated that physical activity and socioeconomic status both were strong predictors of insulin resistance, following BMI, in adult men observed for 20 years.[22]

Considering the available evidence, Bogardus and colleagues concluded that obesity, along with physical inactivity, may account for approximately one-half of the variability in insulin sensitivity in healthy individuals who don't have diabetes.[19]

Genetics

Since the completion of the Human Genome Project in 2003, genetics has played an increasingly important role in disease diagnosis and treatment. In fact, genetic scientists have come to believe that many, if not all, diseases have a genetic component. While some diseases develop directly from a single, inherited genetic mutation, others develop as a genetic response to environmental stressors such as poor diet, viruses, or toxins.[5]

Many common diseases, including type 2 diabetes, seem to be multifactorial in origin, meaning that genetics as well as environmental and behavioral factors combine to produce disease.[5] According to Wood, insulin resistance also may be one of those multifactorial diseases that result from a genetic domino effect: Genes that promote higher blood levels of triglycerides may be triggered by a poor diet and/or sedentary lifestyle and consequently may create the conditions for developing insulin resistance.[5]

In research that was part of the Tufts Twin Study, Elder and colleagues attempted to determine the genetic heritability of components of the metabolic syndrome, which includes insulin resistance.[23] Heritability is defined as the relative influence of genetic factors on the expression of a disease or disease trait. Elder and colleagues connected every component of the metabolic syndrome, including insulin resistance, with a genetic link and determined that genetics had more of an influence on the development of the metabolic syndrome than did environmental influences.

The study's results suggest that, despite established relationships between environmental factors and the metabolic syndrome, genetic variation may be an important and possibly primary determinant of the expression of insulin resistance.

The Effect of Diet

Some research suggests that a diet high in total, trans, and saturated fat may promote insulin resistance.[24–26] Studies also indicate that replacing saturated fat with polyunsaturated or monounsaturated fat may improve insulin sensitivity, but only if total fat intake also is controlled.[25]

According to a recent review by Risérus and colleagues of literature examining the role of different types of fat on insulin resistance, studies comparing insulin sensitivity and fatty acid composition in skeletal muscle (a reflection of the fatty acid composition of the diet) have found a direct, positive relationship between the proportion of long-chain polyunsaturated fatty acids and insulin sensitivity.[26] In addition, evidence suggests the more saturated fatty acids in the muscle cell membrane, the more insulin-resistant the individual.[24]

In the KANWU study, a three-month controlled, parallel, multicenter study performed at five different centers: Kuopio, Finland; Aarhus, Denmark; Naples, Italy; Wollongong, Australia; and Uppsala, Sweden, 162 subjects from these countries received isocaloric diets that differed only in fat quality, not quantity.[25] Researchers found that insulin sensitivity was impaired in individuals on the higher saturated fat diet and improved in those on the higher monounsaturated fat diet. However, substituting monounsaturated fat for saturated fat improved insulin sensitivity only if total fat intake remained at no more than 37% of calories. The authors concluded that the type of fat in the diet impacted insulin resistance, but quantity of fat also was important.

In the SLIM study (Lifestyle Intervention on Postprandial Glucose Metabolism), researchers also demonstrated improved glucose tolerance and insulin sensitivity among participants who reduced their intake of both saturated fat and total fat.[27] Again, the benefits of reduced saturated fat intake were noted only in those with a total fat intake of less than 35% of calories.

All these studies suggest that a diet low in saturated fat but also moderate in total fat content improves insulin sensitivity.

Role in CVD

Insulin resistance is a central part of a cluster of metabolic abnormalities called the metabolic syndrome. Originally discovered and labeled by Reaven as syndrome X,[28] metabolic syndrome is described as the concurrence of conditions, including elevated triglycerides, central obesity, low levels of HDL cholesterol, hypertension, and impaired fasting glucose.[5,29]

According to Reaven, individuals with the metabolic syndrome also may experience impaired clearance of fat from the blood after meals; elevated levels of small, dense lipoproteins; and hypercoagulation resulting from elevated levels of plasma fibrinogen.[28] Insulin resistance is directly implicated in the development of several of these abnormalities, all of which may be considered independent risk factors of CVD.[28,30]

For example, elevated levels of insulin resulting from insulin resistance stimulate the liver to increase its production of triglyceride-rich very-low-density lipoproteins, thus causing blood triglyceride levels to rise.[28,30] Insulin-resistant adipose tissue undergoes lipolysis in the fed and fasting state, also adding to the plasma triglyceride load.[5,28] Insulin resistance may reduce the body's ability to clear fat from the blood after a meal.[28] As Reaven's research demonstrates, all these factors contribute to the development of CVD and an increased risk of heart attack.

Some long-term studies have demonstrated that insulin resistance increases the risk of CVD. In the San Antonio Heart Study, individuals with insulin resistance had a twofold to 2.5-fold increased risk of CVD at eight years.[31] Insulin-resistant individuals without diabetes in the Botnia Study also experienced a twofold increased incidence of CVD at seven years.[32]

In a 2010 review published in *Diabetologia,* DeFronzo summarized research that suggests additional links between insulin resistance and CVD. In vivo and in vitro animal and human studies have demonstrated that insulin, especially at high doses, promotes LDL cholesterol transport into cultured arterial smooth muscle cells, augments collagen synthesis and arterial smooth muscle cell proliferation (thus increasing carotid intimal media thickness and reducing vascular elasticity), and may turn on genes that promote inflammation, which is known to accelerate atherogenesis. According to DeFronzo, the increased risk of CVD in people with insulin resistance can't be completely explained by changes in plasma lipids and fibrinolysis;

instead, insulin's effect on smooth muscle cell proliferation and inflammation likely may be a primary driver of the disease.[30]

Role in Prediabetes and Type 2 Diabetes

According to the National Institutes of Health, insulin resistance is a risk factor for developing both prediabetes and type 2 diabetes.[33] Prediabetes, also known as impaired glucose tolerance or impaired fasting glucose, currently is diagnosed when hemoglobin A1c (HbA1c) levels fall between 5.7% and 6.4%.[34] Individuals with prediabetes are known to have an increased risk of converting to type 2 diabetes.[34]

According to the American Diabetes Association (ADA), the continuum of risk is curvilinear, indicating that as HbA1c rises, the risk of diabetes rises at a disproportionately greater rate.[34]

The Insulin Resistance Atherosclerosis Study is a large epidemiological investigation into the relationship between insulin resistance and cardiovascular risk factors among individuals of three ethnic groups (blacks, Hispanics, and whites). In this study, researchers measured insulin sensitivity and first-phase insulin response in 557 participants with normal glucose tolerance and 269 individuals with impaired glucose tolerance. At five years, both insulin sensitivity and first-phase insulin response predicted conversion to diabetes, regardless of ethnic group. While individuals with a family history of diabetes and those with a higher BMI and larger waist circumference also were more likely to develop diabetes, insulin sensitivity, and first-phase insulin response still were more significantly correlated.[35]

Similarly, results from the Diabetes Prevention Program (DPP) showed that participants who improved insulin sensitivity and insulin secretion through lifestyle change or treatment with metformin experienced a reduction in the conversion to type 2 diabetes. The DPP Research Group concluded that "analysis of the changes in plasma glucose and insulin during the first year of the study suggests that development of diabetes . . . resulted from continued decreases in insulin sensitivity and beta-cell function, whereas reduction in the incidence of diabetes observed in the two active interventions was due to their ability to increase insulin sensitivity and improved beta-cell function." In other words, lifestyle change alone as well as treatment with metformin appeared to reduce insulin resistance and improve insulin secretion. The researchers drew no conclusions regarding the exact physiologic mechanisms involved.[36]

Although it's commonly accepted that insulin resistance usually precedes the development of type 2 diabetes by many years, the physiologic mechanisms that promote the progression of insulin resistance to type 2 diabetes in some individuals are still under investigation. Unger and Grundy were the first to postulate that continuous overstimulation of pancreatic beta cells resulting from insulin resistance and hyperglycemia eventually could lead to beta-cell failure.[37] These investigators also were the first to introduce the terms "glucotoxicity" and "lipotoxicity," which describe the deleterious effects of chronically elevated blood glucose and triglyceride levels on beta-cell function. Researchers have continued to implicate the direct toxic effects of hyperglycemia and hyperlipidemia on beta-cell function as well as the effects of whole-body oxidative stress resulting from hyperglycemia in the conversion of insulin resistance to overt diabetes. However, the exact physiologic processes involved haven't been determined and are still under scientific debate.[38]

Reversing Insulin Resistance

Research shows that weight loss and physical activity can play an important role in improving insulin resistance.

Weight Loss and Improved Insulin Sensitivity

Several studies have demonstrated the importance of weight loss, especially when resulting from a reduction in visceral fat mass, on the reversal of insulin resistance. A four-year intervention involving participants in the Finnish Diabetes Prevention Study demonstrated a strong correlation between changes in insulin resistance and weight. Although this study was small (researchers could follow only 52 people for the entire length of the study), the results were remarkable. In the entire group, insulin sensitivity improved by up to 64% among participants with the highest degree of weight loss (up to 17.2% of body weight) and deteriorated by 24% in those who gained weight (up to 10%). Participants who lost weight generally followed a diet plan that was low fat (fewer than 30% of calories from fat and fewer than 10% of calories from saturated fat) and high fiber (15 g fiber/1,000 kcal).[39]

Interestingly, some research also suggests that caloric restriction promoting visceral fat loss may reduce or even override the impact of dietary fat type on insulin resistance. Researchers in a randomized controlled study compared the effects of a low-carbohydrate diet (20% of energy from carbohydrate and 60% of energy from fat) with a low-fat diet (60% of energy from carbohydrate and 20% of energy from fat) on weight reduction and insulin resistance in adults who were overweight or obese.[40]

In this study, diets were designed on an individual basis to facilitate a weekly 0.5-kg weight loss. At the end of eight weeks, both groups lost an average of 7% of their initial body weight and demonstrated similar reductions in both waist circumference and percent body fat. Both groups experienced comparable improvements in insulin sensitivity, and researchers attributed this improvement to weight loss alone, not to the specific macronutrient makeup of the diets. Because this study implies that dietary fat levels may not be as important as weight loss for reducing insulin resistance, it's evident that questions remain regarding the relative contributions of macronutrients and weight loss to the reversal of insulin resistance.

Effect of Exercise

There's substantial literature showing improved insulin sensitivity after exercise, both with and independent of weight loss.[41–47] There's debate about the best exercise prescription to maximize insulin sensitivity in different populations, but both regular aerobic exercise and resistance training seem to confer beneficial results.

In 2003, Goodpaster and colleagues demonstrated that a regular, moderate-to-high intensity exercise program (a 40-minute workout at up to 75% maximum heart rate, four to six times per week for 16 weeks) enhanced not only insulin sensitivity but also the capacity of obese, middle-aged individuals to burn fat, especially in those who also lost weight.[41] Since sedentary, obese individuals with insulin resistance exhibit a reduced capacity to burn both fat and glucose for energy, enhancing mitochondrial fat and glucose oxidation may reduce insulin resistance.[5] Evidence from this study suggests that exercise is a potential means to that end.[41]

In a randomized 12-week trial designed to examine the effect of exercise (EX group) or exercise combined with moderate caloric restriction (EX + CR group) on insulin resistance and other measurements of the metabolic syndrome, Yassine and colleagues found that exercise alone had a significant impact on insulin resistance in a population of older (65.5 ± 5 years) obese adults. A caloric restriction of 500 kcal/day in the EX + CR group didn't lead to any greater improvement in insulin resistance, despite greater weight loss (7.4% of initial body weight).[47]

The exercise intervention in this study was a simple walking program, although participants were gradually (at the end of four weeks) exercising at a relatively high level of intensity (80% to 85% of maximum heart rate) for 50 to 60 minutes per day, five days per week. Level of fitness, as measured by aerobic capacity, was strongly correlated with insulin sensitivity in this study group.

While dieting can reduce visceral fat mass and improve insulin sensitivity, caloric restriction also results in the loss of some lean body mass. In fact, a recent review estimates that reduced muscle mass can account for 14% to 23% of total weight lost.[48] Results from the Healthy Aging and Body Composition Study indicate that older adults experience greater loss of muscle mass with intentional caloric restriction than do younger individuals.[49] Because skeletal muscle plays an important role in glucose metabolism, muscle wasting from dieting or aging may have a significant impact on the development of insulin resistance.[50] Researchers suggest that the effect of exercise on muscle mass may be an important modulator of insulin sensitivity, especially in older adults.[50,51]

Additional Dietary Considerations

The following are additional dietary considerations in relation to their impact on insulin sensitivity:

- **Fat:** Research shows possible insulin sensitivity improvements with a reduction in saturated, trans, and/or total fat.[24–27]
- **Vegan diet:** One study by Barnard and colleagues demonstrated the effects of a 14-week, low-fat vegan diet on weight loss and insulin sensitivity. In this study, 64 overweight, postmenopausal women were randomly assigned to a low-fat vegan diet group or a control diet group following National Cholesterol Education Program guidelines. Neither group had calorie restrictions. Participants who ate the vegan diet lost 5.8 ± 3.2 kg compared with 3.8 ± 2.8 kg among controls. Insulin sensitivity improved in both groups, with no significant difference between the two.[52]

In a separate study, researchers at the Imperial College School of Medicine in London showed the positive effects of a vegan diet on lowering plasma triglycerides, fasting glucose, and systolic blood pressure compared with controls who ate an omnivorous diet.[53]

With results similar to those of Barnard, these researchers also discovered a nominal improvement in insulin sensitivity in the vegan diet group. However, the vegan group demonstrated significantly improved pancreatic beta-cell function and a reduction in intramuscular fat deposits, both indirect indicators of improved glycemic control and insulin sensitivity.

- **Carbohydrates:** Choosing carbohydrate-dense foods that are low on the glycemic index also may have beneficial effects, especially when combined with a reduction in calories and regular exercise. A study by Kirwan and colleagues demonstrated that combining a low-glycemic diet with exercise resulted in a greater decrease in insulin resistance in older obese adults than did exercise and calorie reduction without regard to glycemic index.[54]
- **Phytochemicals:** In a study that considered the impact of dietary components other than macronutrient content, Minich and Bland recommend examining the diet's phytochemical content for clues to the etiology of insulin resistance.[55] These researchers postulated that a plant-based diet containing significant levels of phytochemicals effectively may prevent insulin resistance. They cited evidence from clinical trials supporting the beneficial effects of fruit and vegetable pigments, bitter melon, green tea, cinnamon, and hops on maintaining normal cellular insulin signaling function, the key to preventing insulin resistance.[55]

Bottom Line

Despite all this research, the ideal diet and lifestyle prescription for the treatment and prevention of insulin resistance is unknown. Moderate caloric restriction that facilitates the loss of abdominal fat seems to be important to improving insulin sensitivity, as does regular aerobic exercise. Some evidence suggests that replacing saturated fat with polyunsaturated fat also may contribute to reduced visceral fat mass.[26]

The ADA has made no specific recommendations for treating insulin resistance, but recommends lifestyle modification for prediabetes, a known insulin-resistant state. In its 2013 Medical Standards of Care Position Statement, the ADA recommended a diet and exercise program that targets and supports a 7% loss of body weight and at least 150 minutes per week of moderate exercise.[34]

Resistance exercise to build muscle mass can be beneficial, especially for older adults. Helping patients devise a diet and exercise program that facilitates the loss of 1 to 2 lbs of body weight per week eventually may help improve their insulin sensitivity.

Saturated and trans fat seem to reduce insulin sensitivity more than poly- and monounsaturated fats, but total fat intake still needs to be controlled. A goal of 30% of calories from fat, mostly plant-based unsaturated fats, can be a reasonable and safe dietary goal for most patients with insulin resistance.

Encouraging patients to follow a plant-based diet featuring vegetables, fruits, beans, whole grains, nuts, and seeds also is a sensible approach. The USDA MyPlate guidelines can be an easy first step many patients can take toward including more phytochemical-packed plants and fewer foods containing saturated fats in their meals. The USDA guidelines also suggest limiting added sugars to no more than 10% of total calories and increasing intake of carbohydrate-dense foods that are also low on the glycemic index, including unrefined grains and grain products. In general, foods that are less processed tend to rate lower on the glycemic index scale. For example, rolled oats have a lower glycemic index than instant oats. However, to more accurately assess glycemic index, it's useful to refer to a glycemic index database, such as the one found at GlycemicIndex.com.

Overall, however, current research seems to indicate that the exact macronutrient balance of the diet may be less important than sustained activity, maintaining a healthy body weight and, perhaps, the micronutrient content of the foods patients consume in preventing and treating insulin resistance.

References

1. Yalow RS, Berson SA. Plasma insulin concentrations in nondiabetic and early diabetic subjects. Determinations by a new sensitive immune-assay technique. *Diabetes.* 1960;4:254–260.
2. Kahn CR, Flier JS, Bar RS, et al. The syndromes of insulin resistance and acanthosis nigricans. Insulin-receptor disorders in man. *N Engl J Med.* 1976;294(14):739–745.
3. Olefsky J, Farquhar JW, Reaven G. Relationship between fasting plasma insulin level and resistance to insulin-mediated glucose uptake in normal and diabetic subjects. *Diabetes.* 1973;22(7):507–513.
4. Reaven GM. Role of insulin resistance in human disease. *Diabetes.* 1988;37(12):1595–1607.
5. Wood PA. *How Fat Works.* Cambridge, MA: Harvard University Press; 2006.
6. Brunzell JD, Ayyobi AF. Dyslipidemia in the metabolic syndrome and type 2 diabetes mellitus. *Am J Med.* 2003;115(Suppl 8A):24S–28S.
7. DeFronzo RA, Tripathy D. Skeletal muscle insulin resistance is the primary defect in type 2 diabetes. *Diabetes Care.* 2009;32(Suppl 2):S157–S163.
8. Bajaj M, Suraamornkul S, Romanelli A, et al. Effect of a sustained reduction in plasma free fatty acid concentration on intramuscular long-chain fatty acyl-CoAs and insulin action in type 2 diabetic patients. ***Diabetes.*** 2005;54(11):3148–3153.
9. Shulman GI. Cellular mechanisms of insulin resistance. ***J Clin Invest.*** 2000;106(2):171–176.
10. Boden G, Shulman GI. Free fatty acids in obesity and type 2 diabetes: defining their role in the development of insulin resistance and beta-cell dysfunction. ***Eur J Clin Invest.*** 2002;32 (Suppl 3):14–23.
11. Shulman GI. Unraveling the cellular mechanism of insulin resistance in humans: new insights from magnetic resonance spectroscopy. ***Physiology.*** 2004;19:183–190.
12. Pagel-Langenickel I, Bao J, Pang L, Sack MN. The role of mitochondria in the pathophysiology of skeletal muscle insulin resistance. ***Endocr Rev.*** 2010;31(1):25–51.
13. Sandeep S, Gokulakrishnan K, Velmurugan K, Deepa M, Mohan V. Visceral and subcutaneous abdominal fat in relation to insulin resistance and metabolic syndrome non-diabetic south Indians. ***Indian J Med Res.*** 2010;131:629–635.
14. Lord J, Thomas R, Fox B, Acharya U, Wilkin T. The central issue? Visceral fat mass is a good marker of insulin resistance and metabolic disturbance in women with polycystic ovary syndrome. ***BJOG.*** 2006;113(10):1203–1209.
15. Preis SR, Massaro JM, Robins SJ, et al. Abdominal subcutaneous and visceral adipose tissue and insulin resistance in the Framingham Heart Study. ***Obesity.*** 2010;18(11):2191–2198.
16. Kershaw EE, Flier JS. Adipose tissue as an endocrine organ. ***J Clin Endocrinol Metab.*** 2004;89(6):2548–2556.
17. Fernandez-Real JM, Ricart W. Insulin resistance and chronic cardiovascular inflammatory syndrome. ***Endocr Rev.*** 2003;24(3):278–301.
18. McLaughlin T, Allison G, Abbasi F, Lamendola C, Reaven G. Prevalence of insulin resistance and associated cardiovascular disease risk factors among normal weight, overweight, and obese individuals. ***Metabolism.*** 2004;53(4):495–499.
19. Reaven GM, Abbasi F, McLaughlin T. Obesity, insulin resistance and cardiovascular disease. ***Recent Prog Horm Res.*** 2004;59:207–223.
20. Abbasi F, Brown BW Jr, Lamendola C, McLaughlin T, Reaven GM. Relationship between obesity, insulin resistance, and coronary heart disease risk. ***J Am Coll Cardiol.*** 2002;40(5):937–943.
21. Bogardus C, Lillioja S, Mott DM, Hollenbeck C, Reaven GM. Relationship between degree of obesity and in vivo insulin action in man. ***Am J Physiol.*** 1985;248(3 Pt 1):E286–E291.
22. Risérus U, Arnlöv J, Berglund L. Long-term predictors of insulin resistance: role of lifestyle and metabolic factors in middle-aged men. ***Diabetes Care.*** 2007;30(11):2928–2933.
23. Elder SJ, Lichtenstein AH, Pittas AG, et al. Genetic and environmental influences on factors associated with cardiovascular disease and the metabolic syndrome. ***J Lipid Res.*** 2009;50(9):1917–1926.
24. Borkman M, Storlien LH, Pan DA, Jenkins AB, Chisholm DJ, Campbell LV. The relation between insulin sensitivity and the fatty-acid composition of skeletal muscle phospholipids. ***N Engl J Med.*** 1993;328(4):238–244.
25. Vessby B, Uusitupa M, Hermansen K, et al. Substituting dietary saturated for monounsaturated fat impairs insulin sensitivity in healthy men and women: the KANWU study. ***Diabetologia.*** 2001;44(3):312–319.
26. Risérus U, Willett WC, Hu FB. Dietary fats and prevention of type 2 diabetes. ***Prog Lipid Res.*** 2009;48(1):44–51.
27. Corpeleijn E, Feskens EJ, Jansen EH, et al. Improvements in glucose tolerance and insulin sensitivity after lifestyle intervention are related to changes in serum fatty acid profile and desaturase activities: the SLIM study. ***Diabetologia.*** 2006;49(10):2392–2401.
28. Reaven GM, Strom TK, Fox B. ***Syndrome X: The Silent Killer: The New Heart Disease Risk.*** New York, NY: Simon & Schuster; 2001.
29. Grundy SM, Brewer HB Jr, Cleeman JI, Smith SC Jr, Lenfant C. Definition of metabolic syndrome: report of the National Heart, Lung and Blood Institute/American Heart Association Conference on Scientific Issues Related to Definition. ***Circulation.*** 2004;109(3):433–438.
30. DeFronzo RA. Insulin resistance, lipotoxicity, type 2 diabetes and atherosclerosis: the missing links. The Claude Bernard Lecture 2009. ***Diabetologia.*** 2010;53(7):1270–1287.
31. Hanley AJ, Williams K, Stern MP, Haffner SM. Homeostasis model assessment of insulin resistance in relation to the

incidence of cardiovascular disease: the San Antonio Heart Study. ***Diabetes Care.*** 2002;25(7):1177–1184.

32. Isomaa B, Almgren P, Tuomi T, et al. Cardiovascular morbidity and mortality associated with the metabolic syndrome. ***Diabetes Care.*** 2001;24(4):683–689.
33. What are the symptoms of insulin resistance and prediabetes? National Diabetes Information Clearinghouse website. http://diabetes.niddk.nih.gov/dm/pubs/insulinresistance/ - relate. Last updated January 22, 2013. Accessed May 7, 2013.
34. American Diabetes Association. Standards of Medical Care in Diabetes 2013. ***Diabetes Care.*** 2013;36(S1):S11–S66.
35. Lorenzo C, Wagenknecht LE, D'Agostino RB Jr, Reuers MI, Karter AJ, Haffner SM. Insulin resistance, beta cell dysfunction, and conversion to type 2 diabetes in a multiethnic population. The Insulin Resistance Atherosclerosis Study. ***Diabetes Care.*** 2010;33(1):67–72.
36. Kitabchi AE, Temprosa M, Knowler WC, et al. Role of insulin secretion and sensitivity in the evolution of type 2 diabetes in the Diabetes Prevention Program: effects of lifestyle intervention and metformin. ***Diabetes.*** 2005;54(8):2404–2414.
37. Unger RH, Grundy S. Hyperglycaemia as an inducer as well as a consequence of impaired islet cell function and insulin resistance: implications for the management of diabetes. ***Diabetologia.*** 1985;28(3):119–121.
38. Poitout V, Robertson RP. Glucolipotoxicity: fuel excess and ß-cell dysfunction. ***Endocr Rev.*** 2008;29(3):351–366.
39. Uusitapa M, Lindi L, Louheranta A, Salopuro T, Lindstrom J, Tuomilehto J. Long-term improvement in insulin sensitivity by changing lifestyles of people with impaired glucose tolerance: 4-year results from the Finnish Diabetes Prevention Study. ***Diabetes.*** 2003;52(10):2532–2538.
40. Bradley U, Spence M, Courtney CH, et al. Low-fat versus low-carbohydrate weight reduction diets: effects on weight loss, insulin resistance and cardiovascular risk: a randomized control trial. ***Diabetes.*** 2009;58(12):2741–2748.
41. Goodpaster BH, Katsiaras A, Kelley DE. Enhanced fat oxidation through physical activity is associated with improvements in insulin sensitivity in obesity. ***Diabetes.*** 2003;52(9):2191–2197.
42. O'Leary VB, Marchetti CM, Krishnan RK, Stetzer BP, Gonzalez F, Kirwan JP. Exercise-induced reversal of insulin resistance in obese elderly is associated with reduced visceral fat. ***J Appl Physiol.*** 2006;100(5):1584–1589.
43. Houmard JA, Tanner CJ, Slentz, CA, Duscha BD, McCartney JS, Kraws WE. Effect of the volume and intensity of exercise training on insulin sensitivity. ***J Appl Physiol.*** 2004;96(1):101–106.
44. Houmard JA, Shaw CD, Hickey MS, Tanner CJ. Effect of short-term exercise training on insulin-stimulated PI-3 kinase activity in human skeletal muscle. ***Am J Physiol.*** 1999; 277(6 Pt 1):E1055–E1060.
45. Kelley DE, Goodpaster B, Wing RR, Simoneau JA. Skeletal muscle fatty acid metabolism in association with insulin resistance, obesity, and weight loss. *Am J Physiol.* 1999; 277(6 Pt 1):E1130–E1141.
46. Hasson RE, Granados K, Chipkin S, Freedson PS, Braun B. Effects of a single exercise bout on insulin sensitivity in black and white individuals. ***J Clin Endocrinol Metab.*** 2010;95(10):E219–E223.
47. Yassine HN, Marchetti CM, Krishnan RK, Vrobel TR, Gonzalez F, Kirwan JP. Effects of exercise and caloric restriction on insulin resistance and cardiometabolic risk factors in older obese adults. A randomized clinical trial. ***J Gerontol A Biol Sci Med Sci.*** 2009;64(1):90–95.
48. Chaston TB, Dixon JB, O'Brien PE. Changes in fat-free mass during significant weight loss: a systematic review. ***Int J Obes (Lond).*** 2007;31(5):743–750.
49. Newman AB, Lee JS, Visser M, et al. Weight change and the conservation of lean mass in old age: the Health, Aging and Body Composition Study. ***Am J Clin Nutr.*** 2005;82(4):872–878.
50. Willey KA, Singh MA. Battling insulin resistance in elderly obese people with type 2 diabetes: bring on the heavy weights. ***Diabetes Care.*** 2003;26(5):1580–1588.
51. Ferrara CM, Goldberg AP, Ortmeyer HK, Ryan AS. Effects of aerobic and resistive exercise training on glucose disposal and skeletal muscle metabolism in older men. ***J Gerontol A Biol Sci Med Sci.*** 2006;61(5):480–487.
52. Barnard ND, Scialli AR, Turner-McGrievy G, Lanou AJ, Glass J. The effects of a low-fat, plant-based dietary intervention on body weight, metabolism, and insulin sensitivity. ***Am J Med.*** 2005;118(9):991–997.
53. Goff LM, Bell JD, So PW, Dornhorst A, Frost GS. Veganism and its relationship with insulin resistance and intramyocellular lipid. ***Eur J Clin Nutr.*** 2005;59(2):291–298.
54. Kirwan JP, Barkoukis H, Brooks LM, Marchetti CM, Stetzer BP, Gonzalez F. Exercise training and dietary glycemic load may have synergistic effects on insulin resistance in older obese adults. ***Ann Nutr Metab.*** 2009;55(4):326–333.
55. Minich DM, Bland JS. Dietary management of the metabolic syndrome beyond macronutrients. ***Nutr Rev.*** 2008;66(8):429–444.

Critical Thinking

1. Define insulin resistance.
2. Evaluate the major risk factors for developing insulin resistance.
3. Explain how central obesity and a high-fat diet may influence the development of insulin resistance.
4. Analyze the role insulin resistance may play in the development of type 2 diabetes and cardiovascular disease.
5. Assess the lifestyle modifications that may improve insulin sensitivity and reduce insulin resistance.

Create Central

www.mhhe.com/createcentral

Internet References

American Diabetes Association
www.diabetes.org

MyPlate
www.MyPlate.gov

Rita Carey Rubin, MS, RD, CDE, is a dietitian and certified diabetes educator practicing in northern Arizona.

Article

Prepared by: Janet Colson, *Middle Tennessee State University*

Sugar Belly

How Much Is Too Much Sugar?

Soft drinks, sports drinks, fruit drinks, energy drinks, coffee drinks, cupcakes, cookies, muffins, doughnuts, granola bars, chocolate, ice cream, sweetened yogurt, cereal, candy. The list of sweet temptations is endless.

The average American now consumes 22 to 28 teaspoons of *added sugars* a day—mostly high-fructose corn syrup and ordinary table sugar (sucrose). That's 350 to 440 empty calories that few of us can afford.

How much added sugar is too much? Cutting back to 100 calories (6½ teaspoons) a day for women and 150 calories (9½ teaspoons) a day for men might mean slimmer waistlines and a lower risk of disease.

BONNIE LIEBMAN

Learning Outcomes

After reading this article, you will be able to:

- Compare and contrast the physiological actions of glucose and fructose in the body.
- Describe the link between the consumption of high-fructose corn sweeteners and increased risk for heart disease, metabolic syndrome, type 2 diabetes, gout, and accumulation of visceral fat.

Obesity

Do sugary foods and drinks deserve more blame for America's obesity epidemic than other foods?

"There is strong evidence linking sugar-sweetened beverages to weight," says Vasanti Malik, a research fellow at the Harvard School of Public Health.

For example, when she and her colleagues tracked more than 50,000 women for four years, they found that weight gain was greatest (about 10 pounds) among women who went from drinking no more than one sugar-sweetened drink a week to at least one a day.[1]

"But most industry-funded studies have reported no association," she notes. "This back-and-forth with industry has been muddying the waters."

For example, a 2009 meta-analysis by scientists with industry ties found no link between soft drinks and weight in children.[2]

"But there were some errors in the way they scaled the data," Malik explains.

What's more, some studies in the industry-funded analysis only compared soda drinkers to non-soda drinkers *who consumed the same number of calories.*

"It doesn't make sense to adjust for total calories because extra calories may explain how sugar-sweetened beverages lead to obesity," says Malik.

"When we re-analyzed the data correctly, there was an association between weight and sugar-sweetened beverages."[3]

What about the added sugars in solid foods? "There's not as much evidence for them," says Malik. "We haven't looked at that carefully yet."

"We focused on sugar-sweetened beverages because they're the largest contributor of added sugar intake," she adds, "and because of the lack of compensation for liquid calories."

Studies find that people may "compensate" for the calories they get from solid foods by eating less later in the day. But that doesn't seem to happen when people drink liquid calories.[4]

"In one study, people given jelly beans consumed less at subsequent meals than those who were given the same calories as liquid sugary beverages," says Malik.

More evidence that sugary beverages can plaster on the pounds: In three studies, scientists randomly assigned people to consume either sugary beverages (made with sugar or high-fructose corn syrup) versus diet beverages (usually made with aspartame) for three to 10 weeks.[5–7] Sure enough, only those who consumed sugar or high-fructose corn syrup gained weight.

Sugars 101

Sucrose (table sugar) is broken down—in the body and (to some extent) in foods—to half fructose and half glucose. At that point it is almost identical to most high-fructose corn syrup. Fruit contains a mixture of fructose, sucrose, and glucose.

But now researchers are hot on the trail of a new lead: Is the fructose that makes up roughly half of most added sugars more likely to migrate to your belly than elsewhere?

A Beeline to the Belly

Clearly, too many calories from anything—sugary beverages, beer, burgers, fries, pizza, ice cream, or dozens of other foods—explains why many American waists have been replaced by a spare tire.

And studies haven't found that you'd gain more pounds from, say, 100 calories of added sugars than from 100 calories of other foods. But calories from fructose (which is found only in added sugars and fruit) may be more likely than other calories to aim for your waist.

To find out if fructose is destined to end up around your midsection, researchers compare fructose to glucose (which is found in added sugars but is also the building block of starches).

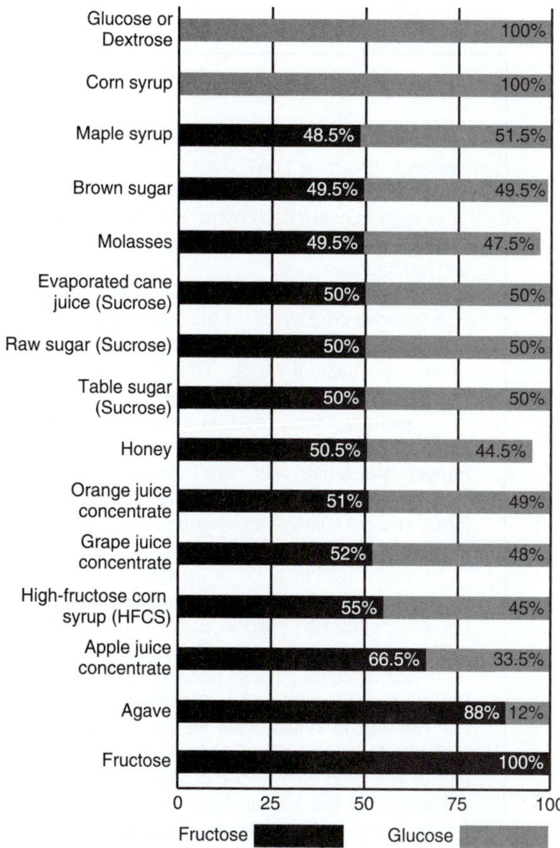

* Sucrose is shown as its component sugars (fructose and glucose). Note: If percentages don't add up to 100, other sugars account for the difference.

Sugar by Any Other Name With a few exceptions (like agave and corn syrup), most sweeteners and the naturally occurring sugars in fruit break down into roughly half fructose and half glucose in the body.* The natural sugar in milk (lactose) breaks down into half glucose and half galactose.

Sources: USDA Nutrient Database and company information.

The first solid evidence came in 2009. Researchers gave 32 overweight or obese middle-aged men and women 25 percent of their calories from beverages sweetened with either fructose or glucose for 10 weeks.[8]

Both groups gained the same weight (about three pounds). But their new fat didn't all go to the same place.

"We saw an increase in visceral fat in people fed fructose," says study author Kimber Stanhope of the University of California, Davis.

Visceral (deep belly) fat is more closely linked to a higher risk of heart disease and diabetes than subcutaneous (just below the skin) fat. (See "Where's the Fat?")

"The high-fructose corn syrup industry's scientific consultants criticized our study," says Stanhope. "They said, 'This is meaningless. No one consumes foods sweetened with pure fructose so no one consumes that much fructose.'"

Now two new studies have reported similar results with less fructose:

- Danish scientists assigned 47 overweight men and women to drink a liter (not quite three 12 oz. cans) a day of one of four drinks: regular cola (sweetened with sucrose), reduced-fat milk, diet cola (sweetened with aspartame), or water.[9] (Sucrose is half glucose and half fructose.)

  After six months, visceral fat went up only in those drinking regular cola. "The increase in visceral fat was quite impressive," says Stanhope.

  And a liter isn't much. Roughly half the population doesn't drink sugary beverages, but among the drinkers, 50 percent swallow at least half a liter a day and 5 percent gulp down at least $1\frac{1}{3}$ liters.[10]

- Swiss researchers assigned 29 healthy, normal-weight men to drink beverages with one of the following: 10 teaspoons of fructose, 20 teaspoons of fructose, 10 teaspoons of glucose, 20 teaspoons of glucose, or 20 teaspoons of sucrose each day.[11]

  "Those aren't large amounts," notes Stanhope. A 12 oz. can of soda has about 10 teaspoons of sugars (roughly half fructose and half glucose). The 10-teaspoon dose was only about 7 percent of the men's calories.

  After just three weeks, waist-to-hip ratio rose slightly only in the men who got fructose (alone or in sucrose), but not glucose. (Measuring waist-to-hip ratio isn't as accurate as measuring visceral fat, but when your waist expands, it's often because visceral fat expands.)

"With three studies now, these data suggest that added sugars cause an increase in visceral fat," says Stanhope.

Where's The Fat?

The fructose in most added sugars appears to boost liver, muscle, and visceral fat. Excess fat anywhere in the body increases the risk of insulin resistance and diabetes. But a fatty liver and visceral fat may increase your risk the most.

And links between visceral fat and sugary foods or drinks are now showing up elsewhere. When University of Minnesota researchers studied nearly 800 men and women, those who drank the most sugar-sweetened beverages had more visceral fat and larger waists.[12]

"We observed greater overall abdominal fat with increasing sugar-sweetened beverage consumption, and the increase in visceral fat was driving it," says Andrew Odegaard, a research associate at the University of Minnesota School of Public Health.

And among roughly 560 teenagers, those who consumed the most fructose (from beverages and food) had the most visceral fat, as well as the most insulin resistance, higher blood pressure, and higher blood sugar levels.[13]

"We took into account a lot of variables that could make this relationship spurious—fiber, calorie intake, fat and lean mass, socioeconomic status, physical activity," says author Norman Pollock, an assistant professor of pediatrics at the Georgia Health Sciences University in Augusta. "But the relationship with visceral fat was still there."

It's not as though added sugars are the only cause of a ballooning belly. Most of our expanding waistlines is due to eating too many calories, period.

But each notch on that belt could have serious consequences for your health.

"From what we understand, visceral fat may be what really drives insulin resistance and cardiometabolic disorders like type 2 diabetes and heart disease," says Odegaard.

Diabetes & Heart Disease

The link between diabetes and sugars is clearest when researchers look at sugary drinks.

"We summarized the results from eight studies," explains Harvard's Vasanti Malik. All told, the meta-analysis pooled data on more than 300,000 people.[14] The results: "For each 12 oz. serving of a sugar-sweetened beverage you drink per day, you're getting about a 15 percent increased risk for diabetes," says Malik. "So it really doesn't take much to increase your risk."

"Fewer studies have looked at cardiovascular disease," she observes. "But we found an increased risk."

When Malik and colleagues tracked 88,000 nurses for 24 years, those who consumed at least two sugar-sweetened beverages a day had a 35 percent higher risk of heart attack than those who drank less than one a month.[15]

Sugar-sweetened-beverage drinkers also have a higher risk of the metabolic syndrome, which can lead to type 2 diabetes or heart disease.[14,16] (You have the metabolic syndrome if you have at least three of the following: elevated blood sugar, blood triglycerides, blood pressure, or waist circumference, or low HDL cholesterol.)

"In our meta-analysis, people who drank two or more sugar-sweetened beverages a day had about a 20 percent increased risk of the metabolic syndrome compared to those who drank none or less than one per month," says Malik.

And it's not just that can of Coke. In 2010, researchers at Emory University reported that among a nationally representative sample of more than 6,000 adults, those who got more sugars from drinks and foods had lower HDL ("good") cholesterol and higher triglyceride levels in their blood.[17]

"Elevated triglycerides, together with elevated LDL ("bad") cholesterol, contributes to changes in our blood vessels that increase the risk of heart disease," explains Emory's Jean Welsh.

"The job of HDL is to carry away the triglycerides and the bad cholesterol so that they don't cause damage."

But none of those studies can prove cause-and-effect. "To find out if fructose is causing adverse effects, you have to give people fructose or glucose drinks for months," says Pollock.

That's just what the latest studies did.

Look to the Liver

In the Danish study, the people who drank a liter a day of sucrose-sweetened cola didn't just have more visceral fat. Their liver and muscle fat more than doubled.[9]

Sugar vs. Sugar

"No High Fructose LOW Corn Syrup," says the Kashi GoLean label.

Is high-fructose corn syrup worse than table sugar (sucrose), even though both are roughly half fructose and half glucose?

"Added sugars—whether they come from sucrose, high-fructose corn syrup, or fruit juice concentrates—all have equal adverse effects metabolically," says Harvard University's Vasanti Malik. "This obsession with high-fructose corn syrup is a little misguided."

In January, researchers at the University of Florida reported that people who were given 24 ounces of Dr Pepper sweetened with high-fructose corn syrup had higher blood sugar levels over the next six hours than those who got sucrose-sweetened Dr Pepper.[1] But other short-term studies have found no difference.[2]

"If you're getting a lot of fructose, it doesn't matter where it's coming from," says the Georgia Health Sciences University's Norman Pollock. "Even 100 percent fruit juice could be bad if you're consuming large quantities."

In fact, in some studies, people who drank more fruit juice had a greater risk of type 2 diabetes or weight gain.[3,4]

"The sugars in juices are natural, but it's still a large amount of sugar," explains Malik. "We saw an increased risk of diabetes with juices but not whole fruit, which suggests that the fiber in fruit—which isn't in the juice—might ameliorate the risk of diabetes."

Her advice: "Drink water, tea, or coffee, keeping the sweeteners and creamers minimal in the coffees and teas. If you want a little flavor, try sparkling waters with a twist of lime or orange. You can cut a little lime or lemon rind or orange peel and add them yourself."

[1] *Metabolism (2011),* DOI:I 10.1016/j.metabol.2011.09.013.
[2] *Am. J. Clin. Nutr 87:* 1194, 2008.
[3] *Diabetes Care 31:* 1311, 2008.
[4] *JAMA 292:* 927, 2004.

Sweet Somethings

Here's how much added sugars you'd get in a sampling of popular foods. (The numbers don't include the naturally occurring sugars in fruit or milk ingredients.)

Most women should get no more than 100 calories (6½ teaspoons) a day from added sugars. Most men should get no more than 150 calories (9½ teaspoons). To convert teaspoons to grams of sugar, multiply by 4. To convert teaspoons to calories from sugar, multiply by 16.

Sweets *(1 cookie, piece of cake, etc., unless noted)*	**Calories**	**Added Sugar *(tsp.)***
Kashi TLC Oatmeal Dark Chocolate Cookies *(1 oz.)*	130	2
Pepperidge Farm Nantucket Dark Chocolate Soft Baked Cookies *(1.1 oz.)*	140	2.5
Krispy Kreme Original Glazed Doughnut *(1.7 oz.)*	190	2.5
Nabisco Chips Ahoy! Original *(3 cookies, 1.2 oz.)*	160	3
Pepperidge Farm Milano Cookies *(3 cookies, 1.2 oz.)*	180	3
Nabisco Oreo *(3 cookies, 1.2 oz.)*	160	3.5
Newman's Own Organics Original Newman-O's *(3 cookies, 1.3 oz.)*	170	3.5
Entenmann's Ultimate Crumb Cake *(1/10 cake, 2 oz.)*	250	4
Entenmann's Rich Frosted Donut *(2.1 oz.)*	300	4.5
Sara Lee All Butter Pound Cake *(¼ cake, 2.7 oz.)*	300	5
Pepperidge Farm Golden 3-Layer Cake *(1/8 cake, 2.5 oz.)*	230	6.5
Krispy Kreme Glazed Chocolate Cake Doughnut *(2.8 oz.)*	300	6.5
Au Bon Pain Chocolate Mocha Whoopie Pie *(3 oz.)*	330	6.5
Marie Calender's Southern Pecan Pie *(1/8 pie, 4 oz.)*	490	6.5
Marie Calender's Lemon Meringue Pie *(1/9 pie, 4.3 oz.)*	320	8.5
Starbucks Marble Pound Cake *(3.8 oz.)*	350	8.5
Panera Chocolate Chipper cookie *(3.3 oz.)*	440	8.5
Entenmann's Cinnamon Danish *(4 oz.)*	460	8.5
Starbucks Cinnamon Chip Scone *(4.2 oz.)*	480	8.5
Entenmann's Jumbo Iced Honey Bun *(5 oz.)*	660	8.5
Au Bon Pain Red Velvet Cupcake *(3.1 oz.)*	400	9
Starbucks Reduced-Fat Cinnamon Swirl Coffee Cake *(4 oz.)*	340	10
Au Bon Pain Hazelnut Mocha Brownie *(4 oz.)*	450	10.5
Dunkin' Donuts Chocolate Chip Muffin	610	14
Panera Chocolate Fudge Brownie with icing *(4.3 oz.)*	470	14.5
Cinnabon Classic Roll	880	15
Cinnabon Caramel Pecanbon	1,080	19
IHOP CINN-A-STACK Pancakes *(4)* with Old Fashioned Syrup *(¼ cup)*	1,110	23.5
The Cheesecake Factory Black-Out Cake	1,330	38
Candy, Chocolate, etc. *(1 bar, box, etc., unless noted)*		
Lindt Excellence 70 percent Cocoa Smooth Dark *(4 squares, 1.4 oz.)*	250	3
Planters Sweet 'N Crunchy Peanuts *(1 oz.)*	140	3.5
Dove Dark Chocolate Silky Smooth Promises *(5 pieces, 1.4 oz.)*	210	5
Hershey's Milk Chocolate Kisses *(9 pieces, 1.4 oz.)*	200	6
Hershey's Milk Chocolate bar *(1.5 oz.)*	210	6
Ghirardelli Chocolate Dark & Mint Squares *(3 squares, 1.6 oz.)*	210	6.5
M&M's Milk Chocolate *(1.7 oz.)*	230	8
Junior Mints, theater size *(4 oz.)*	480	22.5
Cereals		
Quaker Lower Sugar Maple & Brown Sugar Instant Oatmeal *(1 pkt., 1.2 oz.)*	120	1
Kellogg's Original All-Bran *(½ cup, 1.1 oz.)*	80	1.5

	Calories	Added Sugar *(tsp.)*
Post Honey Roasted Honey Bunches of Oats *(¾ cup, 1 oz.)*	120	1.5
General Mills Honey Nut Cheerios *(¾ cup, 1 oz.)*	110	2.5
Kellogg's Vanilla Almond Special K *(¾ cup, 1 oz.)*	110	2.5
Quaker Maple & Brown Sugar Instant Oatmeal *(1 pkt, 1.5 oz.)*	160	2.5
Kellogg's Raisin Bran *(1 cup, 2.1 oz.)*	190	2.5
Bear Naked Maple Pecan Granola *(½ cup, 2.2 oz.)*	260	2.5
Kellogg's Frosted Mini-Wheats Bite Size *(21 biscuits, 1.9 oz.)*	190	3
Kashi GoLean Crunch! *(1 cup, 1.9 oz.)*	190	3.5
Post Just Bunches! Honey Roasted Honey Bunches of Oats *(2/3 cup, 2 oz.)*	250	3.5
Cereal & Granola Bars *(1 bar)*		
Kashi TLC Honey Almond Flax Chewy Granola Bar *(1.2 oz.)*	140	1.5
Fiber One Oats & Chocolate Chewy Bar *(1.4 oz.)*	140	2.5
Nature Valley Vanilla Chewy Yogurt Bar *(1.2 oz.)*	140	3.5
Quaker Dark Chocolatey Chewy Dipps Granola Bar *(1.1 oz.)*	140	3.5
Kellogg's Special K Chocolate Caramel Protein Meal Bar *(1.6 oz.)*	170	4
Kashi GoLean Chocolate Malted Crisp Bar *(1.9 oz.)*	190	4.5
Clif Bar Maple Nut *(2.4 oz.)*	250	5.5
Beverages		
Silk Vanilla Soymilk, refrigerated *(8 fl. oz.)*	100	2
Starbucks Caramel Macchiato *(grande, 16 fl. oz.)*	240	4*
Starbucks Vanilla Latte *(grande, 16 fl. oz.)*	250	4*
Silk Chocolate Soymilk, refrigerated *(8 fl. oz.)*	140	5
Starbucks Tazo Black Shaken Iced Tea *(grande, 16 fl. oz.)*	80	5.5
Ocean Spray Cranberry Juice Cocktail *(8 fl. oz.)*	120	5.5*
Schweppes Tonic Water *(12 fl. oz.)*	130	8
Gatorade Perform Lemon-Lime *(20 fl. oz.)*	130	9
Starbucks White Chocolate Mocha *(grande, 16 fl. oz.)*	470	9*
Coca-Cola *(12 fl. oz.)*	140	10
AriZona Extra Sweet Green Tea *(23.5 fl. oz.)*	260	17
McDonald's Sweet Tea *(large, 32 fl. oz.)*	280	17.5
Starbucks Java Chip Frappuccino *(venti, 24 fl. oz.)*	560	18.5*
Dairy		
Häagen-Dazs Chocolate Ice Cream *(3.7 oz.)*	260	3*
Dannon All Natural Vanilla Yogurt *(6 oz.)*	150	4*
Häagen-Dazs Zesty Lemon Sorbet *(4 oz.)*	120	7
Cold Stone Creamery Sweet Cream Ice Cream *(Love it, 8 oz.)*	530	8.5*
TCBY Golden Vanilla Yogurt *(large, 13.4 fl. oz.)*	400	9.5*
Pinkberry Original Frozen Yogurt *(large, 13 oz.)*	370	14.5*
Cold Stone Creamery Very Vanilla Shake *(Gotta Have It, 24 fl. oz.)*	1,550	32.5*
Other		
Wholesome Sweeteners Organic Raw Blue Agave *(1 Tbs.)*	60	4
Honey *(1 Tbs.)*	60	4.5
Betty Crocker Rich & Creamy Chocolate Frosting *(2 Tbs.)*	130	4.5
Nutella *(2 Tbs.)*	200	5*

*Estimate. Note: added sugars are rounded to the nearest half teaspoon.
Source: Company information.

"That's a substantial increase," notes Stanhope. "We had suggested that consuming high amounts of fructose-containing sugars could lead to an increase in liver fat. This is the first well-controlled study to show it."

Why does liver fat matter? When the body stores fat anywhere but in fat cells, it's called "ectopic" fat. And ectopic fat, especially in the liver, means trouble.

"When liver fat levels go up, that may trigger the sequence of events that leads to insulin resistance," says Stanhope. That's when insulin loses its ability to admit blood sugar into cells. It's often the first step on the road to diabetes or heart disease.

The liver may also explain why fructose leads to higher levels of triglycerides.

"Fructose gets metabolized by the liver very quickly," says Welsh. "When there is more sugar than the liver can process, it converts the sugar to fat. Some of the fat goes into the bloodstream, and that's why we get elevated triglycerides."

What's more, in Stanhope's study, the fructose drinkers burned less fat (and more carbohydrate).[18] "The body doesn't make fat and burn fat at the same time," she explains.

"In our study, fat oxidation got blocked every time people drank the fructose drink because that fructose is getting turned into fat."

Also troubling: "We saw an increase in small, dense LDL when people drank fructose," says Stanhope. Those are cholesterol-carrying particles that are more damaging to arteries than fluffy, large LDL.

And Stanhope noticed something else. "LDL increased as much in the high-fructose corn syrup group as in the pure fructose group. That was surprising because the high-fructose corn syrup group got less fructose."[19]

"Do fructose and glucose together exacerbate the problems?" she asks. "We can't say at this point. But it's possible that because fructose is activating the pathways by which sugar gets turned into fat, more of the glucose is getting turned into fat, too."

As if that weren't enough, fructose may also lead to gout, a painful inflammation due to a buildup of uric acid in joints.

"Fructose has been shown to increase uric acid," says Malik. "And gout has also been associated with sugar-sweetened beverages."[20]

The problem isn't just that fructose boosts several risk factors for diabetes and cardiovascular disease.

"It's that those risk factors—abdominal obesity, high triglycerides, and insulin resistance—all exacerbate each other," says Stanhope. "You get a vicious circle going."

A case in point: "Some researchers argue that if you increase visceral fat, it sends out more inflammatory factors, which go back to the liver, where they promote more insulin resistance," she explains.

Another example: "Fructose-containing sugars increase fat-making in the liver, which causes insulin resistance," says Stanhope. "But insulin resistance also increases fat-making in the liver, so all the processes get revved up."

Healthier? A slice of Starbucks Reduced-Fat Cinnamon Swirl Coffee Cake has 10 teaspoons of added sugars.

"That's why the metabolic syndrome is so difficult to treat with one medication," she adds. "Everything is feeding on everything else."

Empty Calories

How much is too much added sugar? In 2009, the American Heart Association suggested a limit: no more than 100 calories a day for women and no more than 150 calories a day for men.[21]

The heart association wasn't just concerned about "the worldwide pandemic of obesity and cardiovascular disease," but also about the healthy foods that added sugar replaces.

"To follow recommendations to lower the risk of heart disease, diabetes, osteoporosis, hypertension, you name it, you have to use most of your calories for fruits, vegetables, grains, milk, meat, fish, poultry, and oils," explains Susan Krebs-Smith of the National Cancer Institute. "Very few calories are left over for empty calories."

In her recent analysis of a nationally representative survey of more than 16,000 people, roughly 78 percent of women and 67 percent of men ate too much added sugar.[22]

"For example, for someone who eats 2,000 calories a day, 'too much' was more than 130 calories' worth of added sugar," she says.

Not surprisingly, more than 90 percent of the people also came up short on green and orange vegetables, beans, dairy, and whole grains. "Most calories need to count for something nutritionally," adds Krebs-Smith.

But growing evidence suggests that added sugars aren't just empty calories. They're harmful calories.

"We saw huge metabolic differences between people who consumed fructose instead of glucose, despite the same weight gain," says Stanhope.

"Many people believe that excess calories are the problem, and it doesn't matter where they come from. But now we know that that's not true."

The Bottom Line

- Shoot for 100 calories (6½ teaspoons) a day of added sugars if you're a woman and 150 calories (9½ teaspoons) a day if you're a man. Even less may be better for your heart. (See "What Should I Eat?" Oct. 2009, p. 1.)
- Don't drink sugar-sweetened beverages. Limit fruit juices to no more than 1 cup a day.
- Limit all added sugars, including high-fructose corn syrup, cane or beet sugar, evaporated cane juice, brown rice syrup, agave syrup, and honey.
- Don't worry about the naturally occurring sugar in fruit, milk, and plain yogurt.
- If a food has little or no milk or fruit (which contain natural sugars), the "Sugars" number on the package's Nutrition Facts panel will tell you how many grams of added sugars are in each serving. Multiply the grams by 4 to get calories from sugar. Divide the grams by 4 to get teaspoons of sugar.

Notes

1. *JAMA 292:* 927, 2004.
2. *Am. J. Clin. Nutn 87:* 1662, 2008.
3. *Am. J. Clin. Nutr. 89:* 438, 2009.
4. *Int. J. Obes. 24:* 794, 2000.
5. *Am. J. Clin. Nutn 51:* 963, 1990.
6. *Am. J. Clin. Nutr. 76:* 721, 2002.
7. *Br. J. Nutr. 97:* 193, 2002.
8. *J. Clin. Invest. 119:* 1322, 2009.
9. *Am. J. Clin. Nutr 95:* 283, 2012.
10. cdc.gov/nchs/data/databriefs/db71.htm.
11. *Am. J. Clin. Nutr. 94:* 479, 2011.
12. *Obesity 20:* 689, 2011.
13. *J. Nutr. 142:* 251,2012.
14. *Diabetes Care 33:* 2477, 2010.
15. *Am. J. Clin. Nutn 89:* 1037, 2009.
16. *Circulation 116:* 480, 2007.
17. *JAMA 303:* 1490, 2010.
18. *Eur. J. Clin. Nutr. 66:* 201,2012.
19. *J. Clin. Endocrinol. Metab. 96:* E1596, 2011.
20. *BMJ 336:* 309, 2008.
21. *Circulation 120:* 1011, 2009.
22. *J. Nutr. 140:* 1832, 2010.

Critical Thinking

1. Describe the conclusions from the research studies conducted in Denmark and Switzerland on the effect of soda on visceral fat.
2. Identify the organs that are impacted by the increased fat accumulation linked to drinking soda.
3. Explain why drinking soda leads to higher levels of fat in the blood and stored in the body.

Create Central

www.mhhe.com/createcentral

Internet References

Center for Science in the Public Interest
www.cspinet.org/about/index.html

Sugar Love: A Not So Sweet Story
http://ngm.nationalgeographic.com/2013/08/sugar/cohen-text

Article

Prepared by: Janet Colson, *Middle Tennessee State University*

A Diabetes Cliffhanger

Researchers are baffled by the worldwide increase in type 1 diabetes, the less common form of the disease.

Maryn McKenna

Learning Outcomes

After reading this article, you will be able to:

- Differentiate between type 1 and type 2 diabetes.
- Explain why the rise in the prevalence of type 1 diabetes has many scientists baffled.

When public health officials fret about the soaring incidence of diabetes in the U.S. and worldwide, they are generally referring to type 2 diabetes. About 90 percent of the nearly 350 million people around the world who have diabetes suffer from the type 2 form of the illness, which mostly starts causing problems in the 40s and 50s and is tied to the stress that extra pounds place on the body's ability to regulate blood glucose. About 25 million people in the U.S. have type 2 diabetes, and another million have type 1 diabetes, which typically strikes in childhood and can be controlled only with daily doses of insulin.

For reasons that are completely mysterious, however, the incidence of type 1 diabetes has been increasing throughout the globe at rates that range from 3 to 5 percent a year. Although the second trend is less well publicized, it is still deeply troubling, because this form of the illness has the potential to disable or kill people so much earlier in their lives.

No one knows exactly why type 1 diabetes is rising. Solving that mystery—and, if possible, reducing or reversing the trend—has become an urgent problem for public health researchers everywhere. So far they feel they have only one solid clue.

"Increases such as the ones that have been reported cannot be explained by a change in genes in such a short period," says Giuseppina Imperatore, who leads a team of epidemiologists in the Division of Diabetes Translation at the U.S. Centers for Disease Control and Prevention. "So environmental factors are probably major players in this increase."

A Challenge of Counting

Type 1 and type 2 diabetes share the same underlying defect—an inability to deploy insulin in a manner that keeps blood sugar from rising too high—but they arise out of almost opposite processes. Type 1, which once was known as juvenile diabetes, is an autoimmune disease in which the body attacks its own cells—namely, the beta cells of the pancreas—destroying their ability to make insulin. In type 2, formerly known as adult-onset diabetes, tissues that need insulin to take up glucose (such as the liver, muscles and fat) become resistant to insulin's presence. The insulin-producing cells respond by going into overdrive, first making more of the hormone than normal and then losing the ability to keep up with the excess glucose in the blood. Some people end up unable to make insulin at all.

The first strong signal that the incidence of type 1 diabetes was on the rise came in 2006, from a World Health Organization project known as DIAMOND (a combination of words in several languages for worldwide diabetes). That survey, which looked at 10 years of records from 112 diabetes research centers in 57 countries, found that type 1 had risen an average of 5.3 percent a year in North America, 4 percent in Asia and 3.2 percent in Europe.

Statistics from Europe—where the single-payer health care systems that care for residents throughout their lives generate rich stores of data—back up that first finding. In 2009 researchers from a second project called EURODIAB compared diabetes incidence across 17 countries and found not only that type 1 was rising—by 3.9 percent a year on average—but also that it was increasing most quickly among children younger than five. By 2020, they predicted, new cases of type 1 diabetes in that age group will nearly double, from 3,600 children to an estimated 7,076 children.

Most assessments of diabetes in the U.S. have been more partial and local. There is one comprehensive national surveillance project, the federally funded SEARCH for Diabetes in Youth study, which published data in 2007. Because that was an initial report, however, researchers could not compare it with earlier years. Still, when looked at against the findings of other studies, it suggests a rising tide. For example, the 2007 study found higher rates of type 1 in the U.S. than did the WHO's worldwide study of the year before. In addition, the SEARCH study results were sharply higher than regional studies from the 1990s in Alabama, Colorado and Pennsylvania.

Annual Percent Change in Type 1 Diabetes Incidence by Region and Age Group (1990–1999)

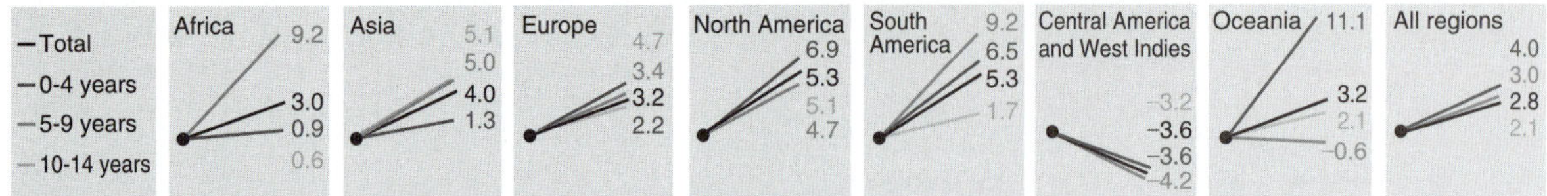

Global mystery: Although some regions (Africa, Asia) are starting from a lower base than others (North America, Europe), the incidence of type 1 diabetes is growing everywhere except the West Indies (where the decline can be traced to one country—Cuba).

Competing Hypotheses

The challenge for explaining the rising trend in type 1 diabetes is that if the increases are occurring worldwide, the causes must also be. So investigators have had to look for influences that stretch globally and consider the possibility that different factors may be more important in some regions than in others.

The list of possible culprits is long. Researchers have, for example, suggested that gluten, the protein in wheat, may play a role because type 1 patients seem to be at higher risk for celiac disease and the amount of gluten most people consume (in highly processed foods) has grown over the decades. Scientists have also inquired into how soon infants are fed root vegetables. Stored tubers can be contaminated with microscopic fungi that seem to promote the development of diabetes in mice.

None of those lines of research, though, have returned results that are solid enough to motivate other scientists to stake their careers on studying them. So far, in fact, the search for a culprit resembles the next-to-last scene in an Agatha Christie mystery—the one in which the detective explains which of the many suspects could not possibly have committed the crime.

The last scene in the drama, unfortunately, still has not been written. Currently the suspects getting the closest scrutiny are infections with bacteria, viruses or parasites. The presumptive etiology: a version of the "hygiene hypothesis" that links clean modern lifestyles and allergies.

The hygiene hypothesis proposes that early exposure to infections or soil organisms teaches the developing immune system how to maintain itself in balance and so keeps it from reacting in an uncontrolled way later in life when it encounters allergens such as dust and ragweed. Living hygienically, it goes on to say, has deprived children of those early exposures, fueling an epidemic of allergies. The diabetes version of the hygiene hypothesis proposes that when the immune system learns not to overreact to allergens, it also learns to tolerate compounds from the body's own tissues—and therefore prevents the autoimmune attack that destroys the ability to make insulin.

Some circumstantial evidence supports that proposal. Children with multiple siblings—who might bring infections home from day care or school—are less likely to be hospitalized for type 1 diabetes (a proxy measure for incidence). The disease is also less common in children who attend day care themselves, and it is more common in specially bred mice that do not encounter infections because they are raised in a sterile environment.

By themselves, however, those findings do not make the case. Christopher Cardwell, a lecturer in medical statistics at Queen's University Belfast, has conducted meta-analyses of associations between type 1 and birth order, maternal age at birth, and birth by cesarean section, all of which affect the organisms to which young children are exposed. "All of these seemed to be associated," he says, "but they all were in my opinion fairly weak associations. None were of a magnitude that could explain the increasing incidence over time."

Back to Fat

Recently the search for a cause behind the rise of type 1 diabetes has taken an unexpected turn. Some investigators are reconsidering the role of an old adversary: being overweight or obese.

That suspicion might seem counterintuitive given that diabetes dogma holds that being overweight tugs the body toward producing large amounts of insulin (as in type 2), not too little insulin. But some contend that the stress of producing all that extra insulin can burn out the insulin-producing beta cells of the pancreas and push a child whose beta cells are already under attack into developing type 1 diabetes. This idea, called the accelerator or overload hypothesis, proposes that "if you have a kid who is chubby, that extra adiposity is going to challenge the pancreatic beta cells," says Rebecca Lipton, an emeritus professor at the University of Chicago. "In a child who has already started the autoimmune process, those beta cells are just going to fail more quickly, because they are being forced to put out more insulin than in a thin child."

Overweight makes a logical perpetrator. People are packing on the pounds in rich countries and poor ones. Of course, investigators want to do more than just to explain the rise of type 1 diabetes; they want to prevent it. Unfortunately, if excess weight is a major contributor to the problem, that task will not be easy. No one, so far, has been able to slow the global obesity epidemic. (By 2048, according to researchers from Johns Hopkins University, all American adults will be at least overweight if present trends continue.) Until societies can ensure that most children (not to mention adults) are more physically active, eat healthfully and maintain a normal weight, diabetes researchers will be in the position of detectives who, having solved a murder, realize they can do nothing to prevent the next one.

Critical Thinking

1. Differentiate the physiological differences between type 1 and type 2 diabetes.
2. Contrast the competing hypotheses that attempt to explain the rise in type 1 diabetes: the hygiene hypothesis and the overload hypothesis.
3. Explain why type 1 is considered an autoimmune disease.

Create Central

www.mhhe.com/createcentral

Internet References

American Diabetes Association
www.diabetes.org

Diabetes Interactive Atlas—Centers for Disease Control and Prevention
www.cdc.gov/diabetes/atlas

Diabetes Programme—TheWorld Health Organization 2013
www.who.int/diabetes/en

The Global Burden. International Diabetes Federation
www.idf.org/diabetesatlas/5e/the-global-burden

Maryn McKenna is a journalist, a blogger and author of two books about public health. She writes about infectious diseases, global health and food policy.

Source: "Incidence and Trends of Childhood Type 1 Diabetes Worldwide 1990–1999," by Diamond Project Group, *In Diabetic Medicine,* Vol. 23, No. 8: August 2006

Article

Prepared by: Janet Colson, *Middle Tennessee State University*

Be Kind to Your Kidneys

GARY CURHAN

Learning Outcomes

After reading this article, you will be able to:

- Outline the functions of the kidneys.
- Describe lifestyle factors that increase the risk of developing chronic kidney disease.
- Explain what causes kidney stone formation.

An estimated one out of five adults in their 60s—and nearly half of those 70 or older—have chronic kidney disease. Many of them don't know it. Your risk is greater if you have diabetes or high blood pressure, though obesity and smoking also play a role.

While most cases never progress to kidney failure, the condition raises the risk of heart attack, stroke, osteoporosis, and anemia.

And kidney stones, which can cause excruciating pain, may also raise the risk of kidney and heart disease. Yet many doctors may not know that kidney stones can be prevented.

Here's how to protect your kidneys.

Chronic Kidney Disease

Q: ***Is chronic kidney disease an under-recognized public health problem?***

A: Absolutely. It's much more common than people had appreciated. That's partly because the population is aging. We know that there is some naturally occurring decline in kidney function with age.

But that doesn't mean that chronic kidney disease is an inevitable part of normal aging. Recent reports from the Nurses' Health Study found that in many healthy people, kidney function didn't change meaningfully over 5–10 years.

Q: ***So it's not just aging, but that people are more likely to have risk factors for kidney disease as they age?***

A: Yes. Two common conditions—high blood pressure and diabetes—increase the risk of developing kidney disease, and people are more likely to get both if they gain weight and as they age.

Some studies estimate that 10 percent of U.S. adults have chronic kidney disease, but it may occur in up to 40 percent of people with diabetes and 18 percent of people with prediabetes. And some studies find reduced kidney function in 28 percent of people with hypertension and 17 percent of those with prehypertension.

Q: ***Those numbers are striking.***

A: Yes, though if you were recently diagnosed with hypertension or diabetes, you are not going to have kidney disease right away. It takes years, sometimes decades, for the disease to show up, and treating somebody for those conditions can make kidney disease much less likely.

Q: ***Why is kidney disease harmful?***

A: Chronic kidney disease can lead to end-stage kidney disease. Your kidneys stop working, and you need either dialysis or a kidney transplant to survive.

Kidneys are important for maintaining optimal health. For example, as your kidney function deteriorates, you're at increased risk for fractures and anemia.

But kidney disease is also a risk factor for heart attack and stroke. In fact, that's what most people with kidney disease die of. And people with kidney disease are also more likely to develop hypertension.

Q: ***Kidney disease causes hypertension and hypertension causes kidney disease?***

A: Yes, it works both ways. If there is some damage to the kidney, you're much more likely to develop high blood pressure. And high blood pressure can harm the kidney.

Q: ***How?***

A: High blood pressure damages the small blood vessels of the kidney, which then damages the glomerulus—the basic filtering unit of the kidney. Each kidney can have up to a million glomeruli.

Kidneys filter about 200 quarts of blood a day. So they are filled with blood vessels, and anything that impairs the blood flow through the kidney reduces the kidney's ability to clean the blood.

Q: ***Do the kidneys keep blood pressure from getting too low?***

A: Yes. If blood pressure starts to drop, the kidneys will try to raise it. In the short term, raising blood pressure is a good thing, because if it's too low, oxygen can't reach the brain. But in the long term, high pressure can damage the kidney's blood vessels.

Q: ***Does diabetes harm the kidneys in the same way?***

A: Not exactly. Diabetes damages not only the small blood vessels in the glomerulus, but also something called the mesangium, which helps support the glomerulus.

What a Kidney Does

Water.

Ensures that there's not too much or too little water in the body.

Blood Pressure.

Makes sure that pressure isn't too high or too low.

Wastes.

Gets rid of urea, uric acid, toxins, and other wastes via urine.

Bones.

Activates vitamin D, which helps the body absorb calcium.

Acid-Base Balance.

Makes sure that the body isn't too acidic or too alkaline.

Heart.

Maintains a balance of electrolytes (like potassium, sodium, and calcium), which is critical for heart rhythm.

Blood.

Releases erythropoietin, which tells bone marrow to make red blood cells.

Q: ***How does kidney disease cause heart attacks and strokes?***

A: It's not completely known. It is likely due in part to higher blood pressure, since even small increases in blood pressure can have a dramatic impact on the risk of cardiovascular disease.

But there are other possibilities. One hypothesis is that with reduced kidney function there is an alteration in calcium and phosphorus metabolism, causing calcium deposits in blood vessels or in the heart muscle itself. And the calcification may lead to heart attacks, strokes, or heart failure.

Q: ***Do kidneys do more than clean blood and control blood pressure?***

A: Yes. Kidneys maintain the internal environment. If you drank a lot of water and your kidneys didn't remove it from the blood, you would basically drown in fluid. And it's the kidneys' job to get rid of almost anything that you ingest that gets absorbed into the bloodstream and that the body doesn't need—say, extra salt, calcium, or phosphorus. Maintaining that balance is critical.

Q: ***How do kidneys protect against anemia and bone fractures?***

A: The kidney produces a hormone—erythropoietin—that leads to the production of red blood cells. And the kidney has an enzyme that activates vitamin D.

When you consume vitamin D or it's made in the skin, it goes to the liver and then to the kidney, where it becomes the active form. The active form is important for absorbing calcium in the intestines, which helps to maintain bone health.

Q: ***Why is obesity bad for kidneys?***

A: Obesity raises blood pressure and the risk of diabetes. Also, as people gain weight, the kidneys have to work harder.

You can imagine that the amount of waste products that need to get removed is far greater for a 250-pound person than for a 150-pound person, especially after we eat a large meal.

So the kidney has to adapt. As people gain weight, the kidney can't make more glomeruli, so the existing ones may start to enlarge and the kidney may start to filter blood at a greater rate, which puts an additional demand on the kidney.

That may lead to damage and the eventual loss of some glomeruli. So the remaining glomeruli have to work that much harder, which leads to more lost glomeruli. It's a vicious cycle.

Q: ***Does excess salt harm kidneys?***

A: Yes. It can raise blood pressure, and it's possible that excess sodium itself may be harmful.

Q: ***Is too much protein harmful?***

A: I wouldn't want someone who already has kidney disease on a diet that's very high in animal protein. But there's still disagreement about whether high-protein diets raise the risk of developing kidney disease. In moderate amounts, it's probably not harmful.

I'd rather that people stop smoking, do more exercise, lose weight, and eat a healthy diet than worry only about how much protein they eat.

Q: ***What else can harm kidneys?***

A: A number of toxins in the environment—lead, mercury, cadmium.

Excessive, long-term use of over-the-counter analgesics like acetaminophen and ibuprofen can also increase the risk of chronic kidney disease, possibly by raising blood pressure and/or by damaging the kidney directly. Studies about aspirin have been inconsistent.

If you take those analgesics on a regular basis, ask your healthcare provider about alternatives. Just because these drugs are available over the counter doesn't mean they're safe.

Q: ***Is exercise good for kidneys?***

A: Exercise helps keep blood vessels healthy, lowers blood pressure, reduces the risk of diabetes, and helps people lose weight. So even without conclusive evidence, I would encourage people to be actiye to protect their kidneys.

Q: ***Does early kidney disease have symptoms?***

A: Most of the time there are none. It's like high blood pressure. The best way to get people diagnosed is by screening people at higher risk for developing kidney disease—those with diabetes or hypertension. We do a blood test for creatinine and check urine for protein. But there's not enough convincing data to demonstrate that we should screen everyone.

Q: ***Can we protect our kidneys?***

A: Yes. Many of the conditions that affect the kidney are preventable. The message is quite similar to what you would do to protect your heart. Lowering your cardiovascular risk goes a long way toward protecting your kidneys.

And kidneys are another reason for people to try to control their blood pressure and blood sugar if they have high levels. The best thing would be to avoid developing high blood pressure and diabetes in the first place.

Kidney Stones

Q: ***What are kidney stones?***

A: Urine is water with a bunch of waste products dissolved in it. As long as they stay dissolved, it's not a problem. But sometimes crystals form in the kidney and grow into a stone.

The lifetime risk of kidney stones in U.S. men is now about 20 percent. In women it's about 10 percent. The risk has increased substantially over time.

Q: ***Why?***

A: Obesity, a higher salt intake, higher sugar and high-fructose corn syrup intake, and maybe higher animal protein intake are associated with a greater risk of forming stones.

In contrast, a diet that's rich in calcium, potassium, fruits, and vegetables is protective. Also, the more you drink, the higher the urine volume and the less concentrated your urine is, so the lower your risk of a stone.

Q: ***More calcium is good?***

A: Yes. Even though the vast majority of stones are made of calcium oxalate, we found out 20 years ago that higher calcium intakes from food are associated with a lower risk. However, individuals who take calcium supplements seem to have a higher risk of stones.

Q: ***Why are supplements different?***

A: When you eat food, some of its calcium will stick to some of its oxalate, and that will keep the oxalate from getting absorbed into the blood and eventually getting into the urine. The calcium and oxalate form a crystal in the intestine and are excreted in the stool, so they don't hurt.

Calcium supplements probably would do the same thing as calcium from foods if people took the supplements with meals, but many people don't. So the calcium gets absorbed into the bloodstream.

If any excess calcium is absorbed, the kidneys remove it from the blood and excrete it in the urine. So you have more calcium in the urine and that would increase the calcium oxalate in the urine, which increases the risk of a stone.

Q: ***Where do we get oxalate?***

A: Oxalate comes from some foods we eat, and the body also produces oxalate. Spinach has a huge amount. We advise people who have formed calcium oxalate stones not to eat spinach.

The Minor Leaks

An estimated 30–40 percent of middle-aged and 50 percent of older women experience urinary leakage. (The problem is less common in men.) But it's a don't ask, don't tell issue.

"Even in our study of nurses, less than 50 percent of the women who had incontinence reported it to their doctors," says Mary Townsend, an epidemiologist at Brigham and Women's Hospital in Boston.

Leaks are more common in women who are older, heavier, or smokers, and in those who have had more children, diabetes, or a hysterectomy.[1]

Caffeine may also play a role.

"We found a moderate increased risk of developing at least weekly incontinence, but only in women who consumed at least 450 milligrams of caffeine a day," says Townsend.[2] (You'd get 420 mg in one Starbucks venti coffee and 520 mg in two tall coffees.)

"Caffeine was only related to urgency incontinence—leaks that occur with a sudden need to go to the bathroom—not with stress incontinence," she notes. That's a leak that typically occurs with coughing or exercise.

How might caffeine cause trouble?

It may be a diuretic. "And in animal studies, caffeine increases the force of muscle contractions in the bladder," says Townsend. "So the combination may lead to urgency."

Other leads have come up empty. "It's a common belief that acidic fruit and tomatoes are bladder irritants," says Townsend.[3] "But we didn't see any association with incontinence."

What may help? Training women to contract their pelvic-floor muscles—using Kegel exercises—makes a difference.[4] So does losing excess weight.[5]

And walking or other moderate exercise may lower the risk, especially of stress incontinence, says Townsend, "in part by maintaining a healthy weight and possibly also by strengthening the pelvic-floor muscles."

[1] *Am. J. Obstet. Gynecol. 194:* 339, 2006.
[2] *J. Urol. 185:* 1775, 2011.
[3] *Int. Urogynecol. J. 24:* 605, 2013.
[4] *Cochrane Database Syst. Rev.*: CD005654, 2010.
[5] *N. Engl. J. Med. 360:* 481, 2009.

Oxalate on Your Plate

Never had a calcium oxalate stone? Enjoy your spinach. If you *have* had one, try other leafy greens instead. And go easy on high-oxalate foods like these.

Food	**Oxalate** *(mg)*
Spinach (½ *cup, cooked*)	755
Spinach *(1 cup, raw)*	656
Rhubarb (½ *cup, cooked*)	541
Almonds *(1 oz., 23 nuts)*	122
Miso soup *(1 cup)*	111
Baked potato with skin *(1)*	97
Beets (½ *cup, cooked*)	76
Navy beans (½ *cup, cooked*)	76
Dates *(3)*	72
Okra (½ *cup, cooked*)	57
Post Wheat'n Bran Shredded Wheat Spoon Size (1¼ *cups*)	53
French fries (4 *oz.,* 1½ *cups*)	51
Cashews (1 *oz.,* 18 *nuts*)	49
Wheat berries (½ *cup, cooked*)	49
Kellogg's Raisin Bran *(1 cup)*	46
Post Original Shredded Wheat Spoon Size *(1 cup)*	45
Bulgur (½ *cup, cooked*)	43
Lentil soup *(1 cup)*	39
Chocolate syrup *(2 Tbs.)*	38
Snickers bar *(1 bar, 1.86 oz.)*	38
Post Bran Flakes (¾ *cup*)	36
Kellogg's All-Bran Complete Wheat Flakes (¾ *cup*)	34
Walnuts *(1 oz., 14 halves)*	31
Orange *(1)*	29
Kellogg's Original Frosted Mini-Wheats Bite Size *(1 cup)*	28
Peanuts *(1 oz., 32 nuts)*	27
Kellogg's All-Bran Original (½ *cup*)	26
Peanut butter *(2 Tbs.)*	26
Raspberries (½ *cup*)	24
Potato chips *(1 oz.)*	21
Kellogg's Müeslix (⅔ *cup*)	17
Tomato sauce (½ *cup*)	17
Red kidney beans (½ *cup, cooked*)	15
Pistachios *(1 oz., 49 nuts)*	14
Brown rice (½ *cup, cooked*)	12
Pecans *(1 oz., 19 halves)*	10

Adapted from Oxalate Content of Foods.xls (regepi.bwh.harvard.edu/health/Oxalate/files).

Potatoes are probably the least appreciated source of oxalate. They're important because Americans eat a lot of potatoes.

Wheat bran and some nuts are also high in oxalate, though the amount differs by type (see "Oxalate on Your Plate," p. 6). But nuts and bran have health benefits, so I tell my patients to eat them in moderation unless they have a very high urine oxalate.

Q: ***Are other greens high in oxalate?***

A: No. There is so much misinformation about the oxalate content of foods. People think, "Spinach is a leafy green so I shouldn't eat anything that is leafy or green." But that's not the case.

Q: ***Why does obesity lead to stones?***

A: People who are overweight or obese have a higher risk of forming uric acid stones. It's not clear why, but larger people generally produce more uric acid, and obesity makes urine more acidic, which is a major driver for forming uric acid stones.

Being overweight may also increase the risk of calcium oxalate stones, but the reason is not clear.

Q: ***What harm do stones cause?***

A: Passing a stone can cause excruciating pain. And in a recent study in Alberta, Canada, researchers found that people who had kidney stones were at higher risk for subsequently developing chronic kidney disease. It seems that in some individuals, crystals get deposited in the kidney and that leads to inflammation and some damage. But it's still very early in that story.

Q: ***Do people with stones have a higher risk of heart disease?***

A: Yes, but the reasons are still being explored. People who form stones and those who have heart attacks or strokes may share risk factors like differences in calcium metabolism. A significant portion of people with kidney stones have high urine calcium that we can't explain.

And whatever is causing that underlying abnormality may also put those people at higher risk for, say, calcification in the blood vessels. But stone disease itself may cause inflammation. Perhaps that's what increases the risk of heart disease.

Q: ***Can stones be prevented?***

A: Yes. That's important for patients and physicians to recognize. My practice is limited to people who have kidney stones. I see people who have had 20, 50, or even more stones, and nobody had ever told them that stones could be prevented.

They were told, "It just happens" or "It's in your genes." Genes do contribute to stone disease, but the vast majority of stones can be prevented.

Q: ***How?***

A: It depends on the type of stone. We ask patients to collect their urine for 24 hours to measure what's in there, and then we make recommendations.

For the most common type, calcium oxalate, avoiding spinach is beneficial. If people have too much calcium in their urine, eating less salt might help, because if your salt intake is very high, that can lead to high calcium in the urine. And eating more fruits and vegetables can help prevent calcium oxalate stones.

Q: ***And uric acid stones?***

A: I recommend eating less meat, poultry, and fish. They contain purines that are metabolized by the body into uric acid, which is then excreted in the urine. And those foods also result in the generation of acid. Acidic urine is a strong risk factor for uric acid stones.

Q: ***Are liquids critical?***

A: It's very important for anyone who's had any kind of stone to drink enough fluid to produce at least two liters of urine

The Bottom Line

To lower your risk of kidney disease:

- Lose (or don't gain) excess weight.
- Minimize sodium and sugar (sucrose and fructose).
- Fill half your plate with vegetables or fruit.
- Exercise for 30–60 minutes a day.
- If necessary, take medicine to lower your blood pressure and blood sugar.
- Eat a diet based on the OmniHeart and DASH studies (see *Nutrition Action,* October 2009, cover story). Some features of a 2,000-calorie diet:
  - *2 servings* of low-fat dairy (milk, yogurt, or cheese)
  - *2 servings* of beans, tofu, or nuts
  - *1 small serving* of fish, poultry, or lean meat.

If you've had a kidney stone, *also:*

- Drink *at least* 8 cups of water or other (not sugar-sweetened) beverages a day.
- If you take a calcium supplement, take it with food.
- Limit high-oxalate foods (see "Oxatate on Your Plate").

a day. Drinking eight cups of liquid a day may be enough, but many patients need more. And some people also need medication.

Q: ***Will any liquids do?***

A: Some are better than others. In general, the more you drink, the higher your urine volume, but sugar-sweetened beverages are actually associated with a higher risk of stones. People shouldn't drink them anyhow, because they're linked to a higher risk of weight gain and diabetes. I recommend fluids without calories.

Some of my patients have been told to avoid alcoholic beverages. While I don't prescribe them, they may help prevent stone formation. And people are often told, "Don't drink coffee or tea because they will dehydrate you." But both decaf and caffeinated coffee and tea are associated with a lower risk of stones.

Critical Thinking

1. Plan a weekly menu that will provide foods to reduce the risk of chronic kidney disease.
2. Gladys is 70 years old with a BMI of 35; she often has a spinach salad with a baked potato for lunch and grilled lean meat or poultry for dinner. To help prevent osteoporosis, she takes 1000 mg of calcium carbonate each day. What changes should Gladys make to her diet and lifestyle to reduce her risk of developing kidney stones?

Create Central

www.mhhe.com/createcentral

Internet References

American Kidney Fund
http://www.kidneyfund.org/

National Kidney Disease Education Program
http://nkdep.nih.gov/

National Kidney Foundation
www.kidney.org/kidneydisease

Gary Curhan is a nephrologist and a professor of medicine at Harvard Medical School and professor of epidemiology at the Harvard School of Public Health. His research has focused on the causes of kidney stones. Curhan is currently editor-in-chief of the *Clinical Journal of the American Society of Nephrology.* He spoke to *NAH*'s Bonnie Liebman by phone from Boston.

Article

Prepared by: Janet Colson, *Middle Tennessee State University*

How to Save Your Brain

It's most people's biggest health fear. But whether you get dementia, scientists now believe, is mostly a matter of lifestyle; it hinges on what you eat every single day. Here's a guide to making the choices that will preserve a healthy mind—starting right now!

NIKHIL SWAMINATHAN

Learning Outcomes

After reading this article, you will be able to:

- Explain the physiology of the mental decline that occurs in Alzheimer's disease.
- List the foods and lifestyle behaviors that may slow the progression of dementia.

When it comes to aging, life can be cruel. There's plenty to . . . well . . . let's come right out and say it: think about. What will happen to my looks? What will happen to my body? Will I still be able to pursue my interests? What will happen to my mind?

That last question is now the second leading health concern (after cancer) among adults in at least four Western countries—France, Germany, and Spain, as well as the United States—according to a recent survey by the Harvard University School of Public Health and the Alzheimer Europe consortium. Fear of developing dementia would likely stir even more concern if Americans didn't mistakenly believe a cure for Alzheimer's disease exists (more than 45 percent of U.S. respondents think there is an effective treatment). Despite the lack of a cure, great progress has been made in the past three decades in understanding the disease.

The most common cause of dementia, or severe cognitive decline, and the sixth leading cause of death in the U. S., Alzheimer's disease is marked by difficulty storing new memories and recalling recent events, loss of ability to track day-to-day information, a disrupted sense of time and space, social withdrawal, irritability, and mood swings. The neurodegenerative condition typically manifests after age 60. Life expectancy in the U.S. is currently about 78 years and rising. The 5.4 million Americans who suffer from the illness include 13 percent of those over age 65.

Scientists attribute the debilitating disorder to the gradual accumulation between brain cells of a toxic protein, beta-amyloid, that blocks the transmission of information from cell to cell, wipes out synapses, and disrupts basic neuron function, leading to cell death. Inflammatory processes are also involved in memory loss.

The vast majority of Alzheimer's cases—over 99 percent—occur spontaneously; they are not linked to genetic factors. But they are linked to obesity. Researchers find that the same lifestyle choices that lead people to become obese or develop heart disease also increase the risk of developing dementia.

It comes down to this: Choices we make throughout life about what we put in our bodies may protect against Alzheimer's, or delay its onset. At the very least, says neuroscientist Gary Wenk, "We can slow down the time that it takes for someone to get symptoms." Professor of psychology, neuroscience, and molecular virology, immunology, and medical genetics at The Ohio State University, Wenk is author of the book *Your Brain on Food.*

Heading off dementia, he insists, starts with what we eat. Food should be thought of the same way as the drugs we put in our body. They're all made up of chemicals. Everything we consume prompts a reaction in the brain. Picking the right foods can minimize damage to neurons and preserve a healthy mind as you age.

Public Enemy Number One

It's oxygen—you know, the molecule without which you can't live. We have a complex relationship with the element: We desperately need it to breathe, and it is absolutely essential for metabolism, that is, converting the food we eat into energy. However, it causes us to age.

Proteins, fats, and carbohydrates are made up of chains of carbon atoms bonded together in a variety of ways. The body is built to break down the chains into the basic sugar glucose, which actually fuels our cells. Left over are carbon bonds that are cleared out by every breath we take—inhale oxygen, which binds with carbon to escort it out the body, exhale carbon dioxide. Biology 101.

Unfortunately, rogue, unbound oxygen molecules—free radicals—that invariably form during energy metabolism are toxic to body cells, essentially causing them to rust over time.

Normally, the hemoglobin molecule in blood regulates oxygen levels throughout the body so that cells are not overexposed to it. Aging also weakens our natural defenses against free radicals, putting all our cells (including neurons) at risk.

Antioxidant molecules are abundant in nature; plants maintain elaborate systems of them, and they are found notably in colorful fruits and vegetables (compounds like vitamins A, C, and E, beta carotene, and capsaicin, the spice in chili peppers). A diet rich in antioxidants combats the oxidative stress we are constantly under.

In the brain, antioxidants slow neurodegeneration. "The chemicals that give fruits their color are exactly what we want to protect us from oxygen," says Wenk. In fact, by eating foods rich in antioxidants, we're taking advantage of the way another life-form has devised to defend itself against environmental harm. From their own sources of proteins and carbohydrates, plant cells synthesize the chemicals we recognize as antioxidants as shields against bacteria, viruses, and the oxidative stress resulting from exposure to ultraviolet light or the toxin ozone.

"EVERY DAY, YOUR BRAIN (AND BODY) AGES A LITTLE BIT, AND EVERYDAY THERE'S AN OPPORTUNITY TO HELP IT NOT TO."

Because of the basic similarities of evolved life processes, the plant protectors can also help human cells from showing the wear and tear of existence. Blueberries, broccoli, grapes, prunes, strawberries, spinach, artichokes, apples—all contain large amounts of antioxidants, as do herbs and spices like rosemary, turmeric, thyme, and oregano. Bright, yellow-orange turmeric is a classic ingredient in the curries that are a staple of Indian cooking. Please note: The incidence of Alzheimer's disease in India is one-sixth that of the U.S.

Adding antioxidant-rich foods to your diet is a fine hedge against dementia. But you need to add more than one. There are thousands of antioxidants—scientists haven't even come close to discovering them all, although they are now testing some of them, including turmeric, as therapeutic agents. Each has a unique combination of chemicals that fight oxidative damage in a distinctive manner.

Regularly consuming a battery of antioxidants through daily diet negates the need for vitamins and supplements, which, Wenk points out, offer little protection against Alzheimer's disease. "There's a parallel between our health and cancer, which, we've learned over the past 50 years, is something people get when they're exposed to low doses of something day after day," he says. "Every day, your brain (and body) ages a little bit, and every day there's an opportunity to help it not to."

What Your Brain Wants

First thing in the morning, after several hours of sleep, the brain is running low on glucose. Once awake, it's on the hunt for exactly the foods that deliver heaps of glucose. In short, it's jonesing for fries.

Fast carbohydrate sources prompt bursts of insulin, a peptide (or small protein) secreted by the pancreas in response glucose. Insulin's job is to get glucose into cells; in the brain, it ushers glucose into needy neurons. Exquisitely sensitive to glucose levels, insulin rushes into the bloodstream; rapid spikes in insulin levels in response to sugary foods are followed just as quickly by rapid declines in the hormone, as it pushes glucose into cells for energy. The result: You're hungry again a couple of hours later. So, you snack. (A bag of potato chips, perhaps?)

"THE PURPOSE OF EATING ANYTIME AFTER 5 P.M. IS TO GET ENOUGH NUTRIENTS TO GET YOU THROUGH THE NIGHT."

Eating big meals loaded with simple carbohydrates (high glycemic meals), a common practice in the U.S., can, over time, undermine the insulin system. So critical is this

What about our Vices?

Don't assume that a brain-saving diet forbids goodies such as alcohol and chocolate. If consumed in moderation—of course—even daily, such indulgences can be beneficial.

Epidemiologists have evidence that alcohol protects against Alzheimer's disease. It's a powerful solute that helps dissolve fat in the body, offering cardiovascular protection that benefits the brain as well. The trick is not to consume so much that the liver becomes fatty. Red wine contains, in addition, the antioxidant resveratrol, effective against aging. Prefer beer? The hops that give beer its color also have antioxidant properties. Have a bite to eat first; it helps slow absorption of alcohol so you don't get drunk.

That bite could be a small bar of chocolate. "There's no better compound in nature in terms of flavonoids," says Wenk. Dark chocolate is best, due to its high cocoa content. Men who eat chocolate regularly, in fact, are known to live longer than men who do not.

As we age, our bodies don't harness the anti-inflammation powers of chocolate and other foods as well as they once did. There is, however, a substitute, shown to protect against Alzheimer's disease among people in their 60s and 70s. It's marijuana, studies in Wenk's lab show. Inhaled, the chemicals in marijuana travel easily into the brain, where they reduce inflammation and also stimulate neurogenesis, the birth of new neurons, another ability that attenuates with age. Wenk finds that a puff a day is sufficiently anti-inflammatory, although he doesn't encourage anyone to start smoking weed. Aside from the fact that it's not legal in most of the U.S., "it might cause the munchies," he says, "and that's not going to help."

metabolic mechanism that the health of the insulin system predicts how well you're aging. When insulin signaling isn't working properly and glucose isn't getting into cells—insulin resistance—neurons are deprived of the fuel they need for cognition and self-control. Insulin resistance is correlated with increased formation of toxic beta-amyloid in the brain and with type 2 diabetes.

Eating several big meals a day compounds the risk. Instead, Wenk suggests eating only one big meal a day, and its timing is crucial: a varied breakfast. Edibles providing a variety of nutrients that are digested slowly yield sustained energy for the day in a way that minimizes wear and tear on the body. That way, you'll require only small refueling bites the rest of the time you're awake. Envision a breakfast that marries complex carbohydrates, such as oatmeal, a whole grain bagel, grapefruit, or low-fat yogurt; a burst of antioxidants, perhaps in the form of orange juice; and eggs or, say, turkey sausage for protein. You could even throw in a doughnut to give your brain the simple sugar punch it so desperately wants.

Don't forget to add coffee or tea. Your brain will also crave caffeine when you wake. Throughout the night, levels build up of the neurotransmitter adenosine, and that buildup blocks the function of neurons that make another neurotransmitter, acetylcholine, which is critical for paying attention and learning. Caffeine frees up acetylcholine neurons to make you more functional. Coffee and tea also contain antioxidant and anti-inflammatory compounds known as flavonoids.

Coffee protects your brain against aging in yet another way. People who drink five or more cups a day are 85 percent less likely to develop Parkinson's disease, which, in addition to its trademark tremors, can also cause dementia. The downside to a lot of caffeine is insomnia, jitteriness, and stomach problems. Good for the brain. Not so good for the body.

A Nibble Here or There

After breakfast, Wenk recommends, graze every hour or half hour, as needed, on fruit or nuts; due to their fiber (fruit) and fat (nuts) content, they release their payload at a stately pace and are metabolized slowly. There's no rush of chemicals to the brain. Lunch, Wenk says, should be low-fat and colorful. Think: chicken salad or fish and steamed vegetables. The afternoon should hold more nibbles followed by a small dinner.

Free yourself from the notion that dinner consists of appetizer, entrée, and dessert. Most calories should be consumed up front, to give the brain the energy it needs to get through the day. Dinner, Wenk explains, is an opportunity to load up on compounds not eaten earlier—foods with omega-3 fats, such as salmon, kiwi, or walnuts, which help neurons maintain their structural integrity. Says Wenk: "As far as the brain is concerned, the purpose of eating after 5 P.M. is to get enough nutrients to get you through the night without waking up."

What to Ditch from Your Diet Now

Obesity is the leading cause of preventable death in the world. According to actuarial charts, body mass index is the most accurate predictor of life span. The excess food it takes to make the normal person obese uses a lot of oxygen for processing. Says Wenk: "First fat ages you, then it kills you."

Once excess calories are turned into fat and stored, fat cells release cytokines, little proteins sent out by the immune system to destroy such interlopers as bacteria. They attack by causing inflammation, which eradicates the foreign bodies. Like much warfare, however, there's collateral damage; neighboring cells are caught in the cross fire. In the brain, inflammation abets dementia—so much so that arthritis sufferers, who typically down lots of anti-inflammatory drugs, tend to bypass dementia.

Taking megadoses of anti-inflammatory drugs has its own risks: gastrointestinal bleeding. Far safer to decrease the size of your belly. A recent report fingered the foods that most lead to long-term weight gain: French fries, potato chips, sugary drinks, red meat, and processed meats such as hot dogs, Eaten regularly, they cause obesity, upping the risk of high cholesterol levels, type 2 diabetes, and dementia.

All in Moderation

Even with the damage oxygen inflicts on the body, you can't not eat. That said, one very workable strategy for avoiding oxygen overexposure is simply to eat less. "Then you don't have to eat so many other things to protect you from the foods you did eat," Wenk observes.

Caloric-restriction diets (eliminating up to 40 percent of food intake per day) not only slow the aging process but offer cognitive benefits. The trade-off, however, is less energy, less activity, weak bone structure, and frailer musculature. To benefit from such a regimen takes a little experimentation. If you typically eat 2,000 calories a day, try cutting back to 1,600 and seeing whether you still have enough energy for some exercise. Since exercise requires energy—and, thus, oxygen—Wenk recommends two hours a week of aerobic exercise, or as little as three 20-minute walks per week.

When epidemiologists interview older people, those who maintain good mental and physical health often don't report being extremely active, which could cause long-term joint pain that also contributes to aging. "What people tell us is they were frequently active, did a little something every day, and that seems to have biased them to live longer," Wenk explains. "They didn't tend to overeat, they didn't tend to overexercise. In fact, they didn't tend to live lives of extremes at all. It was always the moderation."

The Age Factor

Your age might also influence the zeal with which you consider adopting Wenk's brain-saving lifestyle. It is, he insists, like investing in the stock market: "If you start early, in your 30s, then you've got time to do the right things. In your 60s, there's less time to invest in your health."

Genetic makeup is a consideration in when to adopt a brain-saving diet. Heritability of Alzheimer's disease, though rare, appears to travel through the female line, Wenk points out. Anyone whose grandmother, mother, or aunt has developed dementia should consider the protective power of immediate lifestyle change.

Since metabolism slows with age, leading many to gain weight later in life, your best brain-saving regimen may be dropping the number of calories you're taking in. Taking weight off is a crucial step in saving one's brain. "The sooner you get started the better," advises Wenk.

In general though, thirtysomethings might begin to incorporate more colorful vegetables into their diet, or shift the bulk of their food intake to earlier in the day. By the time people hit 60, they might do well to remember the lyrics to the Rolling Stones' hit "Ruby Tuesday":

"There's no time to lose, I heard her say/Catch your dreams before they slip away/Dying all the time/Lose your dreams and you will lose your mind/Ain't life unkind?"

Critical Thinking

1. Describe the physiological events in the brain that lead to the decline in mental acuity associated with Alzheimer's disease.
2. Identify the antioxidant nutrients that may slow the progression of dementia.
3. Explain why coffee and tea may enhance attention, learning, and overall brain function.

Create Central

www.mhhe.com/createcentral

Internet References

Alzheimer's Association
www.alz.org

Alzheimer's Disease. Centers for Disease Control and Prevention
www.cdc.gov/features/alzheimers

Alzheimer's Fact Sheet
www.nia.nih.gov/alzheimers/publication/alzheimers-disease-fact-sheet

Medline Plus
www.nlm.nih.gov/medlineplus

NIKHIL SWAMINATHAN is an editor at *Archaeology Magazine* in New York.

Article

Prepared by: Janet Colson, *Middle Tennessee State University*

Soothe the Fire in Your Belly

When to treat heartburn on your own and when to get help.

CONSUMER REPORTS ON HEALTH

Learning Outcomes

After reading this article, you will be able to:

- Summarize the physiology of heartburn and identify the foods and lifestyle behaviors that increase the risk of heartburn.
- Compare the differences between GERD and heartburn and a heart attack and heartburn.

Nearly everyone has experienced heartburn after eating a sumptuous or simply oversized meal. For many, the distress dies down within an hour or so—with or without the help of Rolaids or Tums—making it seem like nothing to worry about.

But the millions who suffer from frequent heartburn might actually have a chronic condition called gastroesophageal reflux disease, or GERD. Left untreated it can damage the esophagus and even lead to cancer.

Lifestyle changes and over-the-counter medication can provide relief for many people, but it's important to know if your symptoms are serious enough to warrant a trip to the doctor. And when should you turn to potent medications called proton pump inhibitors (PPIs) to extinguish the flames?

More than 50 million people in the United States experience heartburn every month, and about 15 million have daily flare-ups, according to the National Institute of Diabetes and Digestive and Kidney Diseases. The cost of treating the condition can quickly add up. The average person with GERD, a related ailment, spends an estimated $3,355 a year on medication and other treatments to help keep symptoms under control. Obese people, smokers, and pregnant women are more likely to suffer from GERD, but it can strike otherwise healthy men and women at any age.

How Heartburn Happens

When you swallow food, it travels down your throat to your esophagus into your stomach, which produces acid to help break it down so that it can be digested. Your lower esophageal sphincter, a muscle at the entrance to your stomach, is supposed to close after the food passes through to keep stomach acid from going into the esophagus. But if it doesn't, and acid reaches the esophagus (along with food), you'll feel a burning sensation. It usually starts just below your breastbone and can radiate into your throat. You might also notice a sour or bitter taste in your mouth or throat.

Occasional heartburn is generally not worrisome or dangerous, and can be relieved with diet and lifestyle changes and, if necessary, over-the-counter antacids or other medications. However, if you have heartburn twice a week or more, and it recurs for weeks or months, or if you frequently regurgitate food (with or without heartburn), consider seeing your doctor to be checked for GERD.

In contrast to occasional heartburn, GERD can be dangerous. Over time, the refluxed acid can inflame and erode the lining of the esophagus, resulting in esophagitis. You may feel a chronic soreness in your lower throat or chest.

Choosing the right remedy

Heartburn medication	When appropriate
Antacids (*Maalox, Mylanta, Rolaids, Tums,* and generics)	For occasional heartburn (less than twice a week). You should also make lifestyle changes, such as avoiding food that triggers heartburn and eating smaller meals.
H2 blockers (*Pepcid, Zantac,* and generics)	For occasional heartburn not relieved by antacids and lifestyle changes, or before eating a known heartburn trigger.
Proton pump inhibitors (*Prevacid, Prilosec,* and generics)	For frequent heartburn not relieved by lifestyle changes, antacids, or H2 blockers. After two weeks of use, check with your doctor to determine if you have GERD.

Most cases of esophagitis are relatively mild, but when it is left untreated, bleeding, scarring, and narrowing of the esophagus can occur, making eating and swallowing painful and difficult. People who have uncontrolled GERD for years have a higher risk of developing cancer of the esophagus, though it's rare.

Fortunately, changes in your diet and lifestyle might be all you need to alleviate the problem. Those measures include eating smaller meals, not lying down for at least three hours after eating, losing weight if needed, and avoiding alcohol.

Certain food and beverages can trigger heartburn in some people, such as citrus fruit, chocolate, coffee or other caffeinated beverages, fried food, garlic, onions, spicy or fatty food, and tomato-rich food, such as marinara sauce, salsa, and pizza.

Drinking alcoholic beverages may increase GERD symptoms, which over time can cause damage to the lining of the esophagus. Symptoms may resolve after you stop drinking.

Smoking weakens the lower esophageal sphincter muscle and increases the risk of GERD (and other diseases), so if you smoke, you should quit. To help reduce heartburn flare-ups while you're asleep, try placing wood blocks beneath your bedposts to raise the head of your bed 6 to 8 inches. Avoid wearing tight clothing or belts that push on your abdomen, since compressing that area can contribute to reflux.

Medication

If diet and lifestyle changes don't help, it might be time to try an antacid, such as *Maalox, Mylanta, Rolaids,* or *Tums.* Some people might need something stronger to relieve their symptoms. In that case, try an acid-reducing H2 blocker such as famotidine (*Pepcid AC* and generic), nizatidine (*Axid AR*), or ranitidine (*Zantac 75, Zantac 150,* and generic). Those drugs help about half of sufferers and can be bought over-the-counter. You might also consider using an over-the-counter PPI, such as lansoprazole (*Prevacid 24HR*), for up to two weeks to see if it eases your symptoms.

If you've tried these options and still have heartburn at least twice a week for several weeks, it's time for a doctor to determine if you have GERD and if it has damaged your esophagus. If you have the condition, he or she will probably recommend that you have an upper endoscopy. This procedure, done under light anesthesia, involves the insertion of a lighted, flexible endoscope tube into your throat and down into the esophagus. The doctor can also use the endoscope to do a biopsy to test for cancer or Barrett's esophagus, which can lead to cancer.

If you have GERD your doctor will probably prescribe a PPI, such as esomeprazole (*Nexium*), lansoprazole (*Prevacid* and generic), or omeprazole (*Prilosec* and generic). Those popular drugs substantially reduce the amount of stomach acid produced, making the contents of your stomach less erosive. If there's already damage to your esophagus, reducing the amount of acid can help it heal.

But many doctors also think that PPIs are overused, a problem that is exacerbated by heavy advertising from pharmaceutical companies. The federal Agency for Healthcare Research and Quality (AHRQ) also noted a widespread overuse of PPIs (as well as other drugs used to treat GERD) in a September 2011 report. Ads have helped propel those drugs to top-selling slots among all prescription medication.

One PPI, *Nexium,* racked up $6.2 billion in sales in 2011, making it the third highest-selling prescription drug in the U.S. last year, according to IMS Health, an industry group that monitors drug sales. But studies have found that up to 70 percent of people who take a PPI may not have GERD and may not need such a potent, expensive medication.

PPIs can also cause serious side effects, including an increased risk of diarrhea associated with *Clostridium difficile,* an acute, sometimes chronic ailment that can lead to severe

Is it heartburn or a heart attack?

It's no surprise that people who have heartburn sometimes fear that they're having a heart attack because the symptoms can be very similar. But delaying treatment for a heart attack can be a matter of life and death. Some typical heart attack signs are listed below. Not all people experience the same ones. If you're in doubt, don't take a chance. Chew and swallow a 325-milligram aspirin tablet and call for emergency help.

	Heart attack	Heartburn
Sensation	Pressure, squeezing, tightness, or pain in the center of the chest. Might last for several minutes or go away and come back.	Burning in throat that generally occurs after eating. Can be accompanied by a bitter or sour taste at the back of throat.
Location	Pain or discomfort generally starts in the center of your chest ond spreads to one or both arms, your back, stomach, neck, or jaw.	Pain is usually felt below the breastbone or ribs. It usually doesn't radiate to your shoulders, arms, or neck, but can.
Quick tests	Pain often goes away quickly after taking nitroglycerin, but not everyone will have this medication readily available.	Sensation often goes away soon after taking an antacid, such as Rolaids or Tums.

Other clues	Breaking into a cold sweat, fainting, light-headedness, nausea, rapid heartbeat, shortness of breath.	Pain tends to increase when bending over, exercising, lifting heavy objects, or lying down.
Action	Call for emergency help if you suspect you're having a heart attack. Also chew and swallow a 325-milligram aspirin tablet.	Make lifestyle changes and, if necessary, take heartburn medication.

intestinal problems and, in rare cases, death. Long-term use can deplete magnesium levels, which can trigger muscle spasms, an irregular heartbeat, and convulsions. Other potential side effects include a higher risk of pneumonia and certain bone fractures, including breaks in the wrist, forearm, and spine.

PPIs can also interact with other medication, so before you take one, make sure it's compatible with other drugs you take. One of the most serious interactions occurs with omeprazole (*Prilosec* and generic) and clopidogrel (*Plavix),* a blood thinner used to reduce the risk of clots that could lead to a heart attack or stroke. According to the U.S. Food and Drug Administration, omeprazole can reduce the effectiveness of *Plavix* by about half, increasing the risk of a heart attack or stroke. *Nexium* and the H2 blocker cimetidine (*Tagamet* and generic) might also interact with *Plavix* in the same way as *Prilosec.*

If you need a PPI, *Consumer Reports*' Best Buy Drugs report recommends first trying an over-the-counter option, such as generic omeprazole, *Prilosec OTC,* or *Prevacid 24HR.* At less than $1 a day, they cost almost one-tenth the price of several of the prescription alternatives. And for most people, they are as effective as the prescription drugs. But check with your insurance provider to see if over-the-counter PPIs are covered. If not, it may be less expensive to get a prescription PPI because it might only cost you a $5 to $10 drug co-payment.

There's no clear answer about when to consider stopping a PPI, because that decision varies. For some people with GERD, symptoms go away after drug treatment and lifestyle changes, or they recur only periodically. Others appear to have a lifelong battle with GERD, so they may need to continue taking a PPI daily to keep symptoms under control. Some people might even need to consider surgery.

If you are diagnosed with GERD and are given a PPI prescription, ask your doctor how long you should take the medicine. After a few weeks or months, you may be able to slowly taper off the drug and eventually stop taking it without issue. If your symptoms return, you can often resume taking the medicine.

Considering Surgery

If lifestyle changes and medication haven't helped, then surgery may be an option. The standard procedure for GERD is laparoscopic fundoplication, in which the upper part of the stomach is sewn around the lower part of the esophagus. This is intended to help strengthen the sphincter muscle. It often helps relieve reflux symptoms and decrease the use of heartburn medication, according to the 2011 report from the AHRQ.

But some people who have surgery may still need to take drugs. Also, serious side effects can arise from the surgery, including infections, a hernia, and difficulty swallowing. So laparoscopic fundoplication should be used only as a last resort.

Critical Thinking

1. Differentiate between heartburn and gastroesophageal reflux disease (GERD).
2. Identify the groups of individuals who are at higher risk of GERD.
3. Describe the physiology of heartburn and GERD.
4. State the differences between the symptoms of heartburn and symptoms of a heart attack.

Create Central

www.mhhe.com/createcentral

Internet References

Academy of Nutrition and Dietetics
www.eatright.org

The Global GERD Epidemic: Definitions, Demographics, and the Clinical Implications of Changing Population Trends (Slides with Transcript)
www.medscape.org/viewarticle/560076

Article

Prepared by: Janet Colson, *Middle Tennessee State University*

Some of My Best Friends Are Germs

MICHAEL POLLAN

Learning Outcomes

After reading the article, you will be able to:

- Describe Michal Pollan's experiences as a participant in the "American Gut" project.
- Outline the benefits of bacteria that reside in a person's gut and how a plant-based diet benefits the bacteria.

I can tell you the exact date that I began to think of myself in the first-person plural—as a superorganism, that is, rather than a plain old individual human being. It happened on March 7. That's when I opened my e-mail to find a huge, processor-choking file of charts and raw data from a laboratory located at the BioFrontiers Institute at the University of Colorado, Boulder. As part of a new citizen-science initiative called the American Gut project, the lab sequenced my microbiome—that is, the genes not of "me," exactly, but of the several hundred microbial species with whom I share this body. These bacteria, which number around 100 trillion, are living (and dying) right now on the surface of my skin, on my tongue and deep in the coils of my intestines, where the largest contingent of them will be found, a pound or two of microbes together forming a vast, largely uncharted interior wilderness that scientists are just beginning to map.

I clicked open a file called Taxa Tables, and a colorful bar chart popped up on my screen. Each bar represented a sample taken (with a swab) from my skin, mouth and feces. For purposes of comparison, these were juxtaposed with bars representing the microbiomes of about 100 "average" Americans previously sequenced.

Here were the names of the hundreds of bacterial species that call me home. In sheer numbers, these microbes and their genes dwarf us. It turns out that we are only 10 percent human: for every human cell that is intrinsic to our body, there are about 10 resident microbes—including commensals (generally harmless freeloaders) and mutualists (favor traders) and, in only a tiny number of cases, pathogens. To the extent that we are bearers of genetic information, more than 99 percent of it is microbial. And it appears increasingly likely that this "second genome," as it is sometimes called, exerts an influence on our health as great and possibly even greater than the genes we inherit from our parents. But while your inherited genes are more or less fixed, it may be possible to reshape, even cultivate, your second genome.

Justin Sonnenburg, a microbiologist at Stanford, suggests that we would do well to begin regarding the human body as "an elaborate vessel optimized for the growth and spread of our microbial inhabitants." This humbling new way of thinking about the self has large implications for human and microbial health, which turn out to be inextricably linked. Disorders in our internal ecosystem—a loss of diversity, say, or a proliferation of the "wrong" kind of microbes—may predispose us to obesity and a whole range of chronic diseases, as well as some infections. "Fecal transplants," which involve installing a healthy person's microbiota into a sick person's gut, have been shown to effectively treat an antibiotic-resistant intestinal pathogen named *C. difficile*, which kills 14,000 Americans each year. (Researchers use the word "microbiota" to refer to all the microbes in a community and "microbiome" to refer to their collective genes.) We've known for a few years that obese mice transplanted with the intestinal community of lean mice lose weight and vice versa. (We don't know why.) A similar experiment was performed recently on humans by researchers in the Netherlands: when the contents of a lean donor's microbiota were transferred to the guts of male patients with metabolic syndrome, the researchers found striking improvements in the recipients' sensitivity to insulin, an important marker for metabolic health. Somehow, the gut microbes were influencing the patients' metabolism.

Our resident microbes also appear to play a critical role in training and modulating our immune system, helping it to accurately distinguish between friend and foe and not go nuts on, well, nuts and all sorts of other potential allergens. Some researchers believe that the alarming increase in autoimmune diseases in the West may owe to a disruption in the ancient relationship between our bodies and their "old friends"—the microbial symbionts with whom we coevolved.

These claims sound extravagant, and in fact many microbiome researchers are careful not to make the mistake that scientists working on the human genome did a decade or so ago, when they promised they were on the trail of cures to many diseases. We're still waiting. Yet whether any cures emerge from the exploration of the second genome, the implications of what has already been learned—for our sense of self, for our definition of health and for our attitude toward bacteria in general—are difficult to overstate. Human health should now "be thought of as a collective property of the human-associated microbiota," as one group of researchers recently concluded in a landmark review article on microbial ecology—that is, as a function of the community, not the individual.

Such a paradigm shift comes not a moment too soon, because as a civilization, we've just spent the better part of a century doing our unwitting best to wreck the human-associated microbiota with a multifronted war on bacteria and a diet notably detrimental to its well-being. Researchers now speak of an impoverished "Westernized microbiome" and ask whether the time has come to embark on a project of "restoration ecology"—not in the rain forest or on the prairie but right here at home, in the human gut.

In March I traveled to Boulder to see the Illumina HiSeq 2000 sequencing machine that had shed its powerful light on my own microbiome and to meet the scientists and computer programmers who were making sense of my data. The lab is headed by Rob Knight, a rangy, crew-cut 36-year-old biologist who first came to the United States from his native New Zealand to study invasive species, a serious problem in his home country. Knight earned his Ph.D. in ecology and evolutionary biology from Princeton when he was 24 and then drifted from the study of visible species and communities to invisible ones. Along the way he discovered he had a knack for computational biology. Knight is regarded as a brilliant analyst of sequencing data, skilled at finding patterns in the flood of information produced by the machines that "batch sequence" all the DNA in a sample and then tease out the unique genetic signatures of each microbe. This talent explains why so many of the scientists exploring the microbiome today send their samples to be sequenced and analyzed by his lab; it is also why you will find Knight's name on most of the important papers in the field.

Over the course of two days in Boulder, I enjoyed several meals with Knight and his colleagues, postdocs and graduate students, though I must say I was a little taken aback by the table talk. I don't think I've ever heard so much discussion of human feces at dinner, but then one thing these scientists are up to is a radical revaluation of the contents of the human colon. I learned about Knight's 16-month-old daughter, who has had most of the diapers to which she has contributed sampled and sequenced. Knight said at dinner that he sampled himself every day; his wife, Amanda Birmingham, who joined us one night, told me that she was happy to be down to once a week. "Of course I keep a couple of swabs in my bag at all times," she said, rolling her eyes, "because you never know."

A result of the family's extensive self-study has been a series of papers examining family microbial dynamics. The data helped demonstrate that the microbial communities of couples sharing a house are similar, suggesting the importance of the environment in shaping an individual's microbiome. Knight also found that the presence of a family dog tended to blend everyone's skin communities, probably via licking and petting. One paper, titled "Moving Pictures of the Human Microbiome," tracked the day-to-day shifts in the microbial composition of each body site. Knight produced animations showing how each community—gut, skin and mouth—hosted a fundamentally different cast of microbial characters that varied within a fairly narrow range over time.

Knight's daily sampling of his daughter's diapers (along with those of a colleague's child) also traced the remarkable process by which a baby's gut community, which in utero is sterile and more or less a blank slate, is colonized. This process begins shortly after birth, when a distinctive infant community of microbes assembles in the gut. Then, with the introduction of solid food and then weaning, the types of microbes gradually shift until, by age 3, the baby's gut comes to resemble an adult community much like that of its parents.

The study of babies and their specialized diet has yielded key insights into how the colonization of the gut unfolds and why it matters so much to our health. One of the earliest clues to the complexity of the microbiome came from an unexpected corner: the effort to solve a mystery about milk. For years, nutrition scientists were confounded by the presence in human breast milk of certain complex carbohydrates, called oligosaccharides, which the human infant lacks the enzymes necessary to digest. Evolutionary theory argues that every component of mother's milk should have some value to the developing baby or natural selection would have long ago discarded it as a waste of the mother's precious resources.

It turns out the oligosaccharides are there to nourish not the baby but one particular gut bacterium called *Bifidobacterium infantis*, which is uniquely well-suited to break down and make use of the specific oligosaccharides present in mother's milk. When all goes well, the bifidobacteria proliferate and dominate, helping to keep the infant healthy by crowding out less savory microbial characters before they can become established and, perhaps most important, by nurturing the integrity of the epithelium—the lining of the intestines, which plays a critical role in protecting us from infection and inflammation.

"Mother's milk, being the only mammalian food shaped by natural selection, is the Rosetta stone for all food," says Bruce German, a food scientist at the University of California, Davis, who researches milk. "And what it's telling us is that when natural selection creates a food, it is concerned not just with feeding the child but the child's gut bugs too."

Where do these all-important bifidobacteria come from and what does it mean if, like me, you were never breastfed? Mother's milk is not, as once was thought, sterile: it is both a "prebiotic"—a food for microbes—and a "probiotic," a population of beneficial microbes introduced into the body. Some of them may find their way from the mother's colon to her milk ducts and from there into the baby's gut with its first feeding. Because designers of infant formula did not, at least until recently, take account of these findings, including neither prebiotic oligosaccharides or probiotic bacteria in their formula, the guts of bottle-fed babies are not optimally colonized.

Most of the microbes that make up a baby's gut community are acquired during birth—a microbially rich and messy process that exposes the baby to a whole suite of maternal microbes. Babies born by Caesarean, however, a comparatively sterile procedure, do not acquire their mother's vaginal and intestinal microbes at birth. Their initial gut communities more closely resemble that of their mother's (and father's) skin, which is less than ideal and may account for higher rates of allergy, asthma and autoimmune problems in C-section babies: not having been seeded with the optimal assortment of microbes at birth, their immune systems may fail to develop properly.

At dinner, Knight told me that he was sufficiently concerned about such an eventuality that, when his daughter was born by emergency C-section, he and his wife took matters into their own hands: using a sterile cotton swab, they inoculated the newborn infant's skin with the mother's vaginal secretions to insure a proper colonization. A formal trial of such a procedure is under way in Puerto Rico.

While I was in Boulder, I sat down with Catherine A. Lozupone, a microbiologist who had just left Knight's lab to set up her own at the University of Colorado, Denver, and who spent some time looking at my microbiome and comparing it with others, including her own. Lozupone was the lead author on an important 2012 paper in *Nature*, "Diversity, Stability and Resilience of the Human Gut Microbiota," which sought to approach the gut community as an ecologist might, trying to determine the "normal" state of the ecosystem and then examining the various factors that disturb it over time. How does diet affect it? Antibiotics? Pathogens? What about cultural traditions? So far, the best way to begin answering such questions may be by comparing the gut communities of various far-flung populations, and researchers have been busy collecting samples around the world and shipping them to sequencing centers for analysis. The American Gut project, which hopes to eventually sequence the communities of tens of thousands of Americans, represents the most ambitious such effort to date; it will help researchers uncover patterns of correlation between people's lifestyle, diet, health status and the makeup of their microbial community.

It is still early days in this research, as Lozupone (and everyone else I interviewed) underscored; scientists can't even yet say with confidence exactly what a "healthy" microbiome should look like. But some broad, intriguing patterns are emerging. More diversity is probably better than less, because a diverse ecosystem is generally more resilient—and diversity in the Western gut is significantly lower than in other, less-industrialized populations. The gut microbiota of people in the West looks very different from that of a variety of other geographically dispersed peoples. So, for example, the gut community of rural people in West Africa more closely resembles that of Amerindians in Venezuela than it does an American's or a European's.

These rural populations not only harbor a greater diversity of microbes but also a different cast of lead characters. American and European guts contain relatively high levels of bacteroides and firmicutes and low levels of the prevotella that dominate the guts of rural Africans and Amerindians. (It is not clear whether high or low levels of any of these is good or bad.) Why are the microbes different? It could be the diet, which in both rural populations features a considerable amount of whole grains (which prevotella appear to like), plant fiber and very little meat. (Many firmicutes like amino acids, so they proliferate when the diet contains lots of protein; bacteroides metabolize carbohydrates.) As for the lower biodiversity in the West, this could be a result of our profligate use of antibiotics (in health care as well as the food system), our diet of processed food (which has generally been cleansed of all bacteria, the good and the bad), environmental toxins and generally less "microbial pressure"—i.e., exposure to bacteria—in everyday life. All of this may help explain why, though these rural populations tend to have greater exposures to infectious diseases and lower life expectancies than those in the West, they also have lower rates of chronic disorders like allergies, asthma, Type 2 diabetes and cardiovascular disease.

"Rural people spend a lot more time outside and have much more contact with plants and with soil," Lozupone says. Another researcher, who has gathered samples in Malawi, told me, "In some of these cultures, children are raised communally, passed from one set of hands to another, so they're routinely exposed to a greater diversity of microbes." The nuclear family may not be conducive to the health of the microbiome.

As it happens, Lozupone and I had something in common, microbially speaking: we share unusually high levels of prevotella for Americans. Our gut communities look more like those of rural Africans or Amerindians than like those of our neighbors. Lozupone suspects that the reasons for this might have to do with a plant-based diet; we each eat lots of whole grains and vegetables and relatively little meat. (Though neither of us is a vegetarian.) Like me, she was proud of her prevotella, regarding it as a sign of a healthy non-Western diet, at least until she began doing research on the microbiota of H.I.V. patients. It seems that they, too, have lots of prevotella. Further confusing the story, a recent study linking certain gut microbes common in meat eaters to high levels of a blood marker for heart disease suggested that prevotella was one such microbe. Early days, indeed.

Two other features of my microbiome attracted the attention of the researchers who examined it. First, the overall biodiversity of my gut community was significantly higher than that of the typical Westerner, which I decided to take as a compliment, though the extravagantly diverse community of microbes on my skin raised some eyebrows. "Where have your hands been, man?" Jeff Leach of the American Gut project asked after looking over my results. My skin harbors bacteria associated with plants, soil and a somewhat alarming variety of animal guts. I put this down to gardening, composting (I keep worms too) and also the fact that I was fermenting kimchi and making raw-milk cheese, "live-culture" foods teeming with microbes.

Compared to a rain forest or a prairie, the interior ecosystem is not well understood, but the core principles of ecology—which along with powerful new sequencing machines have opened this invisible frontier to science—are beginning to yield some preliminary answers and a great many more intriguing hypotheses. Your microbial community seems to stabilize by age 3, by which time most of the various niches in the gut ecosystem are occupied. That doesn't mean it can't change after that; it can, but not as readily. A change of diet or a course of antibiotics, for example, may bring shifts in the relative population of the various resident species, helping some kinds of bacteria to thrive and others to languish. Can new species be introduced? Yes, but probably only when a niche is opened after a significant disturbance, like an antibiotic storm. Just like any other mature ecosystem, the one in our gut tends to resist invasion by newcomers.

You acquire most of the initial microbes in your gut community from your parents, but others are picked up from the environment. "The world is covered in a fine patina of feces," as the Stanford microbiologist Stanley Falkow tells students. The new sequencing tools have confirmed his hunch: Did you know that house dust can contain significant amounts of fecal particles? Or that, whenever a toilet is flushed, some of its contents are aerosolized? Knight's lab has sequenced the bacteria on toothbrushes. This news came during breakfast, so I didn't ask for details, but got them anyway: "You want to keep your toothbrush a minimum of six feet away from a toilet," one of Knight's colleagues told me.

Some scientists in the field borrow the term "ecosystem services" from ecology to catalog all the things that the microbial community does for us as its host or habitat, and the services rendered are remarkably varied and impressive. "Invasion resistance" is one. Our resident microbes work to keep pathogens from gaining a toehold by occupying potential niches or otherwise rendering the environment inhospitable to foreigners. The robustness of an individual's gut community might explain why some people fall victim to food poisoning while others can blithely eat the same meal with no ill effects.

Our gut bacteria also play a role in the manufacture of substances like neurotransmitters (including serotonin); enzymes and vitamins (notably Bs and K) and other essential nutrients (including important amino acid and short-chain fatty acids); and a suite of other signaling molecules that talk to, and influence, the immune and the metabolic systems. Some of these compounds may play a role in regulating our stress levels and even temperament: when gut microbes from easygoing, adventurous mice are transplanted into the guts of anxious and timid mice, they become more adventurous. The expression "thinking with your gut" may contain a larger kernel of truth than we thought.

The gut microbes are looking after their own interests, chief among them getting enough to eat and regulating the passage of food through their environment. The bacteria themselves appear to help manage these functions by producing signaling chemicals that regulate our appetite, satiety and digestion. Much of what we're learning about the microbiome's role in human metabolism has come from studying "gnotobiotic mice"—mice raised in labs like Jeffrey I. Gordon's at Washington University, in St. Louis, to be microbially sterile, or germ-free. Recently, Gordon's lab transplanted the gut microbes of Malawian children with kwashiorkor—an acute form of malnutrition—into germ-free mice. The lab found those mice with kwashiorkor who were fed the children's typical diet could not readily metabolize nutrients, indicating that it may take more than calories to remedy malnutrition. Repairing a patient's disordered metabolism may require reshaping the community of species in his or her gut.

Keeping the immune system productively engaged with microbes—exposed to lots of them in our bodies, our diet and our environment—is another important ecosystem service and one that might turn out to be critical to our health. "We used to think the immune system had this fairly straightforward job," Michael Fischbach, a biochemist at the University of California, San Francisco, says. "All bacteria were clearly 'nonself' so simply had to be recognized and dealt with. But the job of the immune system now appears to be far more nuanced and complex. It has to learn to consider our mutualists"—e.g., resident bacteria—"as self too. In the future we won't even call it the immune system, but the microbial interaction system." The absence of constructive engagement between microbes and immune system (particularly during certain windows of development) could be behind the increase in autoimmune conditions in the West.

So why haven't we evolved our own systems to perform these most critical functions of life? Why have we outsourced all this work to a bunch of microbes? One theory is that, because microbes evolve so much faster than we do (in some cases a new generation every 20 minutes), they can respond to changes in the environment—to threats as well as opportunities—with much greater speed and agility than "we" can. Exquisitely reactive and adaptive, bacteria can swap genes and pieces of DNA among themselves. This versatility is especially handy when a new toxin or food source appears in the environment. The microbiota can swiftly come up with precisely the right gene needed to fight it—or eat it. In one recent study, researchers found that a common gut microbe in Japanese people has acquired a gene from a marine bacterium that allows the Japanese to digest seaweed, something the rest of us can't do as well.

This plasticity serves to extend our comparatively rigid genome, giving us access to a tremendous bag of biochemical tricks we did not need to evolve ourselves. "The bacteria in your gut are continually reading the environment and responding," says Joel Kimmons, a nutrition scientist and epidemiologist at the Centers for Disease Control and Prevention in Atlanta. "They're a microbial mirror of the changing world. And because they can evolve so quickly, they help our bodies respond to changes in our environment."

A handful of microbiologists have begun sounding the alarm about our civilization's unwitting destruction of the human microbiome and its consequences. Important microbial species may have already gone extinct, before we have had a chance to learn who they are or what they do. What we think of as an interior wilderness may in fact be nothing of the kind, having long ago been reshaped by unconscious human actions. Taking the ecological metaphor further, the "Westernized microbiome" most of us now carry around is in fact an artifact of civilization, no more a wilderness today than, say, the New Jersey Meadowlands.

To obtain a clearer sense of what has been lost, María Gloria Dominguez-Bello, a Venezuelan-born microbiologist at New York University, has been traveling to remote corners of the Amazon to collect samples from hunter-gatherers who have had little previous contact with Westerners or Western medicine. "We want to see how the human microbiota looks before antibiotics, before processed food, before modern birth," she told me. "These samples are really gold."

Preliminary results indicate that a pristine microbiome—of people who have had little or no contact with Westerners—features much greater biodiversity, including a number of species never before sequenced, and, as mentioned, much higher levels of prevotella than is typically found in the Western gut. Dominguez-Bello says these vibrant, diverse and antibiotic-naïve microbiomes may play a role in Amerindians' markedly lower rates of allergies, asthma, atopic disease and chronic conditions like Type 2 diabetes and cardiovascular disease.

One bacterium commonly found in the non-Western microbiome but nearly extinct in ours is a corkscrew-shaped inhabitant of the stomach by the name of *Helicobacter pylori*. Dominguez-Bello's husband, Martin Blaser, a physician and microbiologist at N.Y.U., has been studying *H. pylori* since the mid-1980s and is convinced that it is an endangered species, the extinction of which we may someday rue. According to the "missing microbiota hypothesis," we depend on microbes like H. pylori to regulate various metabolic and immune functions, and their disappearance is disordering those systems. The loss is cumulative: "Each generation is passing on fewer of these microbes," Blaser told me, with the result that the Western microbiome is being progressively impoverished.

He calls H. pylori the "poster child" for the missing microbes and says medicine has actually been trying to exterminate it since 1983, when Australian scientists proposed that the microbe was responsible for peptic ulcers; it has since been implicated in stomach cancer as well. But H. pylori is a most complicated character, the entire spectrum of microbial good and evil rolled into one bug. Scientists learned that H. pylori also plays a role in regulating acid in the stomach. Presumably it does this to render its preferred habitat inhospitable to competitors, but the effect on its host can be salutary. People without H. pylori may not get peptic ulcers, but they frequently do suffer from acid reflux. Untreated, this can lead to Barrett's esophagus and, eventually, a certain type of esophageal cancer, rates of which have soared in the West as H. pylori has gone missing.

When after a recent bout of acid reflux, my doctor ordered an endoscopy, I discovered that, like most Americans today, my stomach has no H. pylori. My gastroenterologist was pleased, but after talking to Blaser, the news seemed more equivocal, because H. pylori also does us a lot of good. The microbe engages with the immune system, quieting the inflammatory response in ways that serve its own interests—to be left in peace—as well as our own. This calming effect on the immune system may explain why populations that still harbor H. pylori are less prone to allergy and asthma. Blaser's lab has also found evidence that H. pylori plays an important role in human metabolism by regulating levels of the appetite hormone ghrelin. "When the stomach is empty, it produces a lot of ghrelin, the chemical signal to the brain to eat," Blaser says. "Then, when it has had enough, the stomach shuts down ghrelin production, and the host feels satiated." He says the disappearance of H. pylori may be contributing to obesity by muting these signals.

But what about the diseases H. pylori is blamed for? Blaser says these tend to occur only late in life, and he makes the rather breathtaking suggestion that this microbe's evolutionary role might be to help shuffle us off life's stage once our childbearing years have passed. So important does Blaser regard this strange, paradoxical symbiont that he has proposed not one but two unconventional therapeutic interventions: inoculate children with H. pylori to give them the benefit of its services early in life, and then exterminate it with antibiotics at age 40, when it is liable to begin causing trouble.

These days Blaser is most concerned about the damage that antibiotics, even in tiny doses, are doing to the microbiome—and particularly to our immune system and weight. "Farmers have been performing a great experiment for more than 60 years," Blaser says, "by giving subtherapeutic doses of antibiotics to their animals to make them gain weight." Scientists aren't sure exactly why this practice works, but the drugs may favor bacteria that are more efficient at harvesting energy from the diet. "Are we doing the same thing to our kids?" he asks. Children in the West receive, on average, between 10 and 20 courses of antibiotics before they turn 18. And those prescribed drugs aren't the only antimicrobials finding their way to the microbiota; scientists have found antibiotic residues in meat, milk and surface water as well. Blaser is also concerned about the use of antimicrobial compounds in our diet and everyday lives—everything from chlorine washes for lettuce to hand sanitizers. "We're using these chemicals precisely because they're antimicrobial," Blaser says. "And of course they do us some good. But we need to ask, what are they doing to our microbiota?" No one is questioning the value of antibiotics to civilization—they have helped us to conquer a great many infectious diseases and increased our life expectancy. But, as in any war, the war on bacteria appears to have had some unintended consequences.

One of the more striking results from the sequencing of my microbiome was the impact of a single course of antibiotics on my gut community. My dentist had put me on a course of Amoxicillin as a precaution before oral surgery. (Without prophylactic antibiotics, of course, surgery would be considerably more dangerous.) Within a week, my impressively non-Western "alpha diversity"—a measure of the microbial diversity in my gut—had plummeted and come to look very much like the American average. My (possibly) healthy levels of prevotella had also disappeared, to be replaced by a spike in bacteroides (much more common in the West) and an alarming bloom of proteobacteria, a phylum that includes a great many weedy and pathogenic characters, including E. coli and salmonella. What had appeared to be a pretty healthy, diversified gut was now raising expressions of concern among the microbiologists who looked at my data.

"Your E. coli bloom is creepy," Ruth Ley, a Cornell University microbiologist who studies the microbiome's role in obesity, told me. "If we put that sample in germ-free mice, I bet they'd get inflamed." Great. Just when I was beginning to think of myself as a promising donor for a fecal transplant, now I had a gut that would make mice sick. I was relieved to learn that my gut community would eventually bounce back to something resembling its former state. Yet one recent study found that when subjects were given a second course of antibiotics, the recovery of their interior ecosystem was less complete than after the first.

Few of the scientists I interviewed had much doubt that the Western diet was altering our gut microbiome in troubling ways. Some, like Blaser, are concerned about the antimicrobials we're ingesting with our meals; others with the sterility of processed food. Most agreed that the lack of fiber in the Western diet was deleterious to the microbiome, and still others voiced concerns about the additives in processed foods, few of which have ever been studied for their specific effects on the microbiota. According to a recent article in *Nature* by the Stanford microbiologist Justin Sonnenburg, "Consumption of hyperhygienic, mass-produced, highly processed and calorie-dense foods is testing how rapidly the microbiota of individuals in industrialized countries can adapt." As our microbiome evolves to cope with the Western diet, Sonnenburg says he worries that various genes are becoming harder to find as the microbiome's inherent biodiversity declines along with our everyday exposure to bacteria.

Catherine Lozupone in Boulder and Andrew Gewirtz, an immunologist at Georgia State University, directed my attention to the emulsifiers commonly used in many processed foods—ingredients with names like lecithin, Datem, CMC and polysorbate 80. Gewirtz's lab has done studies in mice indicating that some of these detergentlike compounds may damage the mucosa—the protective lining of the gut wall—potentially leading to leakage and inflammation.

A growing number of medical researchers are coming around to the idea that the common denominator of many, if not most, of the chronic diseases from which we suffer today may be inflammation—a heightened and persistent immune response by the body to a real or perceived threat. Various markers for inflammation are common in people with metabolic syndrome, the complex of abnormalities that predisposes people to illnesses like cardiovascular disease, obesity, Type 2 diabetes and perhaps cancer. While health organizations differ on the exact definition of metabolic syndrome, a 2009 report from the Centers for Disease Control and Prevention found that 34 percent of American adults are afflicted with the condition. But is inflammation yet another symptom of metabolic syndrome, or is it perhaps the cause of it? And if it is the cause, what is its origin?

One theory is that the problem begins in the gut, with a disorder of the microbiota, specifically of the all-important epithelium that lines our digestive tract. This internal skin—the surface area of which is large enough to cover a tennis court—mediates our relationship to the world outside our bodies; more than 50 tons of food pass through it in a lifetime. The microbiota play a critical role in maintaining the health of the epithelium: some bacteria, like the bifidobacteria and *Lactobacillus plantarum* (common in fermented vegetables), seem to directly enhance its function. These and other gut bacteria also contribute to its welfare by feeding it. Unlike most tissues, which take their nourishment from the bloodstream, epithelial cells in the colon obtain much of theirs from the short-chain fatty acids that gut bacteria produce as a byproduct of their fermentation of plant fiber in the large intestine.

But if the epithelial barrier isn't properly nourished, it can become more permeable, allowing it to be breached. Bacteria, endotoxins—which are the toxic byproducts of certain bacteria—and proteins can slip into the blood stream, thereby causing the body's immune system to mount a response. This resulting low-grade inflammation, which affects the entire body, may lead over time to metabolic syndrome and a number of the chronic diseases that have been linked to it.

Evidence in support of this theory is beginning to accumulate, some of the most intriguing coming from the lab of Patrice Cani at the Université Catholique de Louvain in Brussels. When Cani fed a high-fat, "junk food" diet to mice, the community of microbes in their guts changed much as it does in humans on a fast-food diet. But Cani also found the junk-food diet made the animals' gut barriers notably more permeable, allowing endotoxins to leak into the bloodstream. This produced a low-grade inflammation that eventually led to metabolic syndrome. Cani concludes that, at least in mice, "gut bacteria can initiate the inflammatory processes associated with obesity and insulin resistance" by increasing gut permeability.

These and other experiments suggest that inflammation in the gut may be the cause of metabolic syndrome, not its result, and that changes in the microbial community and lining of the gut wall may produce this inflammation. If Cani is correct—and there is now some evidence indicating that the same mechanism is at work in humans—then medical science may be on the trail of a Grand Unified Theory of Chronic Disease, at the very heart of which we will find the gut microbiome.

My first reaction to learning all this was to want to do something about it immediately, something to nurture the health of my microbiome. But most of the scientists I interviewed were reluctant to make practical recommendations; it's too soon, they told me, we don't know enough yet. Some of this hesitance reflects an understandable abundance of caution. The microbiome researchers don't want to make the mistake of overpromising, as the genome researchers did. They are also concerned about feeding a gigantic bloom of prebiotic and probiotic quackery and rightly so: probiotics are already being hyped as the new panacea, even though it isn't at all clear what these supposedly beneficial bacteria do for us or how they do what they do. There is some research suggesting that some probiotics may be effective in a number of ways: modulating the immune system; reducing allergic response; shortening the length and severity of colds in children; relieving diarrhea and irritable bowel symptoms; and improving the function of the epithelium. The problem is that, because the probiotic marketplace is largely unregulated, it's impossible to know what, if anything, you're getting when you buy a "probiotic" product. One study tested 14 commercial probiotics and found that only one contained the exact species stated on the label.

But some of the scientists' reluctance to make recommendations surely flows from the institutional bias of science and medicine: that the future of microbiome management should remain firmly in the hands of science and medicine. Down this path—which holds real promise—lie improved probiotics and prebiotics, fecal transplants (with better names) and related therapies. Jeffrey Gordon, one of those scientists who peers far over the horizon, looks forward to a time when disorders of the microbiome will be treated with "synbiotics"—suites of targeted, next-generation probiotic microbes administered along with the appropriate prebiotic nutrients to nourish them. The fecal transplant will give way to something far more targeted: a purified and cultured assemblage of a dozen or so microbial species that, along with new therapeutic foods, will be introduced to the gut community to repair "lesions"—important missing species or functions. Yet, assuming it all works as advertised, such an approach will also allow Big Pharma and Big Food to stake out and colonize the human microbiome for profit.

When I asked Gordon about do-it-yourself microbiome management, he said he looked forward to a day "when people can cultivate this wonderful garden that is so influential in our health and well-being"—but that day awaits a lot more science. So he declined to offer any gardening tips or dietary advice. "We have to manage expectations," he said.

Alas, I am impatient. So I gave up asking scientists for recommendations and began asking them instead how, in light of what they've learned about the microbiome, they have changed their own diets and lifestyles. Most of them have made changes. They were slower to take, or give their children, antibiotics. (I should emphasize that in no way is this an argument for the rejection of antibiotics when they are medically called for.) Some spoke of relaxing the sanitary regime in their homes, encouraging their children to play outside in the dirt and with animals—deliberately increasing their exposure to the great patina. Many researchers told me they had eliminated or cut back on processed foods, either because of its lack of fiber or out of concern about additives. In general they seemed to place less faith in probiotics (which few of them used) than in prebiotics—foods likely to encourage the growth of "good bacteria" already present. Several, including Justin Sonnenburg, said they had added fermented foods to their diet: yogurt, kimchi, sauerkraut. These foods can contain large numbers of probiotic bacteria, like *L. plantarum* and bifidobacteria, and while most probiotic bacteria don't appear to take up permanent residence in the gut, there is evidence that they might leave their mark on the community, sometimes by changing the gene expression of the permanent residents—in effect turning on or off metabolic pathways within the cell—and sometimes by stimulating or calming the immune response.

What about increasing our exposure to bacteria? "There's a case for dirtying up your diet," Sonnenburg told me. Yet advising people not to thoroughly wash their produce is probably unwise in a world of pesticide residues. "I view it as a cost-benefit analysis," Sonnenburg wrote in an e-mail. "Increased exposure to environmental microbes likely decreases chance of many Western diseases, but increases pathogen exposure. Certainly the costs go up as scary antibiotic-resistant bacteria become more prevalent." So wash your hands in situations when pathogens or toxic chemicals are likely present, but maybe not after petting your dog. "In terms of food, I think eating fermented foods is the answer—as opposed to not washing food, unless it is from your garden," he said.

With his wife, Erica, also a microbiologist, Sonnenburg tends a colony of gnotobiotic mice at Stanford, examining (among other things) the effects of the Western diet on their microbiota. (Removing fiber drives down diversity, but the effect is reversible.) He's an amateur baker, and when I visited his lab, we talked about the benefits of baking with whole grains.

"Fiber is not a single nutrient," Sonnenburg said, which is why fiber supplements are no magic bullet. "There are hundreds of different polysaccharides"—complex carbohydrates, including fiber—"in plants, and different microbes like to chomp on different ones." To boost fiber, the food industry added lots of a polysaccharide called inulin to hundreds of products, but that's just one kind (often derived from the chicory-plant root) and so may only favor a limited number of microbes. I was hearing instead an argument for a variety of whole grains and a diverse diet of plants and vegetables as well as fruits. "The safest way to increase your microbial biodiversity is to eat a variety of polysaccharides," he said.

His comment chimed with something a gastroenterologist at the University of Pittsburgh told me. "The big problem with the Western diet," Stephen O'Keefe said, "is that it doesn't feed the gut, only the upper G I. All the food has been processed to be readily absorbed, leaving nothing for the lower G I. But it turns out that one of the keys to health is fermentation in the large intestine." And the key to feeding the fermentation in the large intestine is giving it lots of plants with their various types of fiber, including resistant starch (found in bananas, oats, beans); soluble fiber (in onions and other root vegetables, nuts); and insoluble fiber (in whole grains, especially bran, and avocados).

With our diet of swiftly absorbed sugars and fats, we're eating for one and depriving the trillion of the food they like best: complex carbohydrates and fermentable plant fibers. The byproduct of fermentation is the short-chain fatty acids that nourish the gut barrier and help prevent inflammation. And there are studies suggesting that simply adding plants to a fast-food diet will mitigate its inflammatory effect.

The outlines of a diet for the new superorganism were coming clear, and it didn't require the ministrations of the food scientists at Nestlé or General Mills to design it. Big Food and Big Pharma probably do have a role to play, as will Jeffrey Gordon's next-generation synbiotics, in repairing the microbiota of people who can't or don't care to simply change their diets. This is going to be big business. Yet the components of a microbiota-friendly diet are already on the supermarket shelves and in farmers' markets.

Viewed from this perspective, the foods in the markets appear in a new light, and I began to see how you might begin to shop and cook with the microbiome in mind, the better to feed the fermentation in our guts. The less a food is processed, the more of it that gets safely through the gastrointestinal tract and into the eager clutches of the microbiota. Al dente pasta, for example, feeds the bugs better than soft pasta does; steel-cut oats better than rolled; raw or lightly cooked vegetables offer the bugs more to chomp on than overcooked, etc. This is at once a very old and a very new way of thinking about food: it suggests that all calories are not created equal and that the structure of a food and how it is prepared may matter as much as its nutrient composition.

It is a striking idea that one of the keys to good health may turn out to involve managing our internal fermentation. Having recently learned to manage several external fermentations—of bread and kimchi and beer—I know a little about the vagaries of that process. You depend on the microbes, and you do your best to align their interests with yours, mainly by feeding them the kinds of things they like to eat—good "substrate." But absolute control of the process is too much to hope for. It's a lot more like gardening than governing.

The successful gardener has always known you don't need to master the science of the soil, which is yet another hotbed of microbial fermentation, in order to nourish and nurture it. You just need to know what it likes to eat—basically, organic matter—and how, in a general way, to align your interests with the interests of the microbes and the plants. The gardener also discovers that, when pathogens or pests appear, chemical interventions "work," that is, solve the immediate problem, but at a cost to the long-term health of the soil and the whole garden. The drive for absolute control leads to unanticipated forms of disorder.

This, it seems to me, is pretty much where we stand today with respect to our microbiomes—our teeming, quasi-wilderness. We don't know a lot, but we probably know enough to begin taking better care of it. We have a pretty good idea of what it likes to eat, and what strong chemicals do to it. We know all we need to know, in other words, to begin, with modesty, to tend the unruly garden within.

Critical Thinking

1. What is the goal of the "American Gut" project?
2. Explain what a fecal transplant is and the purpose in the procedure.
3. What are the benefits of bacteria that reside an individual's gut?
4. What type diet promotes growth of the good bacteria that reside in our guts?

Create Central

www.mhhe.com/createcentral

Internet References

American Gut—Human Food Project
http://humanfoodproject.com/americangut

Oral Probiotics: An Introduction—National Center for Complementary and Alternative Medicine
http://nccam.nih.gov/health/probiotics/introduction.htm

Michael Pollan is the Knight professor of journalism at the University of California, Berkeley, and the author, most recently, of *Cooked: A Natural History of Transformation*.

Unit 5

UNIT

Prepared by: Janet Colson, *Middle Tennessee State University*

Obesity and Weight Control

Overweight and obesity have become epidemic in the United States during the last century and are rising at a dangerous rate worldwide. According to the National Health and Nutrition Examination Survey, 35% of U.S. adults (78 million people) have a body mass index (BMI) over 30, which is the cut-off for a diagnosis of obesity. Another third of the U.S. population is considered overweight, with BMI of 25–29.9. Therefore, by these definitions, two-thirds of the U.S. population is overweight or obese.

Reports suggest that by the year 2050, half of the U.S. population will be considered obese if current trends continue; however, recent analysis indicate that the rate of increase in overweight and obesity in the United States is nearing a plateau rather than the upward slope. The latest statistics from the Centers for Disease Control and Prevention suggest that there has been only a slight increase in obesity rates since 2005 compared to the significant increase climb in obesity rates from 1980 to 2005.

Overweight and obesity is prevalent in males and females of all ages, races, and ethnic groups. Data from the National Health and Nutrition Examination Survey (NHANES) have shown that obesity rates among non-Hispanic black women and Mexican American women have increased since 2004. More adult men are now overweight or obese as compared to women. From this data, 74% of men and 64% of women are overweight or obese.

Prevention efforts are geared toward curtailing obese children from maturing into obese adults. Overweight and obesity burdens our current healthcare system and government supported healthcare reimbursement programs with exorbitant costs of obesity-related chronic diseases. The major health consequences of obesity are heart disease, diabetes, gallbladder disease, osteoarthritis, and some cancers. The cost for treating the degenerative diseases secondary to obesity is approximately $100 billion per year in the United States.

Even though health and nutrition professionals have tried to prevent and combat obesity with behavior modification, a healthy diet, and exercise, it seems that these traditional ways have not proven effective. Fast-food restaurants are the mainstay for many Americans because they offer quick, inexpensive food. Supersizing has become the norm because, in many instances, it's cheaper to order a biggie combo than smaller items individually. Americans are so accustomed to our fast food nation that many people become infuriated when asked to pull up and wait an extra minute for a 2,400-kcal. meal. The problem is exacerbated by the food industry's historical plight to earn profit and market share by providing U.S. consumers with the fatty, sugary, and salty foods that we demand.

Food companies spend millions of dollars in advertising foods loaded with simple sugars, fat, and salt. Their aggressive advertising, coupled with food accessibility and large portion sizes, have impacted the current obesity pandemic. Other obstacles to maintaining a healthy diet are low accessibility and the high cost of eating a healthy diet.

Scientists have reported that adipose tissue is a dynamically active endocrine organ that releases hormones and inflammatory proteins that may predispose a person to chronic diseases such as heart disease. In addition, research has discovered the role of the "hunger hormone" and how individual differences affect our ability to lose weight. A positive association was recently found between obesity, especially central obesity, and different types of cancer. Thus, there is a great need for a multifaceted public health approach that would involve mobilization of private and public sectors and focus on building better coping skills and increasing activity.

Globalization is causing the rest of the world and especially developing third world countries to mimic the unhealthy Western diet that contributes to obesity. Obesity and its health consequences are now becoming a global epidemic. Sweetened beverages and the sedentary Western way of life that has been adopted by many developing countries are some of the major contributors of this epidemic.

Intervention and prevention should be the top priorities of policymakers. At the public sector, inclusion of health officials, researchers, educators, legislators, transportation experts, urban planners, and businesses to cooperate in formulating ways to combat obesity is crucial. A sound public health policy would require that weight-loss therapies have long-term maintenance and relapse-prevention measures built into them. Healthy People 2010 is the U.S. government's prevention agenda designed to ensure high quality of life and reduce health risks. One of the 28 areas it focuses on is overweight and obesity. Its main objectives are to reduce the proportion of overweight and obese children, teens, and adults by half and to increase the proportion of adults who are at a healthy weight.

Another perspective to consider about the obesogenic environment in the United States is the influence it is having on people who have or may develop disordered eating. An obesogenic environment provides inadequate opportunities for physical activity, offers unlimited access to high calorie foods, and has a large number of obese residents. People who live in this type environment are often predisposed to weight challenges, food addictions, and societal discrimination. Additionally, this environment may contribute to disordered eating behavior that result by being exposed to conflicting messages such as very thin is beautiful and eating energy-dense foods is attractive and desirable; these messages can lead to feelings of helplessness, psychological distress, and self-dislike.

The articles in this unit may be used to supplement information presented in the energy balance and weight control section of general nutrition courses.

Article

Prepared by: Janet Colson, *Middle Tennessee State University*

Can Skinny Fat Beat Obesity?

Newly discovered in adult mammals, beige fat cells can switch between accumulating fat and burning it, depending on metabolic needs.

PHILIP A. REA, PETER YIN, AND RYAN ZAHALKA

Learning Outcomes

After reading this article, you will be able to:

- Describe the three types of adipose tissue cells.
- Discuss the role that the uncoupling protein 1 (UCP1) plays in brown and beige fat.
- Explain what irisin is and its relationship to brown fat.

When we hear the word *fat,* most of us think of ice cream, French fries, or the greasy white stuff in a rasher of streaky bacon. We associate becoming fat with an increased risk of cardiovascular disease, metabolic syndrome, and type 2 diabetes. These risks are real enough, but they pertain to only one of the several types of fat that are found in the human body.

White adipose tissue (or, in non-technical terms, fat), the main culprit in weight gain, tends to accumulate under the skin and as visceral-deposits around internal organs. By contrast, brown adipose tissue usually appears as deposits in the neck area and between the shoulders. Medical researchers first described brown fat in hibernating mammals and, among our own species, in newborn babies.

Until recently, brown fat was thought to exist in humans for only a short time after birth to serve as a stopgap for the maintenance of body temperature, in lieu of the shivering reflex that develops later in life. It was not until 2002, with the large-scale adoption of positron emission tomography (PET) scans, that areas resembling brown fat were recognized in the medical images of adults as well. However, the discoveries related to fat did not end there. The complex biology of adipose tissue continues to yield surprises, including the insight that a newly characterized type of body fat could ultimately play a major role in fighting obesity.

Why Must We Have Fat?

Both white and brown adipose tissue are fat depots—that is, they hold the body's fat reserves—but they differ radically in their composition and function. A white fat cell is made up of a single fat droplet surrounded by a wafer-thin ring of cytoplasm, which in turn contains only a scattering of mitochondria, the powerhouse organelles that burn fats, carbohydrates, and protein down to carbon dioxide and water. A brown fat cell, on the other hand, is made up of several smaller fat droplets embedded in a more extensive cytoplasm containing a large number of mitochondria. Whereas white fat gets its off-white color from the fat that is its main component, brown fat is full of mitochondria rich in iron- and heme-containing respiratory enzymes that give it a rusty brown coloration; moreover, brown fat is infiltrated by a much denser network of blood vessels and capillaries. Brown fat is a heat generator and distributor; white fat is a fuel depot and heat capacitor.

Although the calorie-dense diet popular in many Western societies, in combination with a sedentary lifestyle, is now leading to an unprecedented epidemic of obesity, we should not lose sight of the fact that throughout most of our evolutionary history the ability to hedge against starvation by laying down white adipose tissue has been crucial to human survival. Without the calorie reserves stored in white fat, our ability to minimize heat loss and to subsist between meals would be severely limited; hibernation, for those species that eke out their stored fat to survive the winter months, would simply not be an option.

To take a very loose analogy, if we think of the mammalian body as a dwelling, white fat is something like a combination of the home's fuel reserve and insulation.

By extension of this analogy, brown fat is the physiological equivalent of the furnace in a home heating system that is switched on when the temperature of the home falls below a set point. Like the thermostat of a home heating system, thermoreceptors under the skin and in the body core transmit an electrical signal—in our case, through thermosensory neurons—to a part of the brain known as the hypothalamus. If it senses a sustained drop below the physiological set point of about 37 degrees Celsius (98.6 degrees Fahrenheit), it sends excitatory signals through the sympathetic nervous system to brown fat reserves. These reserves then respond like a furnace switched on by a signal from the thermostat: the hormone noradrenalin, released from the terminals of sympathetic nerves, binds to receptors on the surface of brown fat cells, prompting them to fire up thermogenesis and distribute the heat generated throughout the body via the bloodstream.

If this process sounds unfamiliar, that's because it takes place continuously and without our conscious participation. The response to cold that we are more likely to notice is shivering, but that is actually a much less efficient process caused by the activation of antagonistic muscle pairs when the usual system of thermogenesis cannot meet the immediate challenge of a sudden blast of cold.

Source of Energy Inside the Cell

Inside the cells of animals and plants, mitochondria—double-membraned, rod-shaped structures—serve as the power plants for turning foodstuffs into respiratory energy. In muscle and most other healthy cells, the energy released by the burning of fats, carbohydrates, and proteins is used, in part, for the synthesis of adenosine triphosphate (ATP), the universal energy currency of living things. The energy released by the oxidation of foodstuffs is used to pump protons across the innermost membrane of the mitochondrion from the inside to the outside to set up a proton gradient. This difference then powers the synthesis of ATP from adenosine diphosphate (ADP) and inorganic phosphate (P_i) when protons come back across the inner membrane through a channel in the enzyme (ATP synthase) that is responsible for catalyzing this reaction. When protons flow back through the ATP synthase, the electrochemical energy (the same type of energy stored in an electrical battery) in the proton gradient is converted to chemical bond energy by the combination of ADP with P_i to give ATP. These mitochondria are said to be coupled, because the combustion of carbon compounds is tightly linked to the production of ATP.

When the mitochondria of brown fat cells engage in thermogenesis, the trick they play is to allow the protons that are pumped out during respiration to move down their inwardly directed gradient through a proton channel distinct from the channel in the ATP synthase. Aptly named *uncoupling protein 1* (UCP1), this channel conducts protons from the outside to the inside of the brown fat cell mitochondrion, thus bypassing proton movement through the ATP synthase. In this way UCP1 accelerates fuel consumption, while at the same time releasing energy as heat instead of storing the energy as ATP.

Why do our brown fat cells engage in such elaborate maneuvers simply in order to generate heat? The true genius of this system is that it is driven by the products of fat breakdown. If UCP1 is to ferry protons across the inner mitochondrial membrane, it must first bind fatty acids—the same fatty acids that are derived from the breakdown of storage fat, which in turn is triggered by the interaction of noradrenalin with its receptors on the surfaces of brown fat cells. In other words, the preferred fuel for thermogenesis and the intracellular signal that initiates it are one and the same thing: fatty acids derived from breakdown of the fat droplets stored in brown fat cells.

Sleeper Cells

What we have described is only one part of the story—the part explaining the function of brown fat in general, along with the relatively recent realization that brown adipose tissue, or something resembling it, exists in human adults. Another, newer part of the story, however, has emerged in just the past couple of years, with the discovery that the tissue hailed as brown fat in healthy adult humans does not have the same composition as the classical brown fat cells of newborn babies. In fact, this third type appears different from the well-known forms of both brown and white adipose tissue. Even more intriguing, the number of such cells can change in response to an individual's metabolic needs. These cells, resembling brown fat embedded in white fat reserves, were first observed in the 1980s, but it was not until 2012 that researchers came to understand their unique nature. The cells look for all intents and purposes like brown fat cells, and like brown fat cells they express UCP1. Because they are embedded within subcutaneous white fat, where they contribute a brown coloration to an otherwise off-white matrix, these have been dubbed "beige" or "brite" (as in *br*own *i*n whi*te*) cells.

For some time, scientists attempted to identify the developmental switch responsible for transforming white fat to brown fat. We now know, however, that no such transformation takes place, for two very good reasons. First, the developmental pathway for brown fat cells is distinct from that for white fat cells. Astonishing as it may seem, brown fat cells share their origins not with white fat but with muscle cells. In an animal model, when one of the genes is blocked that ordinarily shows high levels of expression in brown fat precursor cells, these cells do not revert to white fat cells—instead they convert to muscle cells. Remarkably, these cells begin to twitch! Harvard medical researcher Bruce Spiegelman, whose laboratory at the Dana-Farber Cancer Institute conducted the study, considers this "the most shocking result in [his] 30 years as a principal investigator."

The second piece of evidence against a white-to-brown-fat switch has just been published. In 2013 another Harvard team, led by Yu-Hua Tseng of the Joslin Diabetes Center, studied mice that have no brown fat cells at all, owing to a mutation in the signaling pathway. By rights, these animals should have to shiver constantly in order to maintain their body temperature, and yet they do not do so. Instead they draw on the beige cells stored in their white fat reserves. As mentioned earlier, the precursors or "sleeper cells" that give rise to beige fat have a different lineage from that of either brown or white fat.

Beige fat cells demonstrate a versatility that classical white and brown fat cells lack: After being recruited for thermogenic purposes, they can switch from burning fat to accumulating fat and back again. In their unstimulated, sleeper state, beige fat cells resemble their white neighbors, with minimal expression of the genes associated with thermogenesis, including UCP1. Under the stimulus of a cold environment, however, beige fat cells increase their expression of UCP1 to levels characteristic of brown fat cells. Moreover, and this is what gives the discovery of beige fat cells such far-reaching implications, the cells found in the supraclavicular regions of healthy human adults—where earlier researchers thought they had found classical brown fat—now turn out to have a gene expression profile more like that of beige fat in mice than that of classical brown fat cells in newborn humans.

Because it has been established that the gene expression profiles of these cells in human adults clearly differ from those found in the corresponding regions of human newborns, we must consider the possibility that many if not most studies thought to have been conducted on human adult brown fat were actually not carried out on classical brown adipose tissue at all, but instead were done on thermogenically active, UCP1-positive, beige fat cells. The bottom line is that the presence of thermogenically active fat cells in adults, once thought to be decided by an all-or-none roll of the genetic dice, may turn out to be more amenable to change than originally thought.

Bright Prospects for Beige Fat

Certain take-home lessons for us humans are already becoming clear. Beige fat in adults likely represents an evolutionarily conserved mechanism for adaptive thermogenesis, by means of the recruitment of this cell type according to need. In more practical terms, beige fat satisfies many of the requirements of a therapeutic target that until recently was not even known to exist. If there is a target for the treatment of obesity and obesity-associated cardiovascular disease and type 2 diabetes that stands out as particularly manipulable and potentially "druggable," it is beige fat, rather than white or brown.

White fat deposition, weight gain, and obesity develop when energy balance is out of whack, because energy intake consistently exceeds expenditure. The discovery of beige fat offers nothing new here: The first line of attack in weight control is still diet and exercise. Two insights, however, are unprecedented. The first is our appreciation that in adult humans, the abundance and activity of what was formerly thought to be classical brown fat but is now known to be beige, are inversely related to total body fat. Skinny types generally have more beige fat than others, and although it decreases with age, those who hold on to their beige fat longer are less likely to put on weight later in life. In short, if changes in lifestyle can be found to have an effect on the recruitment or activation of beige fat, or if drugs can be developed that have the same effect, it may someday become possible to halt unwanted weight gain, or even to reverse it.

The second insight to be gained from the discovery of beige fat concerns two unfortunate aspects of adulthood: diet-induced weight gain and middle-age spread. Specifically, we now have a better understanding of what it is about regular exercise that makes it such a potent antidote to the downside of aging.

These results are promising, but it remains to be determined if they will prove as applicable to older people or to those whose health is compromised (for example, because of weight problems) as they are to the healthy subjects of these studies. Other questions remain, such as how long the effects may last and whether there are harmful repercussions. Patrick Seale (who, with his colleague Spiegelman, first demonstrated the common origin of brown fat and muscle cells), points out that finding the answers to these questions may not be as simple as it appears, because increasing the activity of beige or brown fat inevitably entails expending more energy and burning more calories in a system that normally is all about energy conservation. In his words, "Our bodies are very smart": The metabolic system can find ways to compensate for a rise in demand, whether through increased appetite or reduced physical activity.

A Crucial Messenger

In the course of millions of years of evolution our ancestors have struggled to take in enough calories for sustenance, so perhaps it is not surprising that today, some of us find it very difficult to lose weight and keep it off. Be that as it may, in the light of our new understanding, lifestyle changes of this type surely warrant further investigation, if only as a way of possibly augmenting more robust regimens to fight obesity.

The search for ways to control obesity has gone on a long time, but in just the past couple of years it may have reached a major turning point: the discovery of the hormone irisin, a polypeptide secreted by muscle cells. First identified in rodents by the Spiegelman research team, irisin increases the expression of UCP1 and other thermogenic genes in white fat deposits, while at the same time increasing dissipative energy expenditure.

If white adipose tissue can be said to have a nemesis, it is this hormone, which has little or no effect on classical brown fat cells but causes a marked increase in the browning of white fat, and whose circulating level in both rodents and humans rises in response to sustained activity. In recognition of its role as a muscle-to-fat go-between, the researchers have named the substance after Iris, the messenger of the Olympian gods. Spiegelman and his colleagues are currently exploring the potential of irisin as a pharmaceutical product for the treatment of type 2 diabetes and obesity through their private company, Ember Therapeutics (with which the authors of this paper have no commercial ties).

In evolutionary terms, the secretion of irisin by muscle cells in response to sustained physical activity may not seem highly adaptive for mammals. If anything, the opposite trait—a capacity to extend energy reserves as far as possible—should be helpful for survival. Why, instead, do we have a regulatory circuit that apparently increases beige fat thermogenesis and dissipative energy expenditure just when energy expenditure by muscle is at its greatest?

The question remains open, but the most reasonable explanation offered so far concerns the balance between two kinds of thermogenesis: the way we warm our bodies by shivering when we're cold and the way we keep warm enough most of the time without shivering. When we undergo a prolonged spell of shivering, the secretion of irisin may perhaps serve to activate beige fat thermogenesis to further enhance heat production. If this hypothesis holds true, the increased energy we expend in maintaining body temperature would eventually be shifted from muscle to fat, the latter of which is calorically richer in energy reserves than the former (which draws on carbohydrate, or glycogen, reserves). Such a system would explain why the benefits of regular endurance exercise far outweigh those expected from the extra calories consumed when actually performing the exercise: There would be a sustained after-burn as a result of exercise-triggered irisin production and beige fat recruitment.

Our understanding of the biochemistry, physiology, and developmental biology of body fat has undergone a radical revision—perhaps not a paradigm shift, but close to it—in a matter of only a few years. First we had brown fat, which we found out was only for babies; then we had beige fat, which is probably what our brown fat is; and now we have muscle-derived factors that can drive the browning/beiging of white fat to potentially tip the scales in favor of thermogenic dissipative fat combustion to melt the white stuff away.

A Deadly Surrogate

To students of dietary history, the idea of combatting obesity by means of uncoupling metabolism is not altogether new. Long before the discovery of thermogenic fats, a yellow phenolic by the name of 2,4-dinitrophenol (2,4-DNP), which in the 19th century had been added to commercial baked products to make them appear buttery or "egg-rich," had been brought to market as a slimming agent in the 1930s.

2,4-DNP was used extensively in the manufacture of explosives, first in France during World War I and then in the late 1920s and early 1930s in Belgium and the United States. The compound was also studied for its toxic properties, specifically the elevation of body temperature associated with its ingestion. The outcome of these inquiries was that 2,4-DNP stimulated metabolism (measured as oxygen consumption) while promoting weight loss and elevation of body temperature.

Appalling as it may seem in the light of what we now know, more than 100,000 people in the United States, and many more in Europe, eventually used these medications. It was only after many fatalities associated with a precipitous elevation of body temperature, innumerable cases of cataracts and blindness (as reported, for example, in this July 9, 1935, item in the *New York Times*) and other adverse reactions that the anti-obesity medications containing 2,4-DNP were banned.

With the benefit of hindsight, we now understand what makes this phenolic so toxic. As an uncoupling agent, 2,4-DNP is a fat-soluble weak acid that rapidly—in some cases, too rapidly—equilibrates protons across the inner mitochondrial membrane with the release of heat.

One might think we have learned from this lesson; yet, to this day, 2,4-DNP can still be purchased on the Internet as an aid to bodybuilding and weight loss. Every so often, there are news reports of overzealous or uninformed bodybuilders or weight-watchers who succumb and die after dosing themselves up with it.

This cautionary tale is not meant to imply, however, that uncoupling agents are inherently hazardous. For irisin and its mimetics, quite the contrary is true, for the simple reason that the effects exerted by irisin are tissue-specific, whereas 2,4-DNP is indiscriminate in its uncoupling action. The feature of 2,4-DNP that makes it so dangerous is that it uncouples electron flow from ATP synthesis indiscriminately in muscle, nerve, epithelial, or any other cell type, to abolish ATP synthesis and impose mock thermogenesis. In strict contrast, irisin is exquisitely specific, with its thermogenic action restricted to UCP1-containing beige fat cells.

Tantalizing as these recent advances are, we should be careful not to overstate the case. The global epidemic of obesity, diabetes, and cardiovascular disease is an inordinately complex issue. Not only does it involve the intricate interplay of many biological factors but it is also rife with gnarly socioeconomic, geopolitical, and psychological ones. Stated plainly, it would be folly to think in terms of diet pills that drive beige fat expansion or activation as a simple fix or cure-all.

In a similar vein, with the all but inexorable development of strategies for playing around with the ratio of beige fat to white fat by means of drugs, surgery, or genetic manipulation, we should be ever mindful of potentially deleterious side effects, either in the short term or in the long term. A case in point is the study published by an international group led by Yihai Cao, of the Karolinska Institute, indicating that when chilling is used as a stimulus to activate brown fat and expand the beige fat cell population in mice with cardiovascular disease, the cold accelerates the growth of atherosclerotic plaque in their arteries instead of halting it. That is, in mice with diseased arteries, a cold environment actually raises the risk of heart attack.

This isolated report has yet to be independently corroborated, but one insight already clear from this work is that knocking out the gene encoding UCP1 in mice with preexisting cardiovascular disease effectively puts the brakes on cold-induced disease progression. It is as if the loss of UCP1 and the resulting abolition of cold-induced thermogenesis collude to bring about a cardioprotective state. This discovery, together with the finding that healthy mice do not appear to be susceptible to the cold-induced progression of cardiovascular disease, indicates that researchers should proceed with caution when it comes to ramping up beige or brown fat-associated thermogenesis in people who already have cardiovascular disease or are predisposed to it. Researchers have not yet determined whether the mouse model of cardiovascular disease is truly equivalent to the disease in humans in this context. If the mouse model proves true, however, its implications will include a bitter irony: Cao's study will indicate that people with preexisting cardiovascular disease, those who stand to gain the most from getting their weight under control through beige fat recruitment, may be poor candidates for an intervention of this type, because they are the ones most at risk of suffering serious side effects.

Clearly, despite these potential concerns, we should make the most of every advantage gained, no matter how small. Irisin is one such advantage, in that it not only has the potential to confer the fat-burning benefits of exercise but also, as shown in just the last few months in mice, appears to stimulate the production of neuroprotective factors in the brain.

Irisin may turn out to be more than just a muscle-to-fat go-between. There is still a lot of work to be done in this area, but the results of some preliminary studies have been intriguing. In the bloodstream of mice that have undergone endurance exercise on a running wheel over the course of 30 days, a rise in irisin levels is associated with an increase in the expression of a brain-health protein in the hippocampus, a part of the brain responsible for memory and learning.

Although it has yet to be determined if this effect is accompanied by improved cognitive function, the implication is obvious. The brain-health protein in question, brain-derived neurotrophic protein, is known to promote the formation of new nerves and neural connections, and there are only two areas in the brain known to generate new nerve cells in an adult. One of these areas is the hippocampus, the structure in which irisin elicits an increase of this neurotrophic factor.

Irisin or its mimetics therefore offer the promise of a surrogate for the weight control and cognitive benefits of regular exercise to the morbidly obese and those who are wheelchair-bound or have advanced cardiovascular disease, for whom exercise is not an option. If safe drugs that specifically target beige fat can be found—something that was not even a remote possibility two or three years ago—they could give hope to those who find themselves in this position.

Bibliography

Boström, P., et al. 2012. A PGC1-α-dependent myokine that drives brown-fat-like development of white fat and thermogenesis. *Nature* 481:463–468.

Dong, M., et al. 2013. Cold exposure promotes atherosclerotic plaque growth and instability via UCP1-dependent lipolysis. *Cell Metabolism* 18:118–129.

Nedergaard, J., T. Bengtsson, and B. Cannon. 2007. Unexpected evidence for active brown adipose tissue in human adults. *American Journal of Physiology, Endocrinology, and Metabolism* 293:E444–E452.

Rajakumari, S., et al. 2013. EBF2 determines and maintains brown adipocyte identity. *Cell Metabolism* 17:562–574.

Seale, P., et al. 2008. PRDM16 controls a brown fat/skeletal muscle switch. *Nature* 454:961–967.

Schultz, T. J., et al. 2013. Brown-fat paucity due to impaired BMP signaling induces compensatory browning of white fat. *Nature* 495:379–383.

Spiegelman, B. M. 2013. Banting Lecture. Regulation of adipogenesis: Toward new therapeutics for metabolic disease. *Diabetes* 62:1774–1782.

Wrann, C. D., et al. 2013. Exercise induces hippocampal BDNF through a PGC-1α/FNDC5 pathway. *Cell Metabolism* 18:1–11.

Wu, J., et al. 2012. Beige adipocytes are a distinct type of thermogenic fat cell in mouse and human. *Cell* 150:366–376.

Wu, J., P. Cohen, and B. M. Spiegelman. 2013. Adaptive thermogenesis in adipocytes: Is beige the new brown? *Genes & Development* 27:234–250.

Yoneshiro, T., et al. 2013. *Journal of Clinical Investigation* 123:3404–34088.

Critical Thinking

1. Compare the effects of irisin to the effects of 2.4 dinitrophenol.
2. Explain the proposed mechanism exercise might have in switching white fat to beige fat.

Create Central

www.mhhe.com/createcentral

Internet References

American College of Sports Medicine
www.acsm.org/

The American Society of Nutrition
www.nutrition.org/

The Nutrition Society
www.nutritionsociety.org/

Philip A. Rea is professor of biology and Rebecka and Arie Belldegrun Distinguished Director of the Roy and Diana Vagelos Program in Life Sciences & Management at the University of Pennsylvania. He has received the President's Medal of the Society for Experimental Biology and has been elected as a Fellow of the American Association for the Advancement of Science for his fundamental research. **Peter Yin** and **Ryan Zahalka** are rising seniors in Penn's College of Arts & Sciences. Yin is majoring in computational biology; Zahalka, in molecular biology. Address: Department of Biology, University of Pennsylvania, Philadelphia, PA 19104. E-mail: parea@sas.upenn.edu

Philip A. Rea, Peter Yin, Ryan Zahalka, "Can Skinny Fat Beat Obesity?," *American Scientist*, vol. 102, 4, July/August 2014, pp. 272–279.

Article

Prepared by: Janet Colson, *Middle Tennessee State University*

The Hungry Brain

The urge to eat too much is wired into our heads. **Tackling obesity may require bypassing the stomach** and short-circuiting our brains.

Dan Hurley

Learning Outcomes

After reading this article, you will be able to:

- Describe how the brain influences what we eat.
- Compare the actions of the hormones that influence food intake.

At 10:19 p.m. on a Monday evening in October, I sat in a booth at Chevys Fresh Mex in Clifton, New Jersey, reviewing the latest research into the neurobiology of hunger and obesity. While I read I ate a shrimp and crab enchilada, consuming two-thirds of it, maybe less. With all this information in front of me, I thought, I had an edge over my brain's wily efforts to thwart my months-long campaign to get under 190 pounds. But even as I was taking in a study about the powerful lure of guacamole and other salty, fatty foods, I experienced something extraordinary. That bowl of chips and salsa at the edge of the table? It was whispering to me: *Just one more. You know you want us. Aren't we delicious?* In 10 minutes, all that was left of the chips, and my willpower, were crumbs.

I am not alone. An overabundance of chips, Baconator Double burgers, and Venti White Chocolate Mochas have aided a widespread epidemic of obesity in this country. Our waists are laying waste to our health and to our health-care economy: According to a study published by the Centers for Disease Control and Prevention in 2010, nine states had an obesity rate of at least 30 percent—compared with zero states some 10 years earlier—and the cost of treatment for obesity-related conditions had reached nearly 10 percent of total U.S. medical expenditure. So-called normal weight is no longer normal, with two-thirds of adults and one third of children and adolescents now classified as overweight or obese. Dubbed the "Age of Obesity and Inactivity" by the *Journal of the American Medical Association,* this runaway weight gain threatens to decrease average U.S. life span, reversing gains made over the past century by lowering risk factors from smoking, hypertension, and cholesterol. We all know what we should do—eat less, exercise more—but to no avail. An estimated 25 percent of American men and 43 percent of women attempt to lose weight each year; of those who succeed in their diets, between 5 and 20 percent (and it is closer to 5 percent) manage to keep it off for the long haul.

The urgent question is, why do our bodies seem to be fighting against our own good health? According to a growing number of neurobiologists, the fault lies not in our stomachs but in our heads. No matter how convincing our conscious plans and resolutions, they pale beside the brain's power to goad us into noshing and hanging on to as much fat as we can. With that in mind, some scientists were hopeful that careful studies of the brain might uncover an all-powerful hormone that regulates food consumption or a single spot where the cortical equivalent of a neon sign blinks "Eat Heavy," all the better to shut it off.

After extensive research, the idea of a single, simple cure has been replaced by a much more nuanced view. The latest studies show that a multitude of systems in the brain act in concert to encourage eating. Targeting a single neuronal system is probably doomed to the same ill fate as the failed diets themselves. Because the brain has so many backup systems all geared toward the same thing—maximizing the body's intake of calories—no single silver bullet will ever work.

The brain's prime directive to eat and defend against the loss of fat emerged early in evolution.

"I call it the 'hungry brain syndrome'," says Hans-Rudolf Berthoud, an expert in the neurobiology of nutrition at the Pennington Biomedical Research Center in Baton Rouge, Louisiana. The brain's prime directive to eat and defend against the loss of fat emerged early in evolution, because just about every creature that ever trotted, crawled, swam, or floated was beset by the uncertainty of that next meal. "The system has evolved to defend against the slightest threat of weight loss, so you have to attack it from different directions at once."

With the obesity epidemic raging, the race for countermeasures has kicked into high gear. Neuroscientists are still seeking hormones that inhibit hunger, but they have other tactics as well. One fruitful new avenue comes from the revelation that hunger, blood sugar, and weight gained per calorie consumed all ratchet up when our sleep is disrupted and our circadian rhythms—the 24-hour cycle responding to light and dark—[are] thrown into disarray. All this is compounded by stress, which decreases metabolism while increasing the yen for high-calorie food. We might feel in sync with our high-tech world, but the obesity epidemic is a somber sign that our biology and lifestyles have diverged.

Seeking Silver Bullets, Shooting Blanks

The path forward seemed so simple back in 1995, when three papers in *Science* suggested a panacea for the overweight: A hormone that made animals shed pounds, rapidly losing body fat until they were slim. Based on the research, it seemed that doctors might soon be able to treat obesity the way they treat diabetes, with a simple metabolic drug.

Fat cells release that "diet" hormone—today named leptin, from the Greek *leptos,* meaning thin—to begin a journey across the blood-brain barrier to the hypothalamus, the pea-size structure above the pituitary gland. The hypothalamus serves as a kind of thermostat, setting not only body temperature but playing a key role in hunger, thirst, fatigue, and sleep cycles. Leptin signals the hypothalamus to reduce the sense of hunger so that we stop eating.

In early lab experiments, obese mice given extra leptin by injection seemed sated. They ate less, their body temperature increased, and their weight plummeted. Even normal-weight mice became skinnier when given injections of the hormone.

Once the pharmaceutical industry created a synthetic version of human leptin, clinical trials were begun. But when injected into hundreds of obese human volunteers, leptin's effect was clinically insignificant. It soon became clear why. In humans, as in mice, fat cells of the obese already produced plenty of leptin—more in fact than those of their thin counterparts, since the level of leptin was directly proportional to the amount of fat. The early studies had worked largely because the test mice were, by experimental design, leptin-deficient. Subsequent experiments showed that in normal mice—as in humans—increases in leptin made little difference to the brain, which looked to *low* leptin levels as a signal to eat more, essentially disregarding the kind of high levels that had caused deficient mice to eat less. This made leptin a good drug for maintaining weight loss but not a great candidate for getting the pounds off up front.

Despite that disappointment, the discovery of leptin unleashed a scientific gold rush to find other molecules that could talk the brain into turning hunger off. By 1999 researchers from Japan's National Cardiovascular Center Research Institute in Osaka had announced the discovery of ghrelin, a kind of antileptin that is released primarily by the gut rather than by fat cells. Ghrelin signals hunger rather than satiety to the hypothalamus. Then, in 2002, a team from the University of Washington found that ghrelin levels rise before a meal and fall immediately after. Ghrelin (from the Indo-European root for the word "grow") increased hunger while jamming on the metabolic brakes to promote the body's storage of fat.

So began another line of attack on obesity. Rather than turning leptin on, researchers began exploring ways to turn ghrelin off. Some of them began looking at animal models, but progress has been slow; the concept of a ghrelin "vaccine" has been floated, but clinical trials are still years off.

Seeking a better understanding of the hormone, University of Washington endocrinologist David Cummings compared ghrelin levels in people who had lost considerable amounts of weight through diet with those who shed pounds by means of gastric bypass surgery—a technique that reduces the capacity of the stomach and seems to damage its ghrelin-producing capacity as well. The results were remarkable. For dieters, the more weight lost, the greater the rise in ghrelin, as if the body were telling the brain to get hungry and regain that weight. By contrast, the big losers in the surgical group saw ghrelin levels fall to the floor. Surgical patients never felt increases in appetite and had an easier time maintaining their weight loss as a result. (A newer weight-loss surgery removes most of the ghrelin-producing cells outright.)

Based on such findings, a ghrelin-blocking drug called rimonabant was approved and sold in 32 countries, though not in the United States. It remained available as recently as 2008, even though it also increased the risk of depression and suicidal thinking; it has since been withdrawn everywhere. The verdict is still out on a newer generation of combination pharmaceuticals, including one that contains synthetic versions of leptin and the neurohormone amylin, known to help regulate appetite. In a six-month clinical trial, the combination therapy resulted in an average weight loss of 25 pounds, or 12.7 percent of body weight, with greater weight loss when continued for a full 52 weeks; those who stopped taking the drug midway regained most of their weight.

The Circadian Connection

The limited results from tackling the hypothalamus sent many scientists looking at the other gyres and gears driving obesity in the brain, especially in regions associated with sleep. The first big breakthrough came in 2005, when *Science* published a landmark paper on mice with a mutated version of the Clock gene, which plays a key role in the regulation of the body's circadian rhythms. The mutant mice not only failed to follow the strict eat-by-night, sleep-by-day schedule of normally nocturnal mice, they also became overweight and developed diabetes. "There was a difference in weight gain based on when the food was eaten, whether during day or night," says the study's senior author, endocrinologist Joe Bass of Northwestern University. "That means the metabolic rate must differ under those two conditions."

Could *my* late-night hours be the undoing of my weight-loss plans? Four days after my humiliating defeat by a bowl of tortilla chips, I met with Alex Keene, a postdoctoral researcher at New York University with a Matisse nude tattooed on his right forearm and a penchant for studying flies. His latest study asked whether a starved fly would take normal naps or sacrifice sleep to keep searching for food. He found that like humans (and most other creatures), flies have a neurological toggle between two fundamental yet incompatible drives: to eat or to sleep. "Flies only live a day or two when they're starved," Keene told me as we walked past graduate students peering at flies under microscopes. "If they decide to sleep through the night when they're starved, it's a bad decision on their part. So their brains are finely tuned to suppress their sleep when they don't have food and to sleep well after a meal."

For a major study published last year, Keene bred flies with dysfunctional mutations of the Clock gene and also of Cycle, another gene involved in circadian rhythms. He found that the genes together regulate the interaction between the two mutually exclusive behaviors, sleep and feeding, kicking in to suppress sleep when a fly is hungry.

Even when fed, flies without working versions of the Clock and Cycle genes tended to sleep poorly—about 30 percent as much as normal flies. "It was as if they were starving right away," Keene explains. Keene went even further, pinpointing where, amid the 100,000 or so neurons in the fly brain, the Clock gene acts to regulate the sleeping-feeding interaction: a region of just four to eight cells at the top of the fly brain.

"My father is an anthropologist," Keene told me as we stood in the fly room, its air pungent with the corn meal and molasses the flies feed on. "It's ironic, right? He looks at how culture determines behavior, while I look at how genes determine behavior. I used to get him so mad he'd storm out of the house."

Perhaps it takes an anthropologist's son to see that the excess availability of cheap, high-calorie chow cannot fully explain the magnitude and persistence of the problem in our culture. The rebellion against our inborn circadian rhythms wrought by a 24-hour lifestyle, lit by neon and fueled by caffeine, also bears part of the blame. The powerful effect of disordered sleep on metabolism has been seen not just in flies but also in humans. A 2009 study by Harvard University researchers showed that in just 10 days, three of eight healthy volunteers developed prediabetic blood-sugar levels when their sleep-wake schedule was gradually shifted out of alignment.

"It's clear from these types of studies that the way we're keeping the lights on until late at night, the way in which society demands that we stay active for so much longer, could well be contributing to aspects of the metabolic disease we're seeing now," says Steve Kay, a molecular geneticist at the University of California, San Diego.

These insights have fostered collaboration between once-diverse groups. "Physicians who specialized in obesity and diabetes for years are now discovering the importance of circadian effects," Kay says. At the same time, "basic research scientists like me, who have been studying the circadian system for so many years, are now looking at its metabolic effects. When so many people's research from so many areas starts to converge, you know we're in the midst of a paradigm shift. This is the slow rumbling before the volcano blows."

This past April, the National Institute of Diabetes and Digestive and Kidney Diseases (NIDDK) of the National Institutes of Health organized a first-ever national conference focused solely on how circadian rhythms affect metabolism. "What has become obvious over the past few years is that metabolism, all those pathways regulating how fats and carbohydrates are used, is affected by the circadian clock," says biochemist Corinne Silva, a program director at the NIDDK. Her goal is to find drugs that treat diabetes and obesity by targeting circadian pathways. "The mechanisms by which circadian rhythms are maintained and the cross talk with metabolic signaling are just beginning to be elucidated," she says, but they should lead to novel therapeutic approaches in the years ahead.

In Keene's view, the newfound link between sleep and obesity could be put to use right now. "People who are susceptible to diabetes or have weight issues might just get more sleep. I get only about six hours of sleep myself. I usually run in the middle of the night. I'm not a morning person," the enviably thin, 29-year-old Keene states.

My visit to his fly room convinced me to try a new angle in my quest to get under 190 pounds: Rather than focus on *how much* food I put in my mouth, I would focus on *when* I eat. I decided I would no longer eat after 10 P.M.

The Pleasure Factor

Timing may be everything for some folks, but it wasn't for me. No wonder: The brain has no shortage of techniques to goad us into eating. Another line of evidence suggests that the brains of overweight people are wired to feel more pleasure in response to food. Sleep deprived or not, they just enjoy eating more. To study such differences, clinical psychologist Eric Stice of the Oregon Research Institute mastered the delicate task of conducting fMRI brain scans while people were eating. The food he chose to give the volunteers inside the tunnel-like scanners was a milk shake. And let the record show, it was a *chocolate* milk shake.

Brains of the overweight are wired to feel more pleasure in response to food.

Obese adolescent girls, Stice found, showed greater activation compared with their lean peers in regions of the brain that encode the sensory experience of eating food—the so-called gustatory cortex and the somatosensory regions, archipelagoes of neurons that reach across different structures in the brain. At the same time, the obese girls sipping milk shakes showed decreased activation in the striatum, a region near the center of the brain that is studded with dopamine receptors and known to respond to stimuli associated with rewards. Stice wondered whether, even among normal-weight girls, such a pattern might predict an increased risk of overeating and weight gain.

To test his hypothesis, he followed a group of subjects over time, finding that those with reduced activation in the dorsal (rear) region of the striatum while sipping a milk shake were ultimately more likely to gain weight than those with normal activation. The most vulnerable of these girls were also more likely to have a DNA polymorphism—not a mutation, per se, but a rather routine genetic variation—in a dopamine receptor gene, causing reduced dopamine signaling in the striatum and placing them at higher risk. "Individuals may overeat," Stice and his colleagues concluded, "to compensate for a hypofunctioning dorsal striatum, particularly those with genetic polymorphisms thought to attenuate dopamine signaling in this region."

Stice was initially surprised by the results. "It's totally weird," he admits. "Those who experienced less pleasure were at increased risk for weight gain." But his more recent studies have convinced him that the reduced pleasure is a result of years of overeating among the obese girls—the same phenomenon seen in drug addicts who require ever-greater amounts of their drug to feel the same reward. "Imagine a classroom of third graders, and everyone is skinny," he says. "The people who initially find that milk shake most orgasmic will want more of it, but in so doing they cause neuroplastic changes that downregulate the reward circuitry, driving them to eat more and more to regain that same feeling they crave."

Even among people of normal weight, individual differences in brain functioning can directly affect eating behaviors, according to a 2009 study by Michael Lowe, a research psychologist at Drexel University. He took fMRI brain scans of 19 people, all of them of normal weight. Nine of the volunteers reported following strict diets; the other 10 typically ate whenever and whatever they wanted. Lowe had all of them sip a milk shake immediately before getting scanned. The brains of the nondieters, he found, lit up just as one would expect, showing activations in areas associated with satiation and memory, as if saying, "Mmmm, that was good." The chronic dieters showed activations in areas of the brain associated with desire and expectation of reward, however. If anything, the milk shake had made them hungrier.

"What we have shown is that these chronic dieters may actually have a reason to restrain themselves, because they are more susceptible than average to overeating," Lowe says.

Yet inborn differences in hunger and desire, too, turn out to be only part of the weighting game. Eating behaviors are also linked to areas of the brain associated with self-control (such as the left superior frontal region) and visual attention (such as the right middle temporal region). A recent fMRI study led by Jeanne McCaffery, a psychologist at Brown Medical School, showed that successful weight losers had greater activation in those regions, compared with normal-weight people and obese people, when viewing images of food.

The effects of stress on eating behaviors also has a neurobiological basis, according to University of Pennsylvania neurobiologist Tracy Bale. She showed that neural pathways associated with stress link directly to areas of the brain associated with seeking rewards. "Few things are more rewarding evolutionarily than calorie-dense food," Bale told me a few days after presenting a seminar on the subject at last fall's Society for Neuroscience meeting in San Diego. "Under stress people don't crave a salad; they crave something high-calorie. It's because those stress pathways in the limbic system feed into the reward centers, and they drive reward-seeking behaviors. What that tells us is that in addition to drug companies' trying to target appetite, they need to look at the reward centers. We're not necessarily fat because we're hungry but because we're looking for something to deal with stress."

Aha! Perhaps it was stress that was messing with my latest, clock-based diet. Back in March 2010, a tree had fallen on my family's home during a major storm, crushing the roof, destroying half the house, and forcing us to flee to a nearby apartment. By November, as I researched this story, we had finally moved back into our rebuilt house. With nerves fully frayed, I found myself drawn as never before to the Tick Tock Diner, where the motto literally is "Eat Heavy," and where the french fries never tasted better. Instead of losing a few pounds to get under 190, by Thanksgiving I had hit 196.

How to Fix a Hungry Brain

Neuroscience has yet to deliver a weight-loss elixir for paunchy 53-year-old journalists like me, much less for those suffering from serious obesity. But that day will come, Steve Kay asserts, once researchers figure out the correct combination of drugs that work simultaneously on multiple triggers of eating and metabolism, just as hypertension is now routinely treated with two- or three-drug combinations.

Some scientists think a more radical approach is called for. Since the triggers of obesity lie in the brain, neurosurgeons at West Virginia University Health Sciences Center are attempting to rewire those triggers directly using deep brain stimulation (DBS). Since 2009 they have performed surgery on three obese patients to implant electrodes that emit rhythmic electric shocks into the hypothalamus. Having failed other medical therapies for obesity, the three agreed to volunteer for DBS, a treatment already approved for treating the tremors and dystonia of Parkinson's disease. "These patients weren't eating all that much; it was mainly a problem of having very slow metabolisms," says Donald M. Whiting, one of the neurosurgeons leading the study. "Our goal was to speed it up." On the basis of successful animal studies, he adds, "we thought we'd switch on the energy and collect our Nobel Prize."

All three patients experienced significantly less hunger when the electrodes were switched on, and all regained their normal hunger when the electrodes were switched off. Unfortunately, none lost a significant amount of weight in the study's first year. The problem, Whiting concludes, is that there are many ways to adjust DBS. With four contact points on the electrodes, each placed half a millimeter apart and each adjustable for voltage, frequency, and pulse width, the research team has been seeking the combination of settings that most effectively rev up metabolism. So far they have found settings that work only temporarily.

"The brain is really pretty smart," Whiting says. "It tends to want to reboot to factory settings whenever it can. We find that we can reset things for a week or two, but then the brain gets back to where it wants." Despite the challenges, Whiting remains convinced that finding a safe and effective medical treatment for weight control will be essential to turn the obesity epidemic around—and that no amount of preaching from Oprah, no behavior program from Weight Watchers nor food from Jenny Craig, will ever suffice.

"This mystification that obesity is caused by a lack of willpower or just eating the wrong foods is simply a misconception," Joe Bass of Northwestern told me. "There is so much social stigma attached to weight that we make a lot of value judgments. The effort in science is to peel back those layers of belief and try to understand things in an experimental, rational mode. Just as we have made progress against heart disease with statins and blood pressure drugs, we will find medications that can safely and substantially lower weight."

Months after my investigation of the brain-gut connection began, I faced the acid test. In early March I stepped back onto my bathroom scale for a final weigh-in. Rather than slip below 190, for the first time in my life I had tipped, by a single pound, over 200. You might blame it on insufficient exercise or on the cheese and crackers I failed to remove from my late-night work ritual. I'm blaming it on my brain.

Critical Thinking

1. Explain what is meant by the "hungry brain syndrome."
2. Describe the hormones that influence food intake and explain their actions in the body.
3. Explain the relationships between sleep and the circadian rhythms influencing feeding behavior.

Create Central

www.mhhe.com/createcentral

Internet References

Calorie Control Council
www.caloriecontrol.org

Centers for Disease Control and Prevention: Overweight & Obesity
www.cdc.gov/obesity

Overweight and Obesity in the U.S.—Food Research Action Center
http://frac.org/initiatives/hunger-and-obesity/obesity-in-the-us

Shape Up America!
www.shapeup.org

Article

Prepared by: Janet Colson, *Middle Tennessee State University*

Obesity Rates in U.S. Appear to Be Finally Leveling Off

After three decades of climbing steadily, obesity rates appear to be stabilizing nationwide. Increases among certain demographic groups are still evident, however.

SHARI ROAN

Learning Outcomes

After reading this article, you will be able to:

- State the groups that have experienced the highest increases in BMI during recent years.
- Outline the most recent obesity rate data from the National Health and Nutrition Examination Survey (NHANES).
- Describe the health implications of the "slowing" of obesity.

After a 30-year, record-shattering rise, U.S. obesity rates appear to be stabilizing.

New statistics cited in two papers report only a slight uptick since 2005—leaving public health experts tentatively optimistic that they may be gaining some ground in their efforts to slim down the nation.

Many obesity specialists say the new data, from the Centers for Disease Control and Prevention, are a sign that efforts to address the obesity problem—such as placing nutritional information on food packaging and revising school lunch menus—are beginning to have an effect in a country where two-thirds of adults and one-third of children and teens are overweight or obese.

"A good first step is to stop the increase, so I think this is very positive news," said James O. Hill, director of the Center for Human Nutrition at the University of Colorado Health Sciences Center in Denver. "It may suggest our efforts are starting to make a difference. The bad news is we still have obesity rates that are just astronomical."

Historically, there was little change in Americans' sizes from 1960 through 1980. But obesity rates soared through the end of the century, for reasons that are still debated.

The new studies reflect 2009–10 data, the most recent available, from the government's National Health and Nutrition Examination Survey, which examined 6,000 adults and 4,111 children, measuring their body mass index, among other items. Though a number of organizations measure obesity rates, the survey's data are considered among the most accurate.

The statistics showed that more than 35 percent of U.S. adults (78 million people) are obese, defined as having a body mass index of 30 or greater. That is similar to the 2005–06 rate. Calculated as weight in kilograms divided by height in meters squared, the BMI is not a perfect measure of fatness but is still viewed as the gold standard in assessing population-wide trends.

An additional third of adults are overweight, the analysis found, also similar to the rates in 2005–06.

Likewise, data in children and teenagers from birth to age 19 reflect little change from the survey's 2007–08 data, according to the reports, which were published online Tuesday in the Journal of the American Medical Assn. Almost 17 percent are obese and 32 percent are overweight or obese.

But though obesity rates may be flattening overall, increases and disparities can still be found in specific racial and ethnic groups.

Rates have risen to 58.5 percent among non-Hispanic black women and to nearly 45 percent among Mexican American women since 2004, for example. And among children and teens, about 21 percent of Hispanics and 24 percent of blacks are obese compared with 14 percent of non-Hispanic whites.

The report also found that gender differences appear to be fading, with percentages of overweight males catching up with or even overtaking those of females.

Among males under 19, obesity rose from 14 percent in 1999–2000 to 18.6 percent in the latest survey; in adult men, the rate jumped from 27.5 percent to 35.5 percent.

In addition, more adult men are now overweight or obese as compared with women—73.9 percent to 63.7 percent. Severe obesity remains more common in women, however.

"We found no indication that the prevalence of obesity is declining in any group," the authors wrote in one of the papers, which looked at obesity rates among adults.

It's not clear why obesity rates are still rising in some groups while stabilizing in others, said Cynthia L. Ogden, a coauthor of the two papers and a researcher at the CDC. But the best bet of some leading obesity experts is that obesity prevention initiatives in some pockets of the country are paying off.

The Let's Move! program founded by First Lady Michelle Obama has raised national awareness through actions such as persuading Wal-Mart to stock more healthful foods and working with professional sports organizations to create public service announcements encouraging children to exercise.

Certain states, including California, have made obesity prevention a major health goal through measures to reduce access to sugary drinks and high-calorie, unhealthful snacks in schools.

A UCLA study released in November showed obesity rates ticking down in some parts of the state between 2005 and 2010, including a decline of 2.5 percent in Los Angeles County. And research published last month found obesity rates in New York City children fell 5 percent between the 2006–07 and 2010–11 school years.

"The places that are making serious changes in the schools and communities can take hope that these changes are starting to have an effect," said Dr. James S. Marks, senior vice president and director of the health group for the Robert Wood Johnson Foundation, a private organization aimed at improving health of Americans.

But, he added, a reduction in obesity rates will probably take many more years and more than the smattering of programs and initiatives so far underway.

The best hope for lowering rates, he said, is to stop people from getting fat to begin with: Experience and studies show that it is difficult for obese adults to permanently shed fat and that children who are already overweight or obese are highly likely to be overweight as adults.

Only one prescription anti-obesity medication is currently approved for long-term use, and researchers have stalled in their efforts to find more. Moreover, most obesity is untreated or under-treated.

Since obesity contributes to joint damage as well as diseases such as diabetes, heart disease and certain cancers, the epidemic truly is a national crisis, said Patrick M. O'Neil, president of the Obesity Society and director of the weight management center at the Medical University of South Carolina in Charleston.

"Even if the statistics stay at current prevalence rates, I see little good news in that," O'Neil said.

People should look to their own lives and individual experiences, and strive for progress by eating more healthfully and exercising more, he said.

"On a population basis you are trying to turn an aircraft carrier, and it's going to take a long time for it to change," he said.

Critical Thinking

1. Interpret the most recent obesity rate data from the National Health and Nutrition Examination Survey (NHANES).
2. Identify the two subgroups that have experienced an increase in obesity since 2005.
3. Define the classifications of obesity and overweight based on body mass index.

Create Central

www.mhhe.com/createcentral

Internet References

Calorie Control Council
www.caloriecontrol.org

Centers for Disease Control and Prevention: Overweight & Obesity
www.cdc.gov/obesity

Let's Move!
www. letsmove.gov

Overweight and Obesity in the U.S.—Food Research Action Center
http://frac.org/initiatives/hunger-and-obesity/obesity-in-the-us

Shape Up America!
www.shapeup.org

Article

Prepared by: Janet Colson, *Middle Tennessee State University*

The Subtle Knife

After weight-loss surgery, strange things start happening to people's minds. Samantha Murphy found out for herself.

SAMANTHA MURPHY

Learning Outcomes

After reading this article, you will be able to:

- Evaluate the possible reasons for changes in taste preferences, food cravings, and mental functions that have been reported by individuals who have had bariatric surgery.
- Compare the actions of the hormones that influence food intake.

It had been so long since I had had anything to drink but water. Finally, the day I had been waiting for arrived and I mixed a glass of my favourite peach iced tea. Anticipating its tart sweetness, I took a big swig of the drink, holding it in my mouth to savour the flavour. My euphoria turned to horror. It tasted like fish.

I spat the foul brew into the sink and tried the raspberry flavour. Fish, again. I slumped dejectedly onto the sofa. Why had no one warned me about this?

Two weeks earlier, I had had surgery to help me lose weight. Eating and drinking had been a struggle ever since: my new hypersensitivity to sweetness was surpassed only by the nausea that hit me when I smelled cooking meat. What was going on?

I hunted for answers in online forums. While my turncoat taste buds seemed to be a common phenomenon after weight-loss or bariatric surgery, no one offered a convincing explanation. But I soon realised that I had got off lucky: the forums were filled with horror stories detailing side effects, from memory loss and anxiety to auditory hallucinations. Even more puzzling were the unexplained mental boosts. About three months after surgery, a significant number of people experienced a sudden burst of "mental clarity".

No obvious thread linked these effects—but it seemed that when surgeons operated on our stomachs, something had happened in our brains, too. Even more intriguing, the surgery seems to work precisely because it creates fundamental changes in the brain. How can this be happening?

For me, surgery was a last resort. I had struggled with my weight since early childhood, and last year I finally opted to have a surgical procedure called a duodenal switch.

Surgery offers many ways to reduce the size of the stomach. Least invasive is a band that constricts it, but if you want to surgically restrict the stomach, the most popular option is Roux-en-Y or "gastric bypass". All such bariatric surgeries work on the same principle: they reduce the amount of food the body can absorb. In the US, where 36 per cent of the population is classified as obese, at least 200,000 people sign up to have the surgery every year, and that number keeps climbing.

Keeping the Weight Off

That's because surgery works. Whatever procedure people have, most find that their excess weight melts away within 18 months (*Obesity Surgery,* vol 6, p 651). For at least 50 per cent of those who choose the more invasive methods like Roux-en-Y, the weight stays off, demolishing the abysmal long-term success rates of diets and pills (*Annals of Surgery,* vol 254, p 272).

Initially, this success was thought to be down to the mechanics—constricting the stomach simply meant a person ate less. There was just one problem with that logic. If it were so simple, 50 per cent of people wouldn't regain their weight, for example by eating high-calorie, liquid foods like heavy cream-based soups and ice cream milkshakes. Those who kept the weight off did so in spite of the availability of such work-arounds. There had to be another reason for their success.

The first clue lay in my taste buds' bizarre behaviour and how that affected my food preferences. Most doctors will tell you that long-term weight loss is only possible with sweeping lifestyle changes: eating foods with less fat and fewer calories. Unfortunately, by definition, most weight-loss methods foster a temporary "dieting" mentality, which is quickly discarded when the goal is reached or when disappointment overtakes motivation.

One reason it is so hard to keep weight off is that we are fighting our very nature. We are all hard-wired to crave unhealthy foods, and these cravings only intensify after we have lost weight by dieting.

But a strange thing was happening after bariatric surgery—food cravings were immediately, massively dampened. "People who have lost weight after surgery don't report a compensatory increase in food cravings or hunger the way dieting people do," says Stephen Benoit, a behavioural neuroscientist at the University of Cincinnati, Ohio, who studies obesity. Quite the opposite: they tend to report reduced levels of hunger, fewer food cravings and an overall altered relationship with food.

Food cravings aren't simply reduced, they are transformed. Within hours of any weight-loss surgery, many people can't stand the taste of sugar or fat and sometimes find the very smell offensive, says Carel le Roux, a bariatric endocrinologist at the Imperial Weight Centre in London. For Roux-en-Y, the effects linger. "In the long-term, we find people shifting their food preferences and going for the salad bar instead of a burger and fries," he says.

Might the switch be psychological? Perhaps, after expensive and physically demanding surgery, people convince themselves they crave only healthy foods. So le Roux and his team devised a test to tease out what lay behind these behavioural changes. They performed Roux-en-Y surgery on rats and then tested their subsequent food preferences. Like so many of their human counterparts, the rats almost instantly shifted their tastes to favour lower-fat, lower-sugar items. "These rats had never met a dietician," says le Roux, "so it wasn't as though they were suddenly more motivated to make healthier choices because they had surgery."

Le Roux had confirmed that these changes were physiological. But what could be causing them? An obvious starting point would be the hormones generated by the digestive system. The upper stomach, for example, produces a powerful hunger-promoter called ghrelin. The small intestine releases a number of appetite-suppressing hormones that promote satiety, including glucagon-like peptide-1 (GLP-1) and peptide YY, or PYY. Even fat cells play a part in regulating appetite, releasing leptin, a hormone that inhibits the desire to eat and regulates metabolism.

Weight-loss surgery cuts into these major hormone manufacturing areas, radically altering their production. "Gastrointestinal hormones and leptin levels change after Roux-en-Y, and do so in a favourable direction," says Lauren Beckman, a researcher at the University of Minnesota in Minneapolis who is studying hormonal changes in people who have had bariatric surgery.

Rearranging the stomach also lowers the production of appetite-stimulating ghrelin, which might explain why many surgery recipients have to force themselves to eat (*Journal of Parenteral & Enteral Nutrition,* vol 35, p 169). Leptin, too, is affected, spiking immediately to damp down hunger (*Journal of Clinical Investigation,* vol 118, p 2380).

Could it be that these hormone changes were triggering the weight loss? Beckman thinks so. If it were the other way around, she explains, "elevated hormone levels would not be expected to occur until at least one month later". Instead, she and other researchers are finding that concentrations of appetite-suppressing GLP-1 and PYY increase within about two days. Not only do these changes happen immediately, but they stay that way, Beckman found, for at least one to two years after surgery.

Intriguingly, the effects of GLP-1 and ghrelin seem to reach beyond the metabolism. Recent animal studies have shown that both hormones can disrupt the nervous system and synaptic plasticity—the very mechanisms that create structural and functional changes in the brain. For example, ghrelin alters the wiring of mouse neurons (*The Journal of Clinical Investigation,* vol 116, p 3229).

Researchers are not completely sure what these fluctuating hormones do to the human brain, but they have a ready-made experimental pool: people who have had weight-loss surgery.

Change Your Stomach, Change Your Brain

After weight-loss surgery, the production of hormones by the digestive system is immediately altered, which seems to affect the way the brain responds to food.

Appetite Regulators

Several hormones produced in the gut affect the brain's satiety centres, particularly the hypothalamus and potentially the thalami.

Ghrelin
Appetite-stimulating hormone
Released by stomach

Glucagon-like peptide-1 (GLP-1):
Appetite-suppressing hormone
Released by small intestine

Peptide YY (PYY)
Appetite-suppressing hormone
Released by small intestine

Leptin
Inhibits the desire to eat
Released by fat cells

Surgery Variants

The three irreversible types of stomach surgery all work on the same principle: reduce the amount of food that can be eaten and absorbed, often by making the stomach smaller.

Roux-en-Y

The stomach is stapled to leave only a small pouch at the top, which is then connected directly to the small intestine.

Vertical Sleeve Gastrectomy

The stomach is cut so that only a long, narrow tube remains.

Duodenal Switch

As in VSG, the stomach is cut into a tube. The intestine is also shortened so it can absorb fewer nutrients.

"Super Normal"

The post-surgical flood of GLP-1, for example, immediately creates changes in the brain's reward centres in the orbitofrontal cortex, says le Roux. Could this explain the permanent shift in food preferences? To test the connection, last year, he and his colleagues at Imperial College London used MRI scanners to look at the brains of people before and after they had Roux-en-Y surgery. The results were staggering. Before surgery, pictures of cakes or burgers caused large areas of their reward centres to light up. But when the experiment was repeated just four days after surgery, their reward centres were impervious to the sight of the tempting foods. "Their exaggerated satiation makes the patient in effect 'super normal'," le Roux says, which accounts for the permanent weight loss. Their brains' circuits were being rewired to make them think like thin people.

That's not all. There is also evidence that changing the gut hormones' balance explains the improved brain function people reported on the weight-loss surgery forums.

GLP-1 is a particularly strong candidate for this effect. Because it suppresses the appetite by lowering blood sugar, it appears to have a strong effect on insulin, whose production drops dramatically within hours of surgery. Lower insulin levels, in turn, reduce the insulin resistance caused by excess weight, which has itself been tied to neurological problems (*Neuroepidemiology,* vol 34, p 222).

Although we don't understand exactly why, most researchers agree that obese volunteers tend to perform less well than leaner people on some learning and memory tasks, specifically ones that measure what is called inhibitory control. This is a subtle measure: your ability to remember where you parked your car this morning depends on your short-term memory. But distinguishing where you parked your car this morning from where you parked it yesterday morning requires inhibitory control, which involves suppressing yesterday's information. So while it is certainly not true that obese people are less smart, it seems they aren't able to distinguish this information as well.

Some researchers think the simple act of balancing insulin levels lifts this cognitive burden. In 2010, Gladys Strain, an obesity researcher at Cornell University's medical college in Ithaca, New York, found that just three months after weight-loss surgery, people scored better on cognitive tests than they did prior to surgery. One year later their test scores were even better (Surgery for Obesity and Related Diseases, vol 4, p 465). Benoit says his group is also finding evidence of cognitive improvements after weight-loss surgery.

But there is a stinging caveat to evidence that the brain is permanently altered by surgery: not all of the changes are positive.

Keith Josephs made the connection by accident. Several years ago, Josephs, a neurologist at the Mayo Clinic in Rochester, Minnesota, began seeing a steady increase in patients with a variety of cognitive problems. Frustrated when batteries of tests revealed nothing amiss, they had turned to him. "They were coming to me with issues like having trouble finding the right word, difficulty concentrating at work, being slow to respond to people talking to them and short-term memory issues," he says. Initially, he was nonplussed. Then he began to see a pattern. All of them had had Roux-en-Y surgery.

"Four days after surgery to lose weight, people were impervious to the sight of tempting food."

Josephs set to work pulling participant records from the hospital database and comparing them against two control groups: obese people who had not had surgery, and people of a normal weight. His results, published late last year, were alarming.

MRI scans revealed that those reporting cognitive problems had 24 per cent less volume in the thalamus, a small area of the brain associated with memory, attention, concentration and sensory information about taste (*Journal of Clinical Neuroscience,* vol 18, p 1671). In particular, the thalamus contains binding sites for ghrelin and GLP-1 (*Brain Research Reviews,* vol 58, p 160).

Large changes in these hormones could affect this brain area in the same way they alter the reward centres. And just as the positive changes in food preference appear not to be temporary, so do these negative changes. "Once the thalami have shrunk, there is nothing we can do to regrow these nerve cells," Josephs says.

Josephs is cautious about the results of his small study, and acknowledges that it needs to be replicated. Nonetheless, he can't ignore or dismiss the results. The group was thorough about checking for confounding factors. For example, because the average age of the participants was 54, they screened for signs of Alzheimer's disease. They also tested rigorously for surgery-related vitamin deficiencies, and found none. Only hormonal changes could explain the shrinkage, he says: "The probability that this occurred just by chance is at best 1 in 1000."

These cognitive problems indicate that the effects of bariatric surgery are far more complicated than most surgeons currently imagine. Even my comparatively harmless fish tea defies explanation. "Taste changes after bariatric surgery in strange ways," le Roux says. "Something is scrambling the signal from the taste buds to the brain."

Are certain populations more susceptible to the positive effects of bariatric surgery? Is one kind of surgery more likely to lead to cognitive decline than the others? Questions like these are only now being asked. The US National Institutes of Health, for example, has just funded a series of longitudinal studies to track the long-term health of people who have had different kinds of bariatric surgery. Some researchers are beginning to wonder whether these changes point to a "knifeless solution" that makes use of these hormonal fluctuations to combat obesity at the neurological level (*International Journal of Obesity,* vol 35, p 40).

Seven months and 45 kilograms later, I find myself benefiting from some of these effects. I still encounter the occasional unexpected cup of fish tea, so I find myself drinking a lot more water. Chocolate remains a joy, but only less sweet dark chocolate, and only in small doses.

There's no question that the possibility of neurological problems is scary. But for me, at least, they are easy to put into perspective. Weight-loss surgery is a life-saving procedure: with a few well-placed cuts, it knocks out diabetes, high blood pressure and sleep apnea, among others. In the context of my new mental clarity, healthier future, and all the small ways my everyday life has been improved, the threat of permanent cognitive effects seems to me a fair trade. Even with the occasional cup of fish tea.

Critical Thinking

1. Differentiate between the three main forms of bariatric weight loss surgery: Roux-en-Y, Vertical Sleeve Gastrectomy, and Duodenal Switch.
2. Identify the hormone appetite regulators that are produced by the gastrointestinal system and fat cells.
3. Evaluate the possible reasons for changes in taste preferences, food cravings, and mental functions that have been reported by individuals who have bariatric surgery.

Create Central

www.mhhe.com/createcentral

Internet References

American Society of Bariatric Surgery
http://asmbs.org

Bariatric Surgery—Obesity Action Coalition
www.obesityaction.org/obesity-treatments/bariatric-surgery

Samantha Murphy is a freelance writer based in Pennsylvania.

Article

Prepared by: Janet Colson, *Middle Tennessee State University*

How Many Bites Do You Take a Day? Try for 100

Researchers are developing tools that count how much or how fast we eat.

SUMATHI READDY

Learning Outcomes

After reading this article, you will be able to:

- Describe what the Bite Monitor is and how it works.
- Explain the proposed benefit of counting the number of times a food is chewed.
- Based on recent studies, state the number of calories an average man consumes and an average woman consumes in one bite of food.

In the never-ending pursuit of weight loss, a number of researchers are developing tools that count how much or how fast we eat.

The Bite Monitor, worn on the wrist like a watch, tallies the number of bites you take. The going assumption is that 100 bites a day is ideal for men and women to lose weight, according to researchers at South Carolina's Clemson University who developed the device. The concept will soon be tested in a study funded by the National Institutes of Health. A commercial product could be ready in about a year and is expected to cost about $195.

Mando Group AB, a Stockholm health-care company, has developed a "talking" plate that measures how fast you eat and assesses your satiety, or fullness. It is expected to be on the market for about $250 this fall.

Already for sale is the HAPIfork, which vibrates and flashes a red signal if a person's bites are spaced apart by less than 10 seconds. The fork, launched last year by Hapilabs Ltd. of Hong Kong, is sold online and in some retail outlets for $99.

"If you're eating too fast, you're probably not chewing and enjoying your food very well and you're probably going to be more likely" to eat too much, said Michael Jensen, an endocrinologist and obesity expert at the Mayo Clinic in Rochester, Minn.

Encouraging people to eat more slowly, take smaller bites and chew each bite more is an important component of weight control and management, experts say. They also believe slowing down while eating benefits digestion, lessens problems like acid reflux and allows for more nutrient absorption.

"There's very strong evidence pointing to the importance of chewing," said Kathleen Melanson, director of the University of Rhode Island's Energy Balance Lab, which researches satiety and other eating issues. "The nerves that feed into the muscles in the jaw connect to satiety areas in the brain," she said.

In a study by Chinese researchers published in the American Journal of Clinical Nutrition in 2011, people who chewed their food 40 times a mouthful—an unusually high number—rather than 15 times ate fewer calories and had lower levels of the hormone ghrelin, which stimulates appetite, and higher levels of a hormone that reduces appetite.

Experts say there isn't a magic number for how many times people should chew their food. Common recommendations range from roughly 10–20 chews per mouthful to help lose weight and improve digestion.

Dr. Melanson's research also suggests part of the reason why solid foods seem to fill us up more. "The higher amount of chewing that's required with more solid foods might contribute to the satiety effect," she said.

Mando Group's talking-plate system consists of a plate, a slender scale and a small computerized screen. You place your plate on the scale and the computer tracks how long it takes to eat the food. If you're eating too fast, a voice reminds you to eat slower. The device also asks at regular intervals how satisfied or full you are to judge satiety. The company's research has found the average eating rate is 300–350 grams, or about 10–12 ounces, in 12–15 minutes. Users who exceed that by about 20 grams a minute are asked to slow down.

"We have found that the eating speed is much, much more important than what you actually put on the plate," said Cecilia Bergh, chief executive and co-founder of Mando Group.

A subsidiary of the company runs weight-loss clinics, including one in New York City, that use the diet-monitoring system in their treatment programs. A new version of the talking plate, expected to be on the market this fall for about $250, will wirelessly connect the scale to a smartphone app.

A randomized controlled study by Dr. Bergh and others found that among 106 obese children, those who used the talking-plate system lost about three times as much weight as others who received only advice on diet and exercise. The study, published in the British Medical Journal in 2010, was funded by the BUPA Foundation, an international health-care insurer and provider.

The Bite Monitor takes a simpler approach to monitoring diet—counting only how many bites a person takes. To arrive at a supposed optimum of 100 bites a day, the Clemson University researchers tracked the number of bites of 77 people over two weeks, according to a study published in March in the Journal of the Academy of Nutrition and Dietetics.

The researchers calculated the average number of calories per bite was 17 for men and 11 for women. If people take 100 bites a day, it makes the daily caloric target roughly 1,700 calories for men and 1,100 calories for women. These targets represent a low-calorie diet according to National Institutes of Health standards. Consumption of calories per bite was the same regardless of whether participants were overweight or not.

"It's a little bit like a pedometer for your mouth," said Eric Muth, a psychology professor at Clemson who created the device with Adam Hoover, a computer-engineering professor. The Bite Monitor, which looks like an ugly watch, measures subtle wrist motions to detect bites with what the researchers say is 90 percent accuracy.

A pilot study at Clemson University and presented at the Obesity Society annual meeting last year seemed to confirm that counting bites helped people lose more weight than others who weren't aware of how many bites they took. Although the difference in weight loss between the two groups wasn't that great, Dr. Muth said the results warranted further research.

Dr. Muth said the research team is now designing a study with National Institutes of Health funding to test the effectiveness of the 100-bite diet. One early finding: Getting people to limit themselves to 100 bites a day doesn't seem to work if they start counting from zero. The researchers instead plan to ask study participants to count down from 100.

"One-hundred bites is really an average starting point," said Dr. Muth. "It's not going to work for everybody."

Dr. Jensen, of the Mayo Clinic, questioned the usefulness of counting bites. A bite of pizza is very different from a bite of salad, he noted. Bites also come in different sizes, and restricting people to 100 bites a day might just encourage them to take bigger mouthfuls, he said.

Dr. Muth said counting bites is a technique that is easy to use. "Our premise with the bite-count diet is we're trying to get you to push the plate away a little bit," he said. "You can do a lot with bites. It's very simple and people understand it."

Still, a more sophisticated version of the Bite Monitor is in the works that would also calculate eating rates by monitoring intervals between bites. Dr. Muth said the research team, working with Dr. Melanson of University of Rhode Island, hopes to launch the new device in about a year. It will be marketed by Bite Technologies, a company co-founded by Drs. Muth and Hoover.

Critical Thinking

1. Design a weight loss program using a Bite Monitor.
2. Calculate the number of calories you consume per bite in a meal. (First, count the number of bites you take during one meal then use a diet analysis program such as the SuperTracker to determine the calories. To determine calories per bite, divide the number of calories by the number of bites.) Does the number of calories you consumed per bite concur with average calories per bite measured by researchers at Clemson University?

Create Central

www.mhhe.com/createcentral

Internet References

Academy of Nutrition and Dietetics
www.eatright.org

Bite Monitor Project of Clemson University
www.ces.clemson.edu/~ahoover/bite-counter/

The Obesity Society
www.obesity.org

Article

Prepared by: Janet Colson, *Middle Tennessee State University*

My Anorexic 9-Year-Old

I never thought this could happen to a child so young, in a body-positive household like ours. Boy, was I wrong.

KRISTI BELCAMINO

Learning Outcomes

After reading this article, you will be able to:

- Recognize signs and symptoms of anorexia nervosa in children.
- Describe treatment strategies for an eating disorder in a school-age child.

My 9-year-old daughter was starving herself to death. And somehow, God forgive me, I didn't notice until it was almost too late.

We were busy running from soccer to swim lessons to play dates. But that's no excuse. The mere idea of a fourth-grader becoming anorexic was so foreign, so wild and so far-fetched, that it never crossed my mind.

My daughter had always been a picky eater and small for her age—less than six pounds at birth. She didn't like to eat much, and I didn't worry about it.

Then one day she asked for help with her sunscreen. She walked up, wearing her purple-and-blue swimsuit, and I squirted a blob of white lotion onto my palms and spread it across her back and shoulders. My fingers felt what had somehow escaped my eyes—pointy bones protruding like little bird wings. Over the bones stretched a thin layer of skin.

What the hell was going on?

Slowly, the pieces fell into place: odd comments over the summer that I had dismissed, thinking if I didn't make a big deal out of them, they would pass like so many other random fears and concerns that my children had.

Questions, such as:

"Are my legs fat?"

"I feel full."

"Do you think I'm fat?"

My response? It was so absurd I laughed and told her if anything she probably didn't eat enough.

I also didn't pay attention when she lost interest in foods she had once loved. I thought it was just a phase. In her short nine years, my complex daughter had brought up unusual fears and concerns. Usually if I didn't make a big deal—took it in stride and gave her a little reassurance—it went away.

This time, it didn't.

When the scale showed she was only 50 pounds—seven pounds less than she'd been during a visit only a few months before—her pediatrician referred us to a children's hospital. There, they diagnosed her as malnourished and suffering from an eating disorder.

My husband and I were stunned—and a little suspicious. She was only in fourth grade, for crying out loud. Didn't this only happen to teenage girls?

But the American Academy of Pediatrics says the prevalence of eating disorders in children and teens is increasing. Although it's still not a large number, the Alliance for Eating Disorders Awareness says 10 percent of those suffering from an eating disorder are 10 or younger. (And boys aren't immune. Up to 15 percent of those suffering an eating disorder are male.) Our doctor has treated a girl as young as 7.

Even so, in my eyes, we seemed the least likely people to have a child with an eating disorder. The word "diet" was pretty much banned from the moment I gave birth to a girl. Same for "skinny." Until my daughter said it, the "F" word—fat—was not heard in our house.

We don't subscribe to fashion magazines and carefully monitor what they watch on TV. Hell, our kids didn't even know there were other channels besides PBS Kids until recently.

I also foolishly thought—in a manner that now seems embarrassingly smug—that by never making my kids "clean their plates" like other parents, I was preventing future issues with food. But that effort didn't make much difference at all, it turns out.

The doctor has told me and my husband, oh I don't know, maybe 25 times, that it is not our fault. But that mother's guilt has a way of creeping right in there. She also said there's no prescribed method of parenting that can prevent a kid from becoming anorexic.

Just like there is no prescribed behavior that guarantees a kid will become anorexic. The only thing people know for sure is that some kids are predisposed to be susceptible to this disorder.

And truly, I don't care where it came from, as long as my daughter gets over it.

She's getting there. We started making weekly visits to Children's Hospital. Along with therapy, those visits included weigh-ins and blood pressure monitoring. Apparently, when you starve yourself, one of the red flag danger signs is low blood pressure. If it's too low, you'll end up in the hospital with a feeding tube and IV.

That image scared the crap out of our daughter. And us.

School was about to start, so we were also directed to bring the school nurse into the plan. At that point, I hadn't really told anyone besides my husband what was going on. So when I walked into the nurse's office with a letter from Children's Hospital, I was nervous but not unduly upset.

However, as soon as the words "eating disorder" came out of my mouth, I surprised myself (and the nurse) by bursting into tears and found myself wiping my tears and snot off a perfect stranger's shoulder.

The nurse organized a plan where staff members covertly monitored my daughter's eating at school. None of her classmates would know it was happening. But this also gave the doctor—and us—a secret weapon: If she didn't eat her lunch, her mother (me) would sit at the school lunch table with her. And her friends. Every day. Needless to say, she ate her lunch.

That was one of the easy battles. Some were much trickier. Every night, we went to bed exhausted from trying to get our increasingly furious kid to take yet another bite at the dinner table. We coaxed her along in the "dolphin" method we'd learned. (Swimming along beside her and gently nudging her in the right direction, as opposed to the "rhino" that bullies the kid into eating or the "kangaroo," which enables the kid along the road to starvation.) No, we had to be the dolphin.

It sucked. Our natural inclination was to say, "Eat your freaking food or the wrath of your parents will rain down on your head with a vengeance you've never imagined in your worst nightmares." Obviously that wouldn't work.

As my husband said when we first found out: "What's the big deal? She just needs to eat."

If only it were so simple. We soon learned that nothing about an eating disorder was rational. And that the more malnourished our daughter became, the more irrationally she behaved. In other words, the voice telling her not to eat was the most powerful thing in her world. In order for her brain to work normally again, she had to gain weight. In order to do that, she needed to eat. A lot.

So instead of threatening her within an inch of her life, we trained ourselves to repeat inane "dolphin" phrases, such as, "We know it's hard, but you can do it. Finish your dinner."

One week during therapy we were told to bring a picnic dinner to the hospital so the doctor could observe the meal. A complete waste of time, I thought. I was convinced that under the spotlight my daughter would act like a perfect little angel and eat every bite.

Instead, during that meal, my daughter gave the girl in "The Exorcist" a run for her money. She glared. She pouted. She ranted. She raved. She acted possessed—the same way she sometimes acted during dinner at home.

The therapist reassured us it wasn't really our daughter. It was the "eating disorder," which she said had a life of its own. Now, that's not something any parent wants to try to wrap their head around.

But slowly our "dolphin" efforts began to have positive effect. We refused to talk about her food or argue with her about what she had to eat. She was only allowed to join in the dinner conversation if she was also taking a bite every few sentences. We also offered rewards. Every time she balked, we reminded her that the fate of a coveted sleepover hung in the balance.

It worked. In one month, she gained five pounds and grew an inch. No shit. An inch. In one month.

Slowly, it stopped being a nightly battle and we leaned back and breathed a sigh of relief. But nothing is ever so easy, is it?

We hit another pothole in the road. My daughter began disappearing into her room, blasting her music and then coming out sweating. She was "Irish dancing" (basically stomping around like a crazy lady for an hour straight). She admitted trying to exercise away the food she had eaten.

Irish dancing was banned.

I should also point out here that my daughter had no clue that some kids vomit to get rid of food in their stomach and there's no way in hell she's going to find out from me.

Now, nearly a year later, after intensive therapy, my daughter is in the moderately healthy weight range, which is still in the 5th percentile. In other words, she's not malnourished anymore.

I don't know if the struggle will ever be over. But I do know how to go to war against the eating disorder now. Meanwhile, I try furiously to hide my gratefulness, relief and joy when my daughter walks into the kitchen and says these simple words that parents around the world hear every day and yet, take for granted, like I will never do:

"Mama, I'm hungry. Can I have a cookie?"

Critical Thinking

1. How common are eating disorders in elementary-school-age children?
2. What medical interventions are used to treat a child who has anorexia nervosa or another eating disorder?
3. Describe how school personnel assist with the treatment of a student who has an eating disorder.
4. Develop a list of signs and symptoms of eating disorders in children.
5. What should teachers and other school personnel do if they suspect a student has an eating disorder?

Create Central

www.mhhe.com/createcentral

Internet References

Academy of Nutrition and Dietetics
www.eatright.org

American Academy of Pediatric
www.aap.org

Anorexia Nervosa and Related Eating Disorders
www.anred.org

Alliance for Eating Disorder Awareness
www.allianceforeatingdisorders.com/portal

Article

Prepared by: Janet Colson, *Middle Tennessee State University*

Prescription Medications for the Treatment of Obesity

U.S. Department of Health and Human Services, WIN *Weight-control Information Network*

Learning Outcomes

After reading this article, you will be able to:

- Describe the type of individuals who are allowed to be prescribed weight loss medications.
- Explain how prescription and over-the-counter drugs promote weight loss and the side effects of each.

Introduction

Obesity is a chronic condition that affects many people. If you are struggling with excess weight, you may find that a healthy eating plan and regular physical activity help you lose weight and maintain weight loss over the long term. But if these lifestyle changes are not enough, prescription medications for obesity treatment may be a helpful part of your weight-control program.

When combined with healthy eating and regular physical activity, prescription obesity drugs may help some people lose weight and improve their health. But these drugs have side effects and may not work for everyone.

This fact sheet will tell you more about the prescription medications that may be used to treat obesity. Talk to your health care provider if you think these medications may help you.

How Do These Drugs Work?

Prescription drugs for the treatment of obesity work in different ways. For example, some drugs may help you feel less hungry or feel full sooner. Others may make it hard for your body to absorb fat from the foods you eat.

These medicines are meant to help people who may be having health problems related to excess weight. See the box "Who may use obesity medications?" for more information. Your doctor will also consider the drugs' side effects, your family's medical history, and your current health issues and medicines.

Who may use obesity medications?

Health care providers often use the body mass index (BMI) to help decide who may benefit from weight-loss drugs. BMI estimates overweight and obesity based on your height in relation to your weight. Your doctor may prescribe a medication to treat your obesity if you are an adult with

- a BMI of 30 or greater OR
- a BMI of 27 or greater and you have obesity-related medical problems, such as high blood pressure, type 2 diabetes, or high cholesterol

To check your BMI, see the Resource section for a link to the Online BMI Calculator. Before using a weight-loss drug, you should first try to lose weight by changing your eating and physical activity habits.

What Are the Benefits?

When combined with changes to eating and physical activity, prescription drugs may help some people lose weight (usually less than 10 percent of their body weight). Results vary by drug and by person. Losing weight may help improve your health by lowering blood sugar, blood pressure, and triglycerides (other fats in the blood). Weight loss of 5 to 10 percent can also improve inflammation profiles and improve how patients feel and their mobility.

Most weight loss takes place in the first 6 months of starting the medicine. After that time, you may lose weight more slowly or begin to regain weight.

What Are the Concerns?

Because obesity drugs are used to treat a condition that affects millions of people, the chance that side effects may outweigh benefits is of great concern. This is why one should never take a weight loss medicine only for cosmetic benefit. In the past, some drugs for obesity treatment were linked to serious health problems. An example is sibutramine (sold as Meridia), recalled in 2010 because of concerns related to heart disease and stroke.

Possible side effects vary by drug and how it acts on your body. See the next section of this fact sheet for the specific side effects of each weight-loss drug. Most side effects are mild and usually improve if you continue to use the drug.

What Drugs Are Available?

The Food and Drug Administration (FDA) is the Government agency that reviews and approves prescription drugs for treating specific health problems. Table 1 ("Prescription Drugs Approved for Obesity Treatment") lists the prescription drugs approved by the FDA for weight control. Three of these drugs—orlistat, lorcaserin, and phenterminetopiramate—are approved for long-term use. This means that you may take them for several months at a time, even years.

Table 1 Prescription Drugs Approved for Obesity Treatment

Weight-loss drug	Approved for	How it works	Common side effects
Orlistat Sold as Xenical by prescription Over-the-counter version sold as Alli	Xenical: adults and children ages 12 and older Alli: adults only	Blocks some of the fat that you eat, keeping it from being absorbed by your body.	Stomach pain, gas, diarrhea, and leakage of oily stools. Note: Rare cases of severe liver injury reported. Should not be taken with cyclosporine.
Lorcaserin Sold as Belviq	Adults	Acts on the serotonin receptors in the brain. This may help you eat less and feel full after eating smaller amounts of food.	Headaches, dizziness, feeling tired, nausea, dry mouth, cough, and constipation. Should not be taken with selective serotonin reuptake inhibitors (SSRIs) and monoamine oxidase inhibitor (MAOI) medications.
Phentermine-topiramate Sold as Qsymia	Adults	A mix of two drugs: phentermine (suppresses your appetite and curbs your desire to eat) and topiramate (used to treat seizures or migraine headaches). May make you feel full and make foods taste less appealing.	Tingling of hands and feet, dizziness, taste alterations (particularly with carbonated beverages), trouble sleeping, constipation, and dry mouth. Note: Sold only through certified pharmacies. MAY LEAD TO BIRTH DEFECTS. DO NOT TAKE QSYMIA IF YOU ARE PREGNANT OR PLANNING A PREGNANCY.
Other appetite suppressant drugs (drugs that curb your desire to eat), which include • phentermine • benzphetamine • diethylpropion • phendimetrazine Sold under many names	Adults	Increase chemicals in the brain that affect appetite. Make you feel that you are not hungry or that you are full. Note: Only FDA approved for a short period of time (up to 12 weeks).	Dry mouth, difficulty sleeping, dizziness, headache, feeling nervous, feeling restless, upset stomach, diarrhea, and constipation.

Other weight-loss drugs that curb appetite are only approved by the FDA for short-term use (a few weeks), but some doctors prescribe them for longer periods (see the box "What is 'off-label' use?"). These medications are also controlled substances because of their potential for abuse. Most weight-loss drugs are only approved for use by adults. Orlistat is approved for children ages 12 and older. **Weight loss medications should never be used during pregnancy, and weight loss is not advised during pregnancy.** Women who are thinking about becoming pregnant should avoid some of these drugs, as they may harm an unborn baby. The drugs outlined in Table 1 are described in more detail in the sections that follow.

Orlistat (Xenical and Alli)

The drug orlistat, sold under the brand name Xenical (pronounced ZEN-i-cal), has been available since 1999. It is approved for use by adults and children ages 12 and older.

The over-the-counter version of orlistat is sold under the brand name Alli. The two drugs contain different amounts of orlistat. Xenical contains 120 mg, while Alli contains 60 mg. Alli is not approved for use by children.

Orlistat will stop about one-third of the fat from the food you eat from being digested. It does so by blocking the enzyme lipase, which breaks down fat. When fat is not broken down, the body cannot absorb it, so fewer calories are taken in. After 1 or 2 years of taking orlistat, patients may lose about 5 to 7 pounds.

Side effects. Common side effects of orlistat include stomach pain, gas, diarrhea, and leakage of oily stool. These side effects are generally mild and temporary, but may be worse when you eat high-fat foods. You should eat a low-fat diet (less than 30 percent of calories from fat) before starting to take this drug. Because orlistat prevents some vitamins from being absorbed, **you should take a multivitamin while using orlistat.**

Rare cases of severe liver injury have been reported. Stop using the drug and see your health care provider immediately if you develop symptoms of liver problems. These symptoms may include dark urine, itching, light-colored stools, loss of appetite, or yellow eyes or skin. Orlistat should not be taken with cyclosporine.

Lorcaserin (Belviq)

Belviq (pronounced BEL-VEEK), works by affecting chemicals in your brain that help decrease your appetite and make you feel full, so you eat less.

In studies done as part of the drug approval process, almost half (47 percent) of patients taking Belviq lost at least 5 percent of their initial body weight at 1 year. If you do not lose 5 percent of your weight within 12 weeks of being on the drug, it is unlikely that the medicine will work for you, and it should be stopped.

Side effects. Common side effects of Belviq include headaches, dizziness, feeling tired, nausea, dry mouth, cough, and constipation. A rare but serious side effect is serotonin syndrome (high fever, muscle rigidity, and confusion), which can occur if the drug is taken along with SSRI antidepressants or MAOI medications. Belviq, as with all weight-loss agents, should not be taken if you are pregnant or planning to become pregnant.

Phentermine-topiramate (Qsymia)

In July 2012, the FDA approved the drug combination phentermine and topiramate, sold as Qsymia (pronounced kyoo-sim-EE-uh) to treat obesity in adults. Qsymia combines two FDA-approved drugs:

- phentermine, a medicine approved to suppress appetite.
- topiramate, a medicine approved to control seizures. It may also be used to prevent migraine headaches. It is in an extended-release form in Qsymia.

Although phentermine when used as a single agent is approved for only a few weeks, the combination has been studied for 2 years and found to be safe for use. Additionally, the doses used in Qsymia are much lower than the usual doses of phentermine and topiramate when prescribed separately.

Qsymia is available in three doses: a starting dose, a recommended dose, and a higher dose. After 1 year of treatment with Qsymia, 62 percent of patients who were prescribed the recommended dose lost at least 5 percent of their weight. If after 12 weeks on the higher dose, you do not lose at least 5 percent of your body weight, it is unlikely that the drug will work for you.

Side effects. Common side effects include tingling of hands and feet, dizziness, taste alterations (particularly with carbonated beverages), trouble sleeping, constipation, and dry mouth. Serious but rare side effects include allergic reactions (such as rash, hives, difficulty breathing), thoughts of suicide, memory problems, mood problems (such as anxiety, depression, panic attacks), and changes to your vision. Rare side effects associated with topiramate include kidney stones and acute glaucoma. **Qsymia must not be used during pregnancy because it may cause harm to the baby.** People with an overactive thyroid gland, glaucoma, or who have recently taken certain antidepressant drugs known as MAOIs should not use Qsymia, although the drug was studied in patients taking SSRI and other antidepressants without adverse events.

Other Appetite Suppressants

These drugs promote weight loss by increasing one or more brain chemicals that affect appetite. You may feel less hungry or feel full sooner when taking these drugs. They are FDA approved only for a short period of time (up to 12 weeks). Some doctors may prescribe them for longer periods of time (see the box "What is 'off-label' use?").

Several appetite suppressants may be used to promote weight loss in adults. They include

- phentermine (sold as Adipex-P, Oby-Cap, Suprenza, T-Diet, Zantryl)
- benzphetamine (sold as Didrex)
- diethylpropion (sold as Tenuate, Tenuate Dospan)
- phendimetrazine (sold as Adipost, Bontril PDM, Bontril Slow Release, Melfiat)

Among these types of drugs, phentermine is the one used most often in the United States.

Side effects. Common side effects of appetite suppressants include dry mouth, difficulty sleeping, dizziness, headache, feeling nervous, feeling restless, upset stomach, and diarrhea or constipation. Severe side effects may include chest pain, fainting, fast heartbeat, shortness of breath, confusion, and swelling in your ankles or feet. People with heart disease, high blood pressure, an overactive thyroid gland, or glaucoma should not use these drugs. These medications are controlled substances because of their potential for abuse.

What Other Prescription Drugs Do Doctors Use "Off-Label" for Obesity Treatment?

Some medicines that have been approved to treat other health problems may also be used for weight loss. Using a medicine for a different purpose from that for which it was approved, in a different population, or for a longer period of time is called using it in an "off-label" way (see box "What is 'off-label' use?").

Other prescription drugs some doctors prescribe off label to promote weight loss include

- bupropion, a drug used to treat depression
- metformin, a drug used to treat type 2 diabetes

The side effects of these medications and the population for whom they might be appropriate vary. Drugs prescribed off label also have not met the rigorous standards of FDA approval as an obesity treatment.

What is "off-label" use?

Health care providers have some leeway in how they may prescribe drugs approved by the FDA. For example, in treating obesity, health care providers may

- prescribe a drug approved for treating another medical problem
- prescribe two or more drugs at the same time
- prescribe a drug for a longer period of time than approved by the FDA

These types of off-label uses are common in treating many health problems. You should feel comfortable asking your doctor if he or she is using a medicine in an off-label way.

What Other Drugs May Be Approved and Available in the Future?

Several new drugs and drug combinations are currently being studied in animals as well as in clinical trials in humans. Research is ongoing to identify more safe and effective medications to help patients with obesity lose weight and maintain a healthy weight for a long time.

Future drugs may use new strategies, such as these:

- combining drugs that affect appetite and those that affect addiction (or craving)
- stimulating gut hormones that reduce appetite
- shrinking the blood vessels that feed fat cells in the body, thereby preventing them from growing
- targeting genes that affect body weight
- using bacteria in the gut to control weight

How can I improve my physical activity levels?

Federal guidelines recommend 300 minutes (5 hours) or more each week of moderate or vigorous aerobic activity for people trying to lose more than 5 percent of their weight or to maintain weight after meeting weight-loss goals. Aerobic activity uses your large muscle groups (chest, legs, and back) to increase your heart rate. This activity may cause you to breathe harder. Examples of moderate aerobic activity are these:

- bicycling (with a helmet)
- brisk jogging or walking
- dancing
- playing basketball or soccer
- swimming

Common Questions and Answers

Q: Can drugs replace physical activity or changes in eating habits as a way to lose weight?

A: No. Studies show that weight-loss drugs work best when used with a weight-control program that helps you improve your eating and physical activity habits. Ask your doctor about ways you can improve your eating plan and add more physical activity to your life.

Q: How do I decide which obesity medication is right for me?

A: Choosing a medication to treat obesity is a decision between you and your health care provider. You will consider the drug's side effects, your family's medical history, and your current health issues and medicines.

Q: How long will I need to take weight-loss drugs?

A: The answer depends upon whether the drug helps you to lose and maintain weight and whether you have any side effects. Because obesity is a chronic condition, changes to diet and physical activity may need to be continued for years, perhaps a lifetime, to improve health and maintain a healthy weight.

Q: Will I regain some weight after I stop taking weight-loss drugs?

A: Probably. Most people who stop taking obesity medications regain the weight they lost. Maintaining healthy eating habits and increasing physical activity may help you regain less weight or keep it off. See the callout box on physical activity for information on recommended types and amounts of physical activity for people trying to lose weight. For tips on healthy eating, check out the Weight-control Information Network (WIN) publication *Just Enough for You: About Food Portions,* listed in the Resources section at the end of this fact sheet.

Q: Can children or teens use obesity medications?

A: Most weight-loss drugs are approved only for use in adults. Prescription orlistat (sold as Xenical) is approved for use in teens ages 12 or older.

Q: Will insurance cover the cost of weight-loss drugs?

A: Some, but not all, insurers cover medications for the treatment of obesity. Contact your insurance provider to find out if these medicines are covered under your plan.

Dos and Don'ts of Using Weight-loss Drugs

- **DO** follow your primary care provider's advice about weight-loss drugs.
- **DON'T** obtain medications over the Internet.
- **DO** use weight-loss medications to reinforce your lifestyle change program.
- **DON'T** think the drugs will work by themselves to replace a diet and physical activity program.
- **DO** know the side effect profiles and precautions in using any medication.
- **DON'T** continue medications if you are not losing weight after a trial (usually 12 weeks).
- **DO** discuss other medications you are taking with your doctor when considering weight-loss medications.
- **DON'T** take weight-loss medications during pregnancy.

Research

The National Institute of Diabetes and Digestive and Kidney Diseases (NIDDK) conducts and supports a broad range of basic and clinical obesity research. More information about obesity research is available at *http://www.obesityresearch.nih.gov.*

Participants in clinical trials can play a more active role in their own health care, gain access to new research treatments before they are widely available, and help others by contributing to medical research. For more information, visit *http://www.clinicaltrials.gov.*

Resources

Additional Reading from the Weight-control Information Network

The following publications are available online at *http://www.win.niddk.nih.gov/publications* and also by calling WIN toll-free at 1–877–946–4627:

- ***Choosing a Safe and Successful Weight-loss Program*** offers guidelines to help readers talk with their health care providers about weight-loss programs.
- ***Just Enough for You: About Food Portions*** explains the difference between a portion and a serving, as well as offers tips to help readers eat healthy portions.
- ***Physical Activity and Weight Control*** explains how regular physical activity may help readers reach and keep a healthy weight.
- ***Understanding Adult Overweight and Obesity*** provides basic information about obesity: What is it? How is it measured? What causes it? What are the health risks? What can you do about it?

Additional Resources

- **Food and Drug Administration.** Provides information about drug approvals, prescription drugs, over-the-counter drugs, drug safety, clinical trials, public health alerts, and other topics. ***http://www.fda.gov***
- **Mayo Clinic.** Offers information about drugs and supplements. ***http://www.mayoclinic.com/health/drug-information/DrugHerbIndex***
- **National Center for Complementary and Alternative Medicine.** Provides information on options other than prescription drugs, such as herbal supplements and acupuncture. ***http://www.nccam.nih.gov***
- **National Library of Medicine Drug Information Portal.** Offers information about specific drugs. ***http://druginfo.nlm.nih.gov/drugportal/drugportal.jsp***
- **Online BMI Calculator for Adults.** ***http://nhlbisupport.com/bmi***

Inclusion of resources is for information only and does not imply endorsement by NIDDK or WIN.

Critical Thinking

1. What three prescription weight-loss drugs are currently approved by FDA for long-term use and what is the mechanism of each?
2. What is meant by "off-label" drugs used for obesity treatment?
3. In the future, what other drugs may be approved by FDA for weight loss?
4. After reading the article, what advice would you give your mother (or a woman about 50 years of age) who thinks she needs to lose 25 pounds?

Create Central

www.mhhe.com/createcentral

Internet References

Food and Drug Administration
www.fda.gov

Weight-control Information Network
www.win.niddk.nih.gov

NIDDK (National Institute of Diabetes and Digestive and Kidney Diseases), March/July 2013.

Article

Prepared by: Janet Colson, *Middle Tennessee State University*

What's behind New Findings That It's Healthy to Be Overweight?

With so much profit to be made from keeping people overweight, the public is not hearing the truth about obesity.

JILL RICHARDSON

Learning Outcomes

After reading this article, you will be able to:

- Explain how a BMI of 25 up to 30 became the weight range used to define an individual as "overweight."
- Explain how the weight-loss industry benefits by setting the BMI to define overweight at 25 instead of 27 or 28.

Did you hear the news? Now it's healthy to be fat! It turns out that your smug skinny friend who eats broccoli and runs marathons should have been eating fast food and watching TV this whole time. Right?

Well, maybe not. A new study published in the *Journal of the American Medical Association* has made headlines because it found that overweight people have lower mortality rates than people with "healthy" weights and that even moderate obesity does not increase mortality.

This means that an overweight 5′4″ woman weighing between 145 and 169 pounds (Body Mass Index of 25 to 29) has less chance of dying than a woman of the same height who weighs less. If she gains weight and falls within the lower obese range (174 to 204 pounds, BMI of 30 to 35), she is equally likely to die as a woman with a "healthy" BMI of 18.5 to 25. Only once her weight exceeds 205 pounds does her risk of mortality increase.

The study made waves when a recent *New York Times* op-ed proclaimed that "baselessly categorizing at least 130 million Americans—and hundreds of millions in the rest of the world—as people in need of 'treatment' for their 'condition' serves the economic interests of, among others, the multibillion-dollar weight-loss industry and large pharmaceutical companies."

So what's the story? Is it healthy to be overweight?

As usual, it's instructive to look back in history—in this case to the mid-1990s when the current standards we use to define "overweight" and "obese" were set. Initially, the U.S. government used a BMI of 27.3 for women and a BMI of 27.8 for men as the lowest BMIs that qualified as overweight.

Across the pond, British scientist Philip James convened the International Obesity Task Force in 1995, and their work, in collaboration with the UN's World Health Organization (WHO), led to an international standard that defined a BMI of 25 or above as overweight for both sexes, and a BMI of 30 or above as obese.

Back in the U.S., the National Institutes of Health put together an expert panel, chaired by Dr. F. Xavier Pi-Sunyer, a recognized expert on obesity, and at the time, the executive director of the Weight Watchers Foundation. In September 1998, they published a document called the "Clinical Guidelines on the Identification, Evaluation, and Treatment of Overweight and Obesity in Adults," which lowered the U.S. standard for overweight to match the international standard.

Suddenly, a 5′4″ woman who weighed 145 or a 5′10″ man who weighed 174 were considered overweight. Newspapers published articles on 29 million Americans who went to bed at a healthy weight one night and woke up the next morning to discover they were overweight—although they had not gained one single pound! At the time, these previously "healthy weight" individuals accounted for nearly 30 percent of the overweight and obese people in America.

In the mainstream media, one of the few opposing voices to this change was former Surgeon General C. Everett Koop, who told the *Washington Post* that, "weight does not increase the risk of death until the BMI reaches 27 or 28." Other critics feared that the new standards would result in an increase in the use of diet drugs or discourage Americans, resulting in them giving up trying to lose weight altogether.

Others point to conflicts of interest among the expert panel that defined 55 percent of the nation (at the time) as overweight or obese, or even data showing that a few extra pounds did not result in increased mortality.

To truly get to the bottom of the issue, one must consider the conflicts of interest on all sides. For example, Pi-Sunyer was tied at the hip with Weight Watchers, he was director of a weight loss clinic, and he served as an advisory board member or paid consultant to several pharmaceutical companies that made diet drugs. Similar accusations have been lobbed at Philip James in the U.K. But on the other side of the coin, nearly every industry in the U.S.—with the exception, no doubt, of the airlines—makes handsome profits from an overweight and obese populace that is desperate to lose weight but continually fails to do so.

Consider a typical American who spends money on large amounts of processed foods at grocery stores and restaurants, and then needs to buy clothing in larger and larger sizes. She even requires more gas to transport her extra weight, and perhaps she and her partner decide they need a larger bed. Desperate to slim down, she enrolls at a gym, buys diet books, special diet foods, and perhaps even weight-loss drugs. Maybe she loses some weight. Maybe she doesn't. But even if she succeeds temporarily, in all but a minority of cases, the weight is back again within a few years and she starts the cycle again. How much money does she spend to get fat and then get thin again?

The industries that sell junk food want Americans to continue buying their products, of course. Many corporations like Coca Cola, Wendy's, Applebees, and Outback Steakhouse fund the so-called Center for Consumer Freedom, which runs the Web site ObesityMyths.com. Visit this site to learn why you should continue drinking Coca-Cola and eating at Applebees without worrying about what the food police tell you. The site devotes a special section to "Myth-Makers" like Philip James, accusing him of conflicts of interest. Often with flimsy evidence, these myth-makers are tarred as being financially tied to the diet drug and weight-loss industries, with the implication that their work lacks credibility because they are being paid off to talk about the global scourge of obesity.

A more reasoned assessment of James' and Pi-Sunyer's conflicts of interest comes from University of Chicago professor J. Eric Oliver, who first points out in his book *Fat Politics,* "It is difficult to find *any* major figure in the field of obesity research or past president of the North American Association for the Study of Obesity who does not have some type of financial tie to a pharmaceutical or weight-loss company." He goes on to acknowledge that, "While the pharmaceutical industry did not necessarily dictate the decisions of the obesity experts, the conflicts of interest among the leading researchers in the obesity field are both undeniable and problematic."

Oliver calls out a "health-industrial complex" which is "built upon a symbiotic relationship between health researchers, government bureaucrats, and drug companies." Each group relies on the others to get what they want, be that drug sales, congressional funding for their government agencies, or prestigious appointments, recognition and lucrative speaking gigs. For each group, adding tens of millions of Americans to the population at risk due to obesity helps them toward their goals. That isn't to say that self-interest was the determining factor in their decision to lower the BMI considered overweight to 25. But it's a possibility that self-interest played a role.

In any case, that's how we got to where we are, with anyone over a BMI of 25 thrown into the "fat" category. But the "news" that being overweight might not increase your risk of mortality is not actually news. The same researcher at the CDC, Katherine Flegal, came to just that conclusion eight years ago, which she explained at length in *Scientific American* in 2007. Even back in the 1990s, there were already some studies with conclusions similar to Flegal's available to the experts setting the weight at which one is considered overweight or obese.

Then and now, these studies provoke some controversy. For one thing, smokers often gain weight when they quit smoking—but quitting smoking is a healthy thing to do. Also, many who are terminally ill are thin and frail—but not healthy! The studies attempt to correct for these issues as much as possible.

Furthermore, as medicine advances, humans are able to live longer with chronic disease. The studies use mortality as their measure, but "not dead" does not indicate that one is healthy. Some even suggest that overweight people might enjoy lower mortality because their doctors screen them for more problems due to their high weights compared to patients with lower weights.

Deb Burgard, an eating disorders specialist, says that Flegal's conclusions make sense, because so many Americans die of diseases that cause them to lose weight while they are ill. An elderly person who has a bit more meat on his or her bones at the beginning of the illness can tolerate the weight loss with less harm to their health.

Linda Bacon, author of *Health at Every Size,* points to other possible discrepancies in our understanding of obesity and health. For one thing, correlation is not causation. Just because many people with a certain disease are also fat, that does not mean that one caused the other. In her book, she points to some evidence that type II diabetes causes obesity, not the other way around.

She also questions the impact of "weight cycling" (repeatedly gaining and then losing weight) on one's health. She says, "weight fluctuation is strongly associated with increased risk for diabetes, hypertension, and cardiovascular diseases, independent of body weight." As many overweight people try to lose weight—sometimes via extreme diets—could the impact of weight cycling confuse our understanding of the health impact of obesity?

Her most convincing point is that sedentary lifestyles and poor eating habits can cause both health problems *and* overweight or obesity. And in fact, Bacon does not encourage readers to sit back and eat endless amounts of junk. She instead counsels them to pay attention to their bodies' signals, eating only when hungry and stopping when full. Don't eat while doing other activities. Pay attention and enjoy your food. Eat whole foods, mostly plants. And be active—but find an activity you enjoy!

Burgard, who worked with Bacon to develop the Health at Every Size model, deals with the fallout of our fat-phobic culture. Whether for health or for beauty reasons, a huge percent of Americans now hate themselves every time they look in the mirror.

"Lots of women wake up in the morning and look in the mirror and say I feel so fat, even though fat's not a feeling," says Burgard. "It's a code word for 'I feel ugly, I feel vulnerable,

I'm going to get rejected socially.' In our culture, that gets connected up to fatness. And so what's fascinating about this is that when people's bodies change, it's not going to be the case that they lose their identification with that part of themselves that feels vulnerable, that feels like a loser."

Often, she finds people with eating disorders try to lose their feelings of vulnerability by losing weight. The pounds may disappear, but the feelings remain. The person tries to lose even more weight to see if that will do the trick, but it never does.

One reason Burgard dislikes the national war on obesity is because it influences people to distrust their appetites. She says, "When people look at their body size, they have this mythology that everybody who eats 'normally' has a thin body and if you don't have a thin body, you must not be eating the right way. It makes you distrust your appetite. They think, 'If you did the right thing you would be thin.' This is the biggest myth of all."

By focusing on weight instead of healthy habits, one is pushed toward the wrong goals. Brand-name diet foods are not always healthy, and extreme starvation diets never are. At the same time, weight-as-a-measure-of-health sends a signal to "normal" weight Americans that they are doing everything right and don't need to change. But healthy diets, regular exercise, good sleep habits, and stress reduction are good for everyone, no matter their weight.

Additionally, the stigmatization overweight people face is 100 percent destructive. In addition to the stress and feelings of shame it engenders, it even drives some people to avoid going to the doctor. Burgard reports that patients tell her they avoid going to the doctor for as long as possible—skipping routine physicals and gynecological visits—because they don't want a lecture about their weight.

She has strong words for the weight loss industry—which she calls the "weight cycling industry"—saying, "That's what happens and that's the way they make money." While some people who lose weight do keep it off, she says they are as rare as people who win the lottery. "OK, they exist," she says, "But if I'm a health care provider, if I know that 98% of the people I send down this road will end up sicker, physically and psychologically, why would I do that?"

Burgard continues, "If you look at the last year, you look at the number of African American and male spokespeople for these companies—there's an explosion of marketing to these communities now—and what we're seeing in the eating disorder community is that the number of boys with body image concerns are going up and up and younger and younger kids are having these concerns. So the eating disorder world and the obesity treatment world are really at odds."

After several months trying to lose weight or keep weight off and failing, many end up in Burgard's office. "We see people who are in dire straits for one reason or another. We see the fallout. We have to speak up because the people who treat obesity have such terrible followup and they blame their patients or their customers for the interventions not working, which is completely unfair and wrong. And they need to understand the suffering that they are causing."

In other words, the new study with not-so-new conclusions does not mean that you can kick back and eat as much junk as your belly can hold—but it does mean we should question the national obsession with losing weight. It also means we should question the motives of the "experts," whether they are having their bread buttered by the weight loss and pharmaceutical industries or they are working on behalf of junk food companies.

Critical Thinking

1. What does J. Eric Oliver mean when he says the "health-industrial complex" is "built upon a symbiotic relationship between health researchers, government bureaucrats, and drug companies"?
2. Other than the weight loss industry, what sectors of the business world gain by having a large percentage of the population obese?
3. How does that stigma of being labeled "overweight" or "obese" affect people who fit into that weight category?

Create Central

www.mhhe.com/createcentral

Internet References

International Obesity Taskforce
www.iaso.org/iotf

The Obesity Society
www.obesity.org

Jill Richardson is the founder of the blog *La Vida Locavore* and a member of the Organic Consumers Association policy advisory board. She is the author of *Recipe for America: Why Our Food System Is Broken and What We Can Do to Fix It.*

Unit 6

UNIT

Prepared by: Janet Colson, *Middle Tennessee State University*

Health Claims

Technological advances in the 21st century have resulted in high-speed communication of results from scientific research and the possibility for miscommunication. Even if the scientific protocol, study, design, data collection, and analysis are impeccable, it is still possible to report the findings in a confusing and biased manner. According to a survey conducted by the Academy of Nutrition and Dietetics (formally the American Dietetic Association), 90% of consumers polled get their nutrition information from television, magazines, and newspapers. Health claims of food is a topic that grasps the attention of readers even if the health claims seem to good to be true. Health claims of food are all over the Internet and communication of a new health claim spreads quickly without much regard to the validity or reliability of the message.

Some Americans are so confused and overwhelmed by the controversies surrounding food and health that they have stopped paying attention to the contradictory claims reported by news media. Which one is better, butter or margarine? Are eggs good or bad for health? The media very frequently misinterpret results, simplify the message, and do not provide the proper context to accurately interpret the information. In addition, the media are eager to publish sensational information and not wait for evidence to be evaluated for validity and reliability. However, some popular heath claims are supported by reputable scientific research. Several of these topics are presented in this unit, including the overall health benefits of dark chocolate and omega 3 fatty acids and certain foods and herbs for brain health.

One of the most popular health messages held in high regard and followed by many is that chocolate is good for the cardiovascular system. Research that supports this theory refers to dark chocolate, which is lower in saturated fat and higher in phytochemicals from the high cocoa content. Milk chocolate, the form most commonly consumed in the United States does not provide the health benefits of dark chocolate.

The health claims of omega-3 fatty acids are based on its beneficial effect on the inflammatory system. Omega-3 fatty acids have been shown to reduce the risk of chronic diseases such as heart disease, certain cancers, and arthritis. Because so many people in the United States suffer from these chronic diseases, the health claims of omega-fatty acids have captured the attention of the U.S. population. Demand for supplements and fortified foods containing omega-3s has culminated in a vast number of products on the market. The information marketed on omega-3 may be confusing to most Americans. Since the metabolic pathways of these PUFAs are complex, there is a great deal of confusion about the best and safest source of omega-3 fatty acids.

Interest in nutrition's impact on brain function and energy level has become a hot topic for the aging baby boomer population. Producers of dietary supplements have responded to this increase in demand by introducing a vast number of dietary supplements to the market that supposedly improve cognitive function and provide energy. Most consumers need advice to help intelligently interpret the claims about nutritional supplements touted to enhance brain function and to help sort information about foods, food components, and other products that are thought to improve mental performance and energy level. Caffeine, caffeine derivatives, glucose, ginkgo biloba, Chinese ginseng, and cocoa flavanols are often considered to be on the "mental menu" as improving brain function.

Our society is inundated with many misleading health claims for foods and dietary supplements. Many people believe the claims because they want an easy fix and the next greatest product that will make them healthy without all the troublesome work of diet and physical activity. The articles in this unit provide practical information about common foods in the typical American diet.

Article

Prepared by: Janet Colson, *Middle Tennessee State University*

What's the Catch?

Why the Latest Study Is Rarely the Final Answer

BONNIE LIEBMAN

Learning Outcomes

After reading this article, you will be able to:

- Explain the differences between a "link" found in a research study and a "cause and effect."
- Outline the steps required for scientists to establish an actual cause and effect relationship between a particular dietary practice and a health outcome.

Do antioxidants lower the risk of cancer, heart disease, or memory loss? Does calcium prevent bone fractures? Is a low-fat (or low-carb) diet the key to weight loss? Does taking vitamin D prevent just about everything?

We're constantly bombarded by headlines about the latest study and its "Surprising! New!" findings that often contradict earlier results. It's enough to make your head spin.

In fact, few studies are game changers. But some results matter more than others. Here's a guide to help you see beyond the headlines.

1. Cause and Effect Might Be Reversed

"Diet drinkers sometimes end up eating more," declared the headline on the CBC News website last January.

The study in question had reported that overweight or obese diet-pop drinkers consumed as many calories as drinkers of sugary pop.[1] Other studies have found that diet-pop drinkers are more likely to be overweight.[2]

But that doesn't mean that diet pop *cause* people to eat more or gain weight.

"People who are overweight tend to consume more diet beverages *because* they're trying to lose weight," says Vasanti Malik, a research associate at the Harvard School of Public Health in Boston, Massachusetts.

"So what you see is an artificial association between consuming these artificially sweetened beverages and body weight. It's a perfect example of what we call reverse causation."

The best evidence that diet pop doesn't cause weight gain: a Dutch trial that randomly assigned 641 children to drink a cup a day of pop sweetened with either sugar or the artificial sweeteners sucralose plus acesulfame potassium for 18 months.[3] Those who got the regular pop gained more weight (and fat).

Why do new studies seem to flip-flip so often? It's partly because old news is no news. A new study that overturns *everything you've ever heard* gets more press than the same old, same old results.

But the headlines can deceive when they play up the "earthshaking" findings and play down the dull, humdrum caveats. We explain some starting on this page.

To learn how researchers hunt for ways to prevent disease, from first hunch to conclusive trials, see below. And see the "Trial & Error" feature for some key trial results.

"This was a double-blind trial with a long-term follow-up, and they measured sucralose in the urine to make sure the children drank the sugar-free beverages," explains Malik. "So it was really well done." Smaller trials on adults have found similar results.[4]

Likewise, when some studies report more diabetes in diet-pop drinkers, it's probably because doctors have told people at risk for diabetes to switch to diet pop.

"In our studies, when we take into account whether people are dieting and changes in their weight, the association between diet pop and diabetes goes away," says Malik.[5]

2. A Link Doesn't Prove Cause and Effect

"Antioxidants block harmful chemical reactions caused by oxidation," explains Dr. Andrew Weil's online Vitamin Library. (Weil recommends that adults take four antioxidants every day: vitamin C, vitamin E, selenium, and mixed carotenoids—including beta-carotene.)

Maybe so, but a new animal study suggests that high-dose antioxidant supplements may make tumors grow by reducing p53, a protein that suppresses tumors.[6] That may explain why more than a dozen trials on thousands of people have found that antioxidant supplements either had no effect on, or, in a few cases, *increased* cancer risk.[7,8]

What led researchers to launch the antioxidant trials in the first place?

"People who had higher intakes or blood levels of beta-carotene or vitamin C had a lower risk of cancer," says JoAnn Manson, chief of preventive medicine at Brigham and Women's Hospital in Boston. Other studies found a lower risk of heart disease in people who took vitamin E supplements.

"But correlation doesn't prove causation," adds Manson. Something else about those people could explain their lower risk.

For example, "blood levels of beta-carotene and vitamin C may be good markers of fruit and vegetable intake," says Manson. "And people who eat more fruits and vegetables or who take vitamin supplements may be more health conscious, may exercise more, and may have an overall healthier diet."

They may also do other things to protect their health. "They may be more likely to take medication if they have high blood pressure, or to take a statin if they have high cholesterol," notes Manson.

Researchers try to adjust for those and other "confounders." For example, they look at whether vitamin E takers have a lower risk of heart disease than vitamin E non-takers who report the same level of exercise.

But scientists can't fully adjust for all confounders, especially the ones they don't know about.

One eye-opening example: there is something different about people in a trial who take nearly all their pills, even if they're taking a (inactive) placebo.[9]

"People who are more likely to take placebos have a lower risk of heart disease and cancer and mortality," says Manson.

And not just *slightly* lower. Among roughly 13,000 people assigned to take a placebo in the Women's Health Initiative, those who took their pills faithfully had a 50 percent lower risk of hip fracture, a 30 percent lower risk of heart attack, a 40 percent lower risk of dying of cancer, and a 35 percent lower risk of dying of any cause than those who took their placebo pills less than 80 percent of the time.[10]

"That's powerful evidence that unmeasured factors and behaviours are linked to a lower risk of chronic disease," says Manson.

3. It's Not Ready for Prime Time

"Not all calories equal," said the headline on ctvnews.ca in June of 2012. "A new study suggests we burn certain kinds of calories more efficiently while on certain diets, making weight loss easier," the network reported.

The study put 21 overweight or obese adults on one of three diets—low fat, low carb, or low glycemie index—for one month each. The diets all had the same number of calories. The authors' conclusion: on the low-carb diet, the people burned 300 more calories a day than on the low-fat diet, and 150 calories more than on the low-glycemic-index diet.[11]

A 300-calorie difference is "roughly equal to an hour of moderate physical activity—without lifting a finger," David Ludwig, lead author and director of the New Balance Foundation Obesity Prevention Center at Boston Children's Hospital, told the *Los Angeles Times.*

What's the catch?

For starters, the diets didn't make a difference in pounds gained or lost, making the results way too early for prime time.

If people burned more calories on the low-carb diet, "it's surprising that the people on the low-carb diet didn't lose more weight after a month," notes Frank Sacks, professor of cardiovascular disease prevention at the Harvard School of Public Health.

Another catch: even if a low-carb diet led to more weight loss over time, it's not clear that people could stick with it. "We did not design the diets for long-term practicality," wrote the authors. For one thing, the researchers served the participants all their meals.

That's not how the Pounds Lost study was designed. It was the largest (811 people) and longest (two-year) trial to test whether people lose more weight on a low-fat or low-carb (or high-protein) diet.[12]

Trial & Error

Here's a sampling of large clinical trials with promising or disappointing results. To be succinct, we omitted many details about the participants, outcomes, and limitations of the studies. We also rounded the number of participants.

1991

MRC Vitmain Study: 1,800 women who had an earlier pregnancy with a neural tube defect (NTD) like spina bifida take folic acid (4,000 mcg a day), a multivitamin, both, or a placebo. Folic acid takers have a 72 percent lower risk of NTDs. Multivitamins have no effect.[1]

2000

Wheat Bran Fibre Trial: 1,400 people with previous colon polyps are told to eat cereal with either 2 grams or 13.5 grams of fibre from wheat bran every day for 3 years. No difference in polyp recurrence.[2]

2001

AREDS: 3,600 people with macular degeneration take vitamin C (500 mg), vitamin E (400 IU), plus beta-carotene (25,000 IU) and/or zinc (80 mg) plus copper (2 mg), or a placebo every day for 6 years. Supplement takers are 28 percent less likely to progress to advanced macular degeneration.[3]

2002

Diabetes Prevention Program: 3,200 people with high fasting blood sugar (but not diabetes) participate in a weight-loss and exercise program for 3 years. Diet-plus-exercise group has 58 percent lower incidence of diabetes than placebo group.[4]

2006

Women's Health Initiative: 48,800 women are told to eat a low-fat diet or their usual diet for 8 years. Low-fat group has no lower risk of breast or colon cancer.[5,6]

2007

Women's Antioxidant Cardiovascular Study: 8,200 women at risk for heart disease take vitamin C (500 mg a day), vitamin E (600 IU on alternate days), and/or beta-carotene (83,000 IU on alternate days), or a placebo for 9 years. No difference in heart attacks, strokes, diabetes, or memory.[7–9]

2009

SELECT: 35,500 men take vitamin E (400 IU a day), selenium (200 mcg a day), both, or a placebo for 5½ years. Vitamin E takers have a 17 percent higher risk of prostate cancer. Selenium has no effect.[10]

2009

Physicians' Health Study II: 14,600 men take vitamin E (400 IU on alternate days), vitamin C (500 mg a day), both, or a placebo for 8 years. No difference in total cancer, prostate cancer, colorectal cancer, lung cancer, macular degeneration, or cataracts.[11–13]

2010

B Vitamin Treatment Trialists Collaboration: 8 trials give 37,500 people at risk for cardiovascular disease folic acid (typically 2,500 mcg), B-12 (typically 1,000 mcg), and B-6 (typically 50 mg) or a placebo every day for 2–7 years. No difference in heart attacks, stroke, or cancers.[14]

2012

Physicians' Health Study II: 14,600 men take a daily multivitamin for seniors (Centrum Silver) or a placebo for 11 years. Vitamin takers have an 8 percent lower risk of total cancers, but no lower risk of heart attack, stroke, or cognitive decline.[15–17]

2012

DRINK: 640 normal-weight children (aged 5–12) who drink sugar-sweetened beverages (SSBs) get 1 cup a day of SSBs or sugar-free beverages. After 1½ years, weight gain, fat gain, and waist size are greater in the sugar-sweetened-beverage drinkers.[18]

2013

Risk and Prevention Study: 12,500 people at high risk for heart attack take 1,000 mg of fish oil or a placebo every day for 5 years. No difference in deaths, heart attacks, or strokes.[19]

1 *Lancet 338:* 131, 1991.
2 *N . Engl. J. Med. 342:* 1156, 2000.
3 *Arch. Ophthalmol. 119:* 1417, 2001.
4 *N. Engl. J. Med. 346:* 393, 2002.
5 *JAMA 295:* 629, 643, 2006.
6 *JAMA 295:* 643, 2006.
7 *Arch. Intern. Med. 167:* 1610, 2007.
8 *Am. J. Clin. Nutr. 90:* 429, 2009.
9 *Circulation 119:* 2772, 2009.
10 *JAMA 306:* 1549, 2011.
11 *JAMA 301:* 52, 2009.
12 *Arch. Ophthalmol. 128:* 1397, 2010.
13 *Ophthalmol. 119:* 1642, 2012.
14 *Arch. Intern. Med. 170:* 1622, 2010.
15 *JAMA 308:* 1871, 2012.
16 *JAMA 308:* 1751, 2012.
17 *Ophthalmol. 121:* 525, 2014.
18 *N. Engl. J. Med. 367:* 1397, 2012.
19 *N. Engl. J. Med. 368:* 1800, 2013.

"No one diet beat the others," says Sacks, the lead author. "The participants lost an average of 13 pounds after six months, and kept off an average of nine pounds after two years, regardless of which diet they were on."

What mattered most was how many calories people ate. "Ignore all the hype about diets that make pounds melt away," says Sacks. "Losing weight comes down to how much food you put in your mouth."

Critics might argue that the Pounds Lost study didn't test a diet that was truly low in fat or carbs (or high in protein) because, after two years, the differences between diets had shrunk.

"It's tough to get hundreds of people to stick with a diet for two years," says Sacks.

But one could also argue that a study like Pounds Lost is a real-world test of the diets. "If participants in a study can't stick with a diet, it's even harder for people to do it on their own," says Sacks.

4. It's Missing the Big Picture

"Study finds calcium supplements don't prevent broken bones," announced the headline in *The New York Times* in 2006.

The *Times* was reporting on the Women's Health Initiative (WHI), a massive clinical trial that randomly assigned roughly 36,000 post-menopausal women to take either calcium (1,000 mg) and vitamin D (400 IU) or a placebo every day. After seven years, the researchers found no fewer fractures in the women who were assigned to take calcium and vitamin D.[13]

What's the catch? The *Times*' headline may have missed the forest for the trees.

The study's overall results compared everyone in the calcium group to everyone in the placebo group, whether or not they took the calcium or placebo pills the researchers gave them. That "intention-to-treat" analysis is legitimate, but sometimes it ignores critical evidence.

"There are three separate lines of strong evidence from the WHI that the calcium-and-vitamin-D supplement was beneficial for bone health," says study co-author JoAnn Manson.

First, "we found significantly higher bone mineral density in the hip, which is the most important area," in women who were assigned to take calcium plus vitamin D, explains Manson. Hip fractures are the most debilitating kind.

"Second, we found a 21 percent lower risk of hip fracture in women aged 60 and older" who took calcium plus D, she notes. And those are the fractures that matter.

"The hip fractures in the women in their 50s were often related to trauma—like skiing accidents—where you wouldn't expect calcium and vitamin D supplements to help," explains Manson. "When you're talking about a hip fracture related to fragility, low bone density, and osteoporosis, those fractures are in women 60 and older."

Third, when the researchers looked only at women of any age who actually took their calcium and vitamin D at least 80 percent of the time—a reasonable group to look at—those women had a 30 percent lower risk of hip fracture than those who took their placebos that often.

"A 30 percent reduction is pretty important," says Manson. "Many people are missing that point."

Taken together, "the evidence is strong that the calcium-and-vitamin-D supplement was beneficial for bone health."

Are there downsides to taking calcium?

"We found a 17 percent increase in kidney stones in women taking calcium supplements," notes Manson.

But the average WHI participant was getting roughly 1,100 mg of calcium from food and the supplements she was taking on her own, so the calcium takers were getting close to 2,100 mg a day. "That could explain the increased risk of kidney stones," suggests Manson.

And contrary to recent reports, "there was no increase in heart disease or stroke or other cardiovascular events" in the calcium-plus-vitamin-D takers, she adds.

Manson doesn't advise all women to take a daily 1,000 mg calcium supplement, like the WHI participants did.

"The Recommended Dietary Allowance for women is 1,000 mg of calcium, and 1,200 mg after menopause," she says. "Women should try to get as much of that as possible from food, because calcium in foods is linked to a lower risk of kidney stones and heart disease. And they should take a supplement only to get up to the RDA. Very often that's just 500 or 800 mg more."

Notes

1. *Am. J. Public Health* 2014. doi:10.2105/AJPH.2013.301556.
2. *Obesity 20:* 118, 2012.
3. *N. Engl. J. Med. 368:* 1279. 2012.
4. *Am. J. Clin. Nutr. 76:* 721, 2002.
5. *Am. J. Clin. Nutr. 93:* 1321, 2011.
6. *Sci. Transl. Med. 6:* 221ra15, 2014.
7. *JAMA 306:* 1549, 2011.
8. *N. Engl. J. Med. 330:* 1029, 1994,
9. *Emerg. Themes Epidemiol. 10:* 1, 2013.
10. *Med. Care 49:* 427, 2011.
11. *JAMA 307:* 2627, 2012.
12. *N. Engl. J. Med. 360:* 859, 2009.
13. *N. Engl J. Med. 354:* 669, 2006.

Critical Thinking

1. Select one recent newspaper article that describes the findings of a peer-reviewed, nutrition-related study. Compare the conclusion outlined in the newspaper article to the conclusion of the peer-reviewed journal article. Describe the differences and similarities between the two.
2. Describe how results of a study may be sensationalized by the media.

Create Central

www.mhhe.com/createcentral

Internet References

Academy of Nutrition and Dietetics
www.eatright.org/

Center for Science in the Public Interest
www.cspinet.org

National Institutes of Health
www.nih.gov

Article

Prepared by: Janet Colson, *Middle Tennessee State University*

Four of the Biggest Quacks Plaguing America with False Claims about Science

From the Food Babe to Dr. Oz, these four are the media's biggest fear-mongers and snake-oil peddlers.

CLIFF WEATHERS

Learning Outcomes

After reading this article, you will be able to:

- Explain the dangers that can result when the public takes health and nutrition advice from quacks.
- List examples of quackery that the author describes about Dr. Mercola, Mike Adams, Vani Hari, and Dr. Oz.

It may be easy to draw a caricature of a "quack" as a cross between the ShamWow pitchman and an alchemist, but they're really not so easy to spot. Modern-day quacks often cherry-pick science and use what suits them as semantic backdrop to fool unsuspecting consumers. Quacks may dazzle people with fanciful research studies or scare them with intimidating warnings before trying to peddle products that make unreasonable promises. And those who use these alternative, unproven products may forego treatments that would be more likely to help them.

In short, quackery is dangerous. It promotes fear, devalues legitimate science and can destroy lives. Here are the four biggest quacks giving dubious health advice in the media and some samples of their detrimental advice.

1. Dr. (of Osteopathy) Joseph Mercola

Mercola is not a strict medical doctor, but an osteopath who practiced in suburban Chicago (according to *Chicago* magazine, he gave up his practice in 2006 to focus on Internet marketing). Mercola has also written several books on health that have become bestsellers.

Mercola operates one of the Internet's largest and most trafficked health and consumer information sites. With an estimated 15.5 million unique monthly visitors, Merola.com dwarfs even ConsumerReports.org and HealthCentral.com. The site vigorously promotes and sells dietary supplements, many of which bear Dr. Mercola's name.

A typical article on Mercola's site touts the wonders of yet another miracle cure or supplement. Some recent articles include "13 Amazing Health Benefits of Himalayan Crystal Salt" and "Your Flu Shot Contains a Dangerous Neurotoxin." His site has also touted Vitamin D as "The Silver Bullet for Cancer."

Many of Mercola's musings clash—sometimes bitterly—with conventional medical wisdom. Mercola advises against immunization, water fluoridation, mammography, and the routine administration of vitamin K shots for newborns.

The medical community says Mercola is dangerous, and he steers patients away from proven medical treatments in favor of unproven therapies and supplements.

"The information he's putting out to the public is extremely misleading and potentially very dangerous," says Dr. Stephen Barrett, who runs the medical watchdog site Quackwatch.org. "He exaggerates the risks and potential dangers of legitimate science-based medical care, and he promotes a lot of unsubstantiated ideas and sells [certain] products with claims that are misleading."

Mercola has been the subject of a number of Food and Drug Administration warning letters about his activities, including marketing products as providing "exceptional countermeasures" against cancer, heart disease, diabetes, and a host of other illnesses. He also has marketed coconut oil to treat heart disease, Crohn's disease, and irritable bowel syndrome. Mercola.com also sold an infrared camera to be used as a cancer screening tool.

Some of Dr. Mercola's wildest claims include:

- HIV may not be the cause of AIDS. Mercola believes that the manifestations of AIDS (including opportunistic infections and death) could result from "psychological stress" brought on by the belief that HIV is harmful. Mercola.com has also featured positive presentations of the claims of AIDS truthers who deny the existence of AIDS or the role HIV has in the disease.
- Mercola has said that microwave ovens emit dangerous radiation and that microwaving food alters its chemistry.
- Commercial sunscreens *increase the likelihood of skin cancer,* instead of protecting from it. Of course, he sells his own natural sunscreens on his website.

2. The "Health Ranger," Mike Adams

Adams runs a website called Natural News that is dedicated to supporting alternative medicine techniques and various conspiracy theories about chemtrails, the link between vaccinations and autism, and the dangers of fluoridated drinking water. Dr. Mercola is a frequent guest blogger on his site.

Natural News, which gets an estimated 7 million unique visitors a month, primarily promotes alternative medicine, raw foods, and holistic nutrition. Adams claims he began the site after curing himself of Type II diabetes by using natural remedies.

Adams seems to revel in going against the grain. He likes to tell readers on his website that if they just exercise, eat the right foods and take the right supplements (he markets supplements on his site) infectious disease cannot harm them. Like Mercola, he is an AIDS denialist, and claims flu vaccines are totally ineffective.

Dr. David Gorski of the Science-Based Medicine website calls Natural News "a one-stop shop, a repository if you will, of virtually every quackery known to humankind, all slathered with a heaping, helping of unrelenting hostility to science-based medicine and science in general."

Adams also considers himself a scientific researcher, but some of his claims are dubious. He has even bought himself a mass spectrometer which he uses to test various products for toxicity. He recently used this device to show that a flu vaccine containing thiomersal registered 51 parts per million of mercury. But that's not the news in his findings: Adams went on to insist that his critics must be brain-damaged (or perhaps brainwashed) by mercury: "The only people who argue with this are those who are already mercury poisoned and thus incapable of rational thought. Mercury damages brain function, you see, which is exactly what causes some people to be tricked into thinking vaccines are safe and effective."

Science-Based Medicine blogger Dr. Steven Novella describes Adams' site as "a crank alt-med site that promotes every sort of medical nonsense imaginable. If it is unscientific, antiscientific, conspiracy-mongering, or downright silly, Mike Adams appears to be all for it—whatever sells the 'natural' products he hawks on his site."

What makes Adams unique is that he likes to mix far-right vitriol and conspiracy theories with his alternative medicine advice. He has come out as a climate-change denialist, *9/11* Truther, and a Birther.

Here's some more quackery from Adams and Natural News:

- Guns don't kill people, medications do. Adam Lanza and Elliot Rodger committed their horrific mass murders because of the medications they were taking.
- A cold fusion device has been invented and will be a game changer for energy. *It wasn't.*
- Americans are constantly bombarded by lead coming from airplane chemtrails. (Actually, *lead levels in blood* have been *falling for years.*)
- Bill Gates and Microsoft are in the process of developing weaponized, ethnically targeted influenza viruses as part of a sinister eugenics plot.

3. The "Food Babe," Vani Hari

She doesn't have a degree in nutrition, chemistry, or medicine, and her work background is as a management consultant. Yet without any serious credentials, Hari—the "Food Babe"—bills herself as a voice of consumer protection on the Internet. In just a few years, she's assembled an army of followers who have joined her on her quest to get hard-to-pronounce ingredients banned from foods.

Hari's acolytes see her as a muckraking reporter, saving us from nefarious chemicals, GMOs and unappetizing ingredients like beaver anus, yoga mat, and fish bladder. The public and the media love her; a "food safety" campaign by the Food Babe can get thousands of signatures, countless media mentions, and guest appearances on television shows such as *Dr. Oz* and *The Doctors.*

But Hari is really more of a fear-mongerer and conspiracy theorist than a safe-food advocate. Her campaigns are born of misinformation and anxiety. Recently, she published a petition on her website demanding that the top beer companies come clean about the ingredients in their beer. Citing a long list of creepy, chemical-sounding ingredients that are allowed in beer, she implied that the industry was flying under the radar and obscuring the additives it puts in its products. It turned out that the beer companies were actually using very few of the ingredients on her list, and some were only used in the production process and were not part of the finished product. When we looked further into it, we found that many of the nefarious ingredients and techniques she described were either misrepresented or entirely misunderstood by her.

However, at Hari's request, the top two breweries in the United States acquiesced and listed their ingredients on their websites, and none of the ingredients would come as a real shock to beer drinkers. Still, Hari continued to insist that GMO corn and other bad ingredients were integral ingredients in beer.

In response to critics who say Hari is not qualified to make hard judgments on food ingredients, Hari says, "I don't think you need to have those degrees to be intellectually honest, to be able to research, to be able to present ideas."

Dr. David Gorski, a cancer surgeon who writes for the website Science-Based Medicine takes offense to Hari's food campaigns: "Her strategy is very transparent, but unfortunately it's also very effective," wrote Gorski. "Name a bunch of chemicals and count on the chemical illiteracy of your audience to result in fear at hearing their very names."

Gorski says since companies live and die by public perception; it's far easier to "give a blackmailer like Hari what she wants than to try to resist or to counter her propaganda by educating the public."

Some of Vani Hari's more specious ideas about food are:

- Microwaves kill food and remove its nutrients. Also, microwaves change the chemical properties of water. She persists with this theory although it has been persistently debunked by science.
- Water, when exposed to the words "Hitler" and "Satan" changes its physical properties.
- Flu shots contain "a bunch of toxic chemicals and additives that lead to several types of Cancers and Alzheimer [sic] disease over time." Actually, flu shots are made up mostly of proteins and preservatives that give no indication of being harmful, despite plenty of medical research.

Hari has not provided any scientific evidence to back her claims as of yet.

4. Dr. Mehmet Oz

What do Vani Hari, Dr. Joseph Mercola and Mike Adams have in common? They're all guest experts appearing on the *Dr. Oz Show.*

Dr. Oz is a media darling and cardiothoracic surgeon who first appeared on the Oprah Winfrey Show in 2004. In 2009, Oprah produced Oz's namesake show focusing on medical issues and personal health.

But before we label Oz a quack, it's only fair that we also should note he's a professor at the Department of Surgery at Columbia University, directs the Cardiovascular Institute and Complementary Medicine Program at New York-Presbyterian Hospital, has authored more than 400 medical research papers and holds several patents.

But unless you've been living under a rock for the last month, you probably know Dr. Oz has been exposed as a daytime-television snake oil peddler, while being shamed during testimony before a U.S. Senate subcommittee last month.

Sen. Claire McCaskill, the chairwoman of the Senate subcommittee on Consumer Protection, took Oz to task over false claims he's made for over-the-counter weight loss cures. For example, Oz proclaims that worthless supplements such as green coffee beans have "miracle" properties.

The Missouri senator made it clear that she thinks Oz abuses his great influence. Products he endorses on his show are almost guaranteed to fly off the shelves. "People want to believe they can take an itty-bitty pill to push fat out of their body," McCaskill chided the celebrity doctor. "I know you know how much power you have."

Oz acknowledged to the subcommittee that while there's no such thing as a "miracle" supplement, and many he touts wouldn't pass scientific muster, he insisted he was comfortable recommending them to his fans.

"My job is to be a cheerleader for the audience," Oz says. "And when they don't think they have hope, when they don't think they can make it happen, I want to look and I do look everywhere, including alternative healing traditions, for any evidence that might be supportive to them."

As McCaskill then pointed out, Oz was giving people false hope. Isn't that what quacks do?

Oz often uses his show as a soapbox for the likes of Hari, Mercola and Adams. And when they're guests on his show, they're handled with kid gloves. Oz even describes Adams as an "activist researcher," a "whistleblower," and a "food safety activist." Viewers then open their wallets to Adams, who is there to promote his website. A similar scenario plays out when Mercola, a frequent guest, joins Oz. Hari, for her part, does not market miracle products on her site. She does, however, seem to make money from affiliate advertising.

Oz's great sin is that he uses his show to promote all types of modern shamanism. Critics find it mystifying that he, a medical doctor, would host and promote people on his show who are anathema to science. It's Oz's instant access to millions and his medical degrees and peer-reviewed research papers that have given him credibility, but critics say he loses all of it when he promotes guests who explicitly reject the tenets of reason. So, can Oz still be considered a serious scientist?

Unlike the other three quacks mentioned in this article, Oz is more a ringmaster than a snake-oil salesman. However, he's not without his list of dubious stances:

- In November 2012, Dr. Oz invited Julie Hamilton, a representative of the National Association for Research and Therapy of Homosexuality, who claimed that she could heal homosexuality with gay reparative therapy. Although the show did include guests who condemned reparative therapy, Dr. Oz never weighed in on the subject, and the audience was led to believe that there were valid arguments on both sides of this issue.
- His proclamation on Oprah that resveratrol is an effective anti-aging supplement sparked a resveratrol marketing craze. Numerous fly-by-night online peddlers used his name and likeness (along with the likenesses of age-defying actresses Jennifer Aniston and Marisa Tomei) to peddle the so-called miracle supplement. But it's anyone's guess what was in those pills.
- Oz has invited a medium on his show who told selected audience members that she was communicating with their lost loved ones.
- Oz once invited a faith healer, Issam Nemeh, to "heal" sick audience members on his show. On his website, Oz bragged about the "Oz Effect": "Dr. Nemeh has received an overwhelming response from the viewers of the Dr. Oz show. Medical office appointments with Dr. Nemeh are already filled for the next four months."

Critical Thinking

1. Of the four individuals described in the article, whose advice is most misleading to the public? Justify your answer with specific examples.
2. Go to the website of one of the "quacks" described in the article. Identify three nutrition-related claims on the site that are misleading. Using reliable sources, explain the accuracy or inaccuracy of each claim.

Create Central

www.mhhe.com/createcentral

Internet References

Food Babe
http://foodbabe.com/

Mercola.com
www.mercola.com

Nutrition Action Healthletter
www.cspinet.org

Quackwatch
www.quackwatch.com

The Dr. Oz Show
http://www.doctoroz.com/

The Health Ranger
http://www.healthranger.com/index.asp

Cliff Weathers is a senior editor at AlterNet, covering environmental and consumer issues. He is a former deputy editor at *Consumer Reports*. His work has also appeared in *Salon, Car and Driver, Playboy, Raw Story* and *Detroit Monthly* among other publications.

Article

Prepared by: Janet Colson, *Middle Tennessee State University*

Beyond the Buzz

Is What You've Heard *True* . . . or Just *New*?

STEPHANIE SCARMO

Learning Outcome

After reading this article, you will be able to:

- Distinguish between valid and invalid nutrition information and current topics related to dairy products, gluten, breakfast, fast foods, and garlic.

Should you drink chocolate milk after your daily brisk walk? Do dairy foods raise the risk of ovarian cancer? If you cut out wheat, will those extra pounds melt away? With so much information—and misinformation—out there, it's hard to know what to believe. Here's the truth about some of the latest buzz.

Drink Chocolate Milk after Exercise?

"Got milk? Try chocolate after your workout," urged the FitnessMagazine.com article.

When it comes to recovering from intense exercise, a classic childhood beverage has taken the spotlight.

When you're inactive or moving slowly, your body gets energy mostly from burning fat (assuming you haven't just eaten). But for more intense activity (brisk walking, running, cycling, etc.), you can't burn fat fast enough to get all the energy you need. So if you're, say, running for several hours, your body is going to rely more on carbs for the *extra* energy it needs.[1]

"When we're talking about recovery from endurance exercise, you're generally trying to restore muscle glycogen," explains Beth Glace, a sports nutritionist at the Nicholas Institute of Sports Medicine and Athletic Trauma at Lenox Hill Hospital in New York City.

Glycogen is essentially a long chain of glucose (blood sugar). The body converts glucose to glycogen in order to store the glucose in muscles and in the liver. But we don't have much glycogen, especially compared to our vast stores of fat.

So during an intense, prolonged activity, you can run out of glycogen. That's what marathoners are talking about when they say they "hit the wall."

"In more seriously trained athletes, let's say a triathlete, they might do a run in the morning and a swim or bike workout later in the afternoon," says Glace. "So it really becomes crucial for them to restore their glycogen reserves quickly. This is where chocolate milk comes in."

In some studies, drinking chocolate milk immediately after a strenuous workout is one of the best ways to recover quickly—better than sugary sports drinks like Gatorade.[2,3] The milk's naturally occurring sugar (lactose) is half glucose, its protein speeds up glycogen synthesis in the body, and its electrolytes (like potassium and, to a lesser extent, sodium) help you rehydrate. Why *chocolate* milk?

"The extra sugar provides more carbohydrates for energy storage," explains Glace. A typical low-fat chocolate milk has roughly four times more carbs than protein, which may be the optimal ratio to rapidly replenish glycogen stores in muscles.[2,4]

Can you get the carbs and protein in your next meal? Probably, if you eat soon. You restore glycogen more quickly if you eat the carbs and protein within an hour.

Of course, most of us aren't running marathons or cycling competitively for two hours and then doing another intense activity within 24 hours. Do *we* need a recovery beverage? Not likely.

"A recovery food or drink becomes important if you're doing another hard workout that day," says Glace. "If you're just going for a walk, it probably doesn't matter because you're not burning that much glycogen."

And if you're taking that brisk walk to lose weight, you don't want the 170 or so calories in a cup of chocolate milk . . . or *any* extra calories, for that matter.

Bottom Line

Unless you're doing prolonged, intense exercise on successive days, or more than one strenuous workout on the same day, you don't need chocolate milk (or any food) to recover.

---

1 *Am. J. Clin. Nutr. 61:* 968S, 1995.
2 *Med. Sci. Sports Exerc. 44:* 682, 2012.
3 *Int. J. Sport Nutr. Exerc. Metab. 16:* 78, 2006.
4 *Int. J. Sport Nutr. Exerc. Metab. 13:* 382, 2003.

Skipping Breakfast Makes You Fatter?

"Skipping breakfast to lose weight makes you fatter," reported the UK's *Daily Mail* in October 2012.

"The idea is that people end up overeating later in the day because they think, 'Oh, I skipped breakfast, so now I can eat more at lunch or dinner,' " explains Rania Mekary, a nutrition researcher at Harvard University.

But in a recent effort to debunk common obesity "myths," researchers concluded that there's not enough evidence to prove that eating breakfast protects against weight gain.[1] They relied largely on one of the only clinical trials—and a weak one, at that—that compared how much weight people lost after they were randomly assigned to either eat or skip breakfast.

Among 50 obese women, those who were told to eat breakfast every day for 12 weeks didn't lose (or gain) more weight than those who were told to skip breakfast.[2] (Interestingly, women who had to change their eating habits for the study—that is, breakfast skippers who were told to eat and breakfast eaters who were told to skip—lost more weight than those who didn't change.)

Some large surveys have reported that breakfast eaters weigh less than skippers, but those kinds of studies can't prove cause and effect.[2,3]

Bottom Line

There's no good evidence that eating—or skipping—breakfast makes you lose or gain weight.

[1] *N. Engl. J. Med. 368:* 446, 2013.
[2] *Am. J. Epidemiol. 158:* 85, 2003.
[3] *Am. J. Clin. Nutr. 88:* 1396, 2008.

Avoid Fast Food to Dodge Asthma?

"Fast food linked to severe asthma in children," said *U.S. News and World Report* in January.

The online news magazine was reporting on a survey of more than half a million children and adolescents in 51 countries. Those who reported eating fast food at least three times a week were 27 to 39 percent more likely to have severe asthma (as well as allergy symptoms and eczema) than those who said that they ate fast food less than once a week or never.[1]

"It's a clue, but it's not nearly the discovery that the media made it out to be," explains Carlos Camargo, an asthma researcher and physician at Massachusetts General Hospital in Boston. "While the study was large, this type of research can't say whether fast food *caused* asthma."

Most asthma gets diagnosed in childhood, but the disease can also strike in adulthood. In fact, asthma affects about 7 percent of U.S. adults aged 18 and over.[2] In 1980, it was just 3 percent.[3] Asthma inflames and narrows the airways in the lungs, which leads to wheezing, coughing, and shortness of breath.

What accounts for the increase in asthma worldwide? It's not clear, although some researchers have speculated that the rise may be due to an increase in "Westernized" diets. But so far, studies haven't found any foods that raise the risk.

Nor do foods seem to help relieve symptoms. "No specific food has been shown to help with asthma control," says Camargo. "It's possible that ensuring adequate intake of specific nutrients, like omega-3 fatty acids or vitamin D, may help," he notes. "But we need large randomized trials to test those possibilities."

One thing that may help control asthma symptoms: losing excess pounds.

In a small trial, 46 overweight or obese adults were divided into three groups. A third were counseled to cut calories to (on average) 1,170 a day, a third were given pedometers and encouraged to take 10,000 steps per day, and a third were asked to do both.

After 10 weeks, people in the groups that lost the most weight—those who cut calories or cut calories and exercised—reported fewer symptoms (like less wheezing and shortness of breath, and fewer puffs from an inhaler).[4]

Bottom Line

There's no good evidence that eating fast food—or any other food—increases your risk of developing asthma. If you have asthma, losing extra weight may help control symptoms.

[1] *Thorax 68:* 351, 2013.
[2] *MMWR Surveill. Summ. 60 Suppl:* 84, 2011.
[3] *MMWR Surveill. Summ. 56:* 1, 2007.
[4] *Clin. Exp. Allergy 43:* 36, 2013.

Taking Garlic Pills Protects Your Heart?

"Supports your cardiovascular system," say the Kyolic bottles.

"Cholesterol's Natural Enemy," boast the Garlique packages.

Sounds like taking garlic supplements keeps heart disease at bay. Not so fast.

People have been eating or using garlic for hundreds of years, trying to ward off everything from gangrene and the plague to vampires. And they've been taking garlic pills since the 1980s to lower their cholesterol.

In a 2007 study, Christopher Gardner, an associate professor of medicine at Stanford University, put raw garlic and two popular garlic-pill formulations to a rigorous long-term test in 192 adults with moderately high LDL ("bad") cholesterol.

Supplement manufacturers market garlic in a dizzying array of formulations. "But the compounds that end up in garlic oil, aged garlic, and garlic powder, for example, wouldn't necessarily be the same compounds or amounts or proportions that are in fresh garlic," explains Gardner.

So his team randomly assigned roughly a quarter of the participants to eat four grams (around 1½ teaspoons) a day of raw garlic. Another quarter were given Garlicin (powdered garlic) pills, while a quarter got Kyolic (aged garlic) pills and a quarter were told to take a placebo.[1] (The garlic-pill takers were given enough Garlicin or Kyolic to match the active compounds in the raw garlic.)

No matter how hard the researchers tried—they mixed the raw garlic into sandwiches—the raw-garlic eaters could tell which group they were in. "Our garlic pills, however, were successfully blinded," notes Gardner.

After six months, LDL cholesterol, HDL ("good") cholesterol, and triglycerides were no different in the garlic eaters and the garlic-pill takers than in those who got the placebo.

"The backlash we got when we published our study! I must have had 50 offers from supplement companies of, 'Hey! I know why your study didn't work. You didn't use my pill,' " recalls Gardner.

"But the industry, they want to sell pills. I wouldn't buy any of these supplements to lower my blood cholesterol."

Bottom Line

Leave the garlic pills on the shelf. If your LDL ("bad") cholesterol is above "optimal" (if it's 100 or more), cut calories (if you need to lose weight), exercise more, and eat a healthy Omni-Heart diet (see "Mediterranean Mix-Up," May 2013).

---

[1] *Arch. Intern. Med. 167:* 346, 2007.

Eating Wheat Packs on The Pounds?

"Lose the wheat, lose the weight, and find your path back to health," proclaims cardiologist William Davis in his best-selling book, *Wheat Belly.*

Wheat consumption and obesity rates have increased in the United States since the mid-1980s, as Davis notes. We're also eating more calories now, although wheat—along with sugars, fats, and oils—accounts for much of the increase.

And cutting bread, bagels, pasta, tortillas, pizza crust, muffins, pancakes, crackers, croissants, cereal, cookies, cakes, doughnuts, pies, pita chips, pretzels, and dozens of other wheat foods out of your diet would certainly make a dent in your weight . . . assuming you didn't replace their calories with calories from other foods.

However, no good studies have tested whether wheatless diets are any better for losing weight—or keeping weight off—than other popular weight-loss diets.

The truth is that you can lose weight on just about *any* diet that cuts calories. Unfortunately, after six months or a year, most people begin to regain the weight they lost, no matter which foods they cut to lose the weight.[1]

"What we're really interested in is a scenario that helps you lose weight and keep it off in the long term," says Julie Jones, professor of foods and nutrition at St. Catherine University in Saint Paul, Minnesota. And there's no good evidence that slashing carbs helps you do that.

"Avoiding wheat isn't the answer," says Jones, who recently reviewed the evidence for many of *Wheat Belly*'s claims.[2]

Some people—those who have celiac disease or gluten intolerance—need to avoid wheat. "But don't do it to lose weight," says Jones. "This, like the rest of all fad diets, will run its course."

Bottom Line

Unless you cut calories, eliminating wheat won't help you lose weight or keep it off.

---

[1] *N. Engl. J. Med. 360:* 859, 2009.

[2] *Cereal Foods World 57:* 177, 2012.

Dairy Foods Cause Ovarian Cancer?

"Milk linked to ovarian cancer," reported CBS News in 2004.

Dairy foods—especially low-fat milk, yogurt, and cheese—supply calcium and vitamin D for bones and may protect against colorectal cancer and high blood pressure.[1] So how did dairy get a bad rap when it comes to the seventh leading cause of cancer deaths among women worldwide?

In 1989, a study reported that women with ovarian cancer were more likely to say that they ate foods that were higher in lactose, the naturally occurring sugar in milk.[2]

But having a disease can color what people remember eating. To avoid that possible bias, researchers pooled the data from 12 studies that asked more than half a million healthy women what they ate and then followed them for the next 7 to 20 years.

Women who consumed the most milk, cheese, yogurt, and ice cream were no more likely to be diagnosed with ovarian cancer than those who ate the least. However, the researchers found a "weak" (their word) 19 percent increased risk in women who consumed at least 30 grams of lactose per day.[3]

To get 30 grams, you'd need to consume roughly 2½ cups of milk, 2 cups of yogurt, 3 cups of ice cream, greek yogurt, or cottage cheese, or 27 pounds of cheddar.

How might lactose raise the risk of ovarian cancer if dairy doesn't? It's not clear. Could dairy foods have some other nutrients that lower risk and counteract the lactose? Could genes play a role? Or could the "weak" link simply be due to chance?

"If there is an increased risk of ovarian cancer, it's only at very high intakes of lactose," says Shelley Tworoger, an ovarian cancer researcher at Harvard University. "Even then, it was still a relatively modest association."

In 2007, the World Cancer Research Fund and the American Institute for Cancer Research declared that there wasn't enough evidence to reach a conclusion about dairy's effect on the risk of ovarian cancer.

So what *does* increase risk? A family history of ovarian cancer, having used hormone therapy, or never having been pregnant. So may excess weight. (Oral contraceptive use can *lower* risk, notes Tworoger.)

One of the reasons the survival rate for ovarian cancer is so low: the disease often causes no noticeable symptoms until it has spread to a distant site, when the five-year survival rate drops to only about 27 percent.

But new advances to detect the cancer early may be coming.

In January, researchers at Johns Hopkins University in Baltimore found that PAP smears, which are routine screening tests for cervical cancer, could detect telltale DNA from endometrial and ovarian cancers as well.[4]

"There's a lot of potential, but more work needs to be done to understand if we can use this to identify tumors in healthy women that you wouldn't otherwise be able to identify," says Tworoger.

Bottom Line

There's only weak evidence that large amounts of lactose (equal to what you'd get in 2½ glasses of milk) increase the risk of ovarian cancer.

---

[1] *Br. J. Nutr. 96 Suppl. 1:* S94, 2006.
[2] *Lancet 2:* 66, 1989.
[3] *Cancer Epidemiol. Biomarkers Prev. 15:* 364, 2006.
[4] *Sci. Transl. Med. 5:* 167, 2013.

Critical Thinking

1. Why do some people consider chocolate milk beneficial as a post-recovery beverage for athletes?
2. Does eating breakfast help you lose weight?
3. What is the relationship between fast food and asthma?
4. Jessica is trying to lose weight. She has decided to cut out all grain products and drink three protein shakes each day made from 12 oz of skim milk with 25 grams of soy protein added to the milk in each shake. What health problems might occur with this type diet?
5. Jerry is 50 years old, his BMI is 33, and he is very concerned about his health. He thinks that walking three miles each day, eating five cloves of garlic, cutting out all grain products, and taking omega-3 supplements will ward off heart problems, cancer, and diabetes. What advice would you tell Jerry about his diet and lifestyle?

Create Central

www.mhhe.com/createcentral

Internet References

Asthma and Allergy Foundation of America
www.aafa.org

Center for Science in the Public Interest
www.cspinet.org/about/index.html

National Cancer Institute
www.cancer.gov

National Dairy Council
www.nationaldairycouncil.org

National Ovarian Cancer Coalition
www.ovarian.org

Article

Prepared by: Janet Colson, *Middle Tennessee State University*

Answers to the Seven Big Questions Everyone Asks about Gluten

JILL RICHARDSON

Learning Outcomes

After reading this article, you will be able to:

- Describe what gluten is and the main source of gluten in the American diet.
- List three forms of cultivated wheat and explain how they differ.
- List the various conditions that necessitate gluten-free diets.

These days, it seems almost easier to find false "information" about gluten than the truth. Gluten-free is trendy, and it's no longer strange to find restaurant menus dotted with "GF" logos next to various items like "polenta lasagna" that have been tweaked to remove any trace of wheat.

Recently, Jimmy Kimmel made fun of people who follow gluten-free diets by asking pedestrians if they were gluten-free and, if so, what is gluten. And . . . they had no idea. Some people even believe that wheat nowadays is genetically engineered (it isn't). And with so much hype and confusion swirling around, others believe that anyone who says they can't have gluten is making it up. So here are some facts about wheat and gluten you should know.

1. What Is It?

What we call "gluten" is made of two separate proteins, gliadin and glutenin, found in wheat and other related grains (barley, rye, and triticale). When water is added, they combine to form gluten, a stretchy, elastic molecule that gives bread its wonderful consistency.

You can often find alternative forms of wheat in natural food stores, like einkorn wheat, emmer, spelt, or kamut. Sometimes people who cannot tolerate most wheat can tolerate these other forms of it, but not always.

2. Is It Genetically Engineered?

Much has been made about human tinkering with wheat DNA, yet so far, commercial wheats are not genetically engineered. This might change in the future—just give Monsanto more time—but so far, there is no genetically engineered wheat legally on the market in the United States.

The rumors that wheat is genetically engineered likely stem from two sources. First, from the ancient breeding that gave us modern wheat. Einkorn and emmer were two of the first forms of cultivated wheat. Einkorn is a diploid, meaning that it has two complete sets of chromosomes (one from the mother and one from the father), just like humans do.

Then, wheat got weird. Emmer and durum wheat are each tetraploid, with four complete sets of chromosomes. And spelt and common bread wheat are hexaploid, with six complete sets of chromosomes. This occurred without any genetic engineering, thousands of years ago.

Humans can't survive with extra sets of chromosomes, but plants can. It's still a bit odd, but it's actually somewhat common in the plant world. Strawberries can have eight sets of chromosomes, and marijuana aficionados found they could increase THC content by tricking the plant into growing with extra sets of chromosomes in it. Still, some marketers are using wheat's extra set of chromosomes as a reason to condemn it.

The extra chromosomes showed up in wheat long before modern science and plant breeding came along. More recently, scientists spent the 20th century fiddling with wheat to see if they could improve yield, disease resistance and other traits, including its ease of use in commercial kitchens.

The idea that modern breeding led to the increase in gluten intolerance has been promoted by books like Wheat Belly by William Davis. And in fact, a 2010 study compared the amount of specific gluten epitope (the part of the antigen recognized by the immune system) known to cause trouble for people with celiac disease in modern wheat and traditional wheat varieties (landraces). Overall, the gluten epitope was more present in modern varieties than traditional ones.

Still, changing wheat varieties is only one potential cause in the increase in gluten intolerance. We also live in a time with increases in all kinds of auto-immune diseases, including many that are entirely unrelated to gluten, like peanut allergies or asthma. Some scientists suspect the increase in auto-immune diseases actually stem from our lack of exposure to common allergens in the first few years of life. A recent study found that children exposed to cockroach droppings and cat and mouse dander as infants had lower rates of wheezing at age three.

In short: maybe it's not all wheat's fault.

3. What is Celiac Disease?

For celiac sufferers like Deanna Askin and Laura Clawson, the health consequences of eating gluten are real and severe. Before her diagnosis, Askin's symptoms parallel *what you'd* expect for a celiac sufferer who consumes gluten regularly. "I think starting around in high school I started having all sorts of digestive problems and breathing problems," Askin recalls. "I was tired all the time. I couldn't make it through class without falling asleep. I was hungry all the time, I was always starving."

Her doctors gave her several diagnoses, like acid reflux, but nothing helped. "It started getting worse and worse. I started getting cold sores, like real bad, taking up half my face. I was so tired and I got diagnosed with narcolepsy by a sleep clinic. I would fall asleep driving to and from work. I felt bloated all the time and my skin felt hard, like expanded but hard."

Then, at 21, she had a blood test to check for celiac and it came out positive. Today, as long as she eats a gluten-free diet, she feels fine. But when she consumes even just a little bit of gluten by accident, she suffers for weeks. "It's just so many odd random symptoms that it's hard to even remember them all until you get them all again at once," she says as she lists several of them, like horrible stomach pains. "I'm really hungry and then I go and eat and it hurts. I'm really fatigued and tired and feel really weak."

Laura Clawson's symptoms were much different. She suffered from anxiety and depression, and she "got every single cold and flu that was going around to the max." About six months after she gave up gluten, she says, "I had this moment where I was walking down the street and realized, I'm kind of happy all the time. What's going on here?" If she accidentally eats a little bit of gluten again, she relapses into anxiety.

4. Does Anyone Else besides Celiac Sufferers Need to Go Gluten Free?

In short, yes. Tricia Thompson, a registered dietitian, provides information on her website about various categories of gluten-free people. Aside from those with celiac disease or wheat allergies, there is another catch-all category referred to as non-celiac gluten sensitivity. This refers to people who do not have a food allergy to wheat or an auto-immune disease related to gluten, but still suffer symptoms like diarrhea when exposed to gluten.

Natasha Chart went gluten-free after a long problem with migraine headaches that began in her teens. In her 20s, the migraines grew even more common, and her doctors were unable to help. Finally, an alternative health provider recommended an elimination diet, a common tactic to identify one's migraine trigger. All migraine patients have one or more triggers, whether it's a food, a smell, or lack of sleep, that sets off their headaches. Removing foods from your diet and adding them back in one at a time is a way to identify food triggers. That's how Chart discovered that gluten and soy were her problems.

That said, not everyone who says they can't eat gluten suffers so severely. Some are told by chiropractors or other alternative health practitioners that they cannot eat gluten after undergoing tests using a practice called "applied kinesiology" that is little more than quackery. Others go gluten-free because it's the latest fad diet.

It's nice to respect your friends' wishes when serving them food, but it's important to know which category they fall into, since gluten restrictions differ if you've got celiac compared to if you're just jumping on the gluten-free band wagon because it sounds like a good idea.

5. Is It Really That Serious or Is It In Their Heads?

The gluten-free crowd is notorious for its strict adherence to avoiding even just a few molecules of gluten. For those with celiac, even the tiniest bit of gluten is a serious matter.

When Askin was first diagnosed with celiac, her doctor told her to avoid bread and pasta, and she did—but continued to be sick. It took her a year or two to learn which foods contained gluten, since oats are typically contaminated, and brewer's yeast can have gluten, and it can pop up in other strange places.

This month, she got sick after eating out, because her gluten-free meal was fried in the same oil as food containing gluten. She only had a few bites before the kitchen realized the mistake, but it made her sick all the same.

"People don't understand the consequences of it," says Askin. "They think it's just a trendy diet. And every time they are careless it has such a huge effect. I have to take off work because I'm too tired, and I have to go to the doctor, and I spend $40 in supplements. Plus it has a correlation with lymphoma and esophageal cancer because it takes a big toll on your body. My lymph nodes swell up like crazy."

Askin obviously has an extreme need to avoid gluten, as do all celiac sufferers. Those who are trying out a gluten-free diet because it's a trend might not. If you are cooking for a friend who is gluten-free, be sure to ask about her needs. Some, like Askin, cannot eat gluten-free hummus after someone else dips a pita chip (made of wheat) in it. That's too much contamination for her already. But others might be okay with that, as long as they avoid the pita chips.

6. Which Foods Contain Gluten?

Tricia Thompson has a list of gluten-containing foods on her website. At its core, being gluten-free means avoiding wheat, barley, rye, malt, brewer's yeast, and in most cases, oats. She also offers articles about foods of concern. Beer, unless it's gluten-free, is out, because it's made with barley. Soy sauce is out, because it's typically made with wheat or barley. The gluten-free alternative is tamari, but make sure to read the label just in case.

Now that so many foods are advertised as gluten-free, Thompson launched a site called Gluten Free Watchdog to test products that claim to be gluten-free to see if they really are.

7. Should I Go Gluten Free?

If you are worried whether you are suffering from a wheat allergy, celiac disease, or a non-celiac gluten sensitivity, the first place to go is to your doctor. Your doctor can perform a blood test to check for celiac, and might also suggest an intestinal biopsy to confirm the diagnosis. It's also possible to try eliminating gluten from your diet on your own, to see if you notice any changes in your health, but then you won't have an official diagnosis and the guidance from your doctor that would come with it.

Gluten-free living is not for everyone. It's not like trans-fat, where the entire world would be better off without it. If you aren't allergic or sensitive to gluten, then keep enjoying crusty sourdough breads, pizza, cookies, and all of the other glutinous goodies the world has to offer.

Critical Thinking

1. Plan a one-day, gluten-free menu that meets MyPlate recommendations.
2. Summarize a peer-reviewed, primary research article related to gluten.
3. Outline the FDA's regulations on the term *gluten-free* on food labels.

Create Central

www.mhhe.com/createcentral

Internet References

Celiac Central
www.celiaccentral.org

Celiac Disease Foundation
http://celiac.org

Celiac Support Association
www.csaceliacs.org

The Gluten Free Society
www.glutenfreesociety.org

The National Association of Wheat Growers
www.wheatworld.org

Jill Richardson is the founder of the blog La Vida Locavore and a member of the Organic Consumers Association policy advisory board. She is the author of *Recipe for America: Why Our Food System Is Broken and What We Can Do to Fix It.*

Article

Prepared by: Janet Colson, *Middle Tennessee State University*

Proposed Changes to the Nutrition Facts Label

Learning Outcomes

After reading this article, you will be able to:

- Outline the changes the FDA is proposing to make on food labels.
- Explain how the FDA decided to make the changes on food labels.

The FDA is proposing to update the Nutrition Facts label found on most food packages in the United States. The Nutrition Facts label, introduced 20 years ago, helps consumers make informed food choices and maintain healthy dietary practices. If adopted, the proposed changes would include the following.

- Greater Understanding of Nutrition Science
- Updated Serving Size Requirements and New Labeling Requirements for Certain Package Sizes
- Refreshed Design

Proposed Nutrition Facts Label At-A-Glance

The FDA is proposing to update the Nutrition Facts label found on most food packages in the United States. The Nutrition Facts label, introduced 20 years ago, helps consumers make informed food choices and maintain healthy dietary practices. If adopted, the proposed changes would include the following.

1. Greater Understanding of Nutrition Science

- Require information about "added sugars." Many experts recommend consuming fewer calories from added sugar because they can decrease the intake of nutrient-rich foods while increasing calorie intake.
- Update daily values for nutrients like sodium, dietary fiber, and Vitamin D. Daily values are used to calculate the Percent Daily Value listed on the label, which help consumers understand the nutrition information in the context of a total daily diet.
- Require manufacturers to declare the amount of potassium and Vitamin D on the label, because they are new "nutrients of public health significance." Calcium and iron would continue to be required, and Vitamins A and C could be included on a voluntary basis.
- While continuing to require "Total Fat," "Saturated Fat," and "Trans Fat" on the label, "Calories from Fat" would be removed because research shows the type of fat is more important than the amount.

2. Updated Serving Size Requirements and New Labeling Requirements for Certain Package Sizes

- Change the serving size requirements to reflect how people eat and drink today, which has changed since serving sizes were first established 20 years ago. By law, the label information on serving sizes must be based on what people actually eat, not on what they "should" be eating.
- Require that packaged foods, including drinks, that are typically eaten in one sitting be labeled as a single serving and that calorie and nutrient information be declared for the entire package. For example, a 20-ounce bottle of soda, typically consumed in a single sitting, would be labeled as one serving rather than as more than one serving.

- For certain packages that are larger and could be consumed in one sitting or multiple sittings, manufacturers would have to provide "dual column" labels to indicate both "per serving" and "per package" calories and nutrient information. Examples would be a 24-ounce bottle of soda or a pint of ice cream. This way, people would be able to easily understand how many calories and nutrients they are getting if they eat or drink the entire package at one time.

3. Refreshed Design

- Make calories and serving sizes more prominent to emphasize parts of the label that are important in addressing current public health concerns such as obesity, diabetes, and cardiovascular disease.
- Shift the Percent Daily Value to the left of the label, so it would come first. This is important because the Percent Daily Value tells you how much of certain nutrients you are getting from a particular food in the context of a total daily diet.
- Change the footnote to more clearly explain the meaning of the Percent Daily Value.

Label Formats

Original vs. Proposed

Proposed Serving Size Changes

What's considered a single serving has changed in the decades since the original nutrition label was created. So now serving sizes will be more realistic to reflect how much people typically eat at one time.

Nutrition Facts

Serving Size 2/3 cup (55 g)
Servings Per Container About 8

Amount Per Serving	
Calories 230	Calories from Fat 72
	% Daily Value*
Total Fat 8 g	**12%**
Saturated Fat 1 g	**5%**
Trans Fat 0 g	
Cholesterol 0 mg	**0%**
Sodium 160 mg	**7%**
Total Carbohydrate 37 g	**12%**
Dietary Fiber 4 g	**16%**
Sugars 1 g	
Protein 3 g	
Vitamin A	10%
Vitamin C	8%
Calcium	20%
Iron	45%

* Percent Daily Values are based on a 2,000 calorie diet. Your daily value may be higher or lower depending on your calorie needs.

	Calories	2,000	2,500
Total Fat	Less than	65 g	80 g
Sat Fat	Less than	20 g	25 g
Cholesterol	Less than	300 mg	300 mg
Sodium	Less than	2,400 mg	2,400 mg
Total Carbohydrate		300 g	375 g
Dietary Fiber		25 g	30 g

Nutrition Facts

8 servings per container
Serving Size 2/3 cup (55 g)

Amount per 2/3 cup
Calories 230

% DV*	
12%	**Total Fat** 8 g
5%	Saturated Fat 1 g
	Trans Fat 0 g
0%	**Cholesterol** 0 mg
7%	**Sodium** 160 mg
12%	**Total Carbs** 37 g
14%	Dietary Fiber 4 g
	Sugars 1 g
	Added Sugars 0 g
	Protein 3 g
10%	**Vitamin D** 2 mcg
20%	**Calcium** 260 mg
45%	**Iron** 8 mg
5%	**Potassium** 235 mg

* Footnote on Daily Values (DV) and calories reference to be inserted here.

Questions & Answers

General

1. What changes are you planning to make on the label and how did you decide to make them?

The FDA's proposed new Nutrition Facts label will make it easier for consumers to make informed decisions about the food they eat. The label reflects the latest scientific thinking about nutrition and the links between what people eat and chronic diseases like obesity and cardiovascular disease. FDA is proposing changes to the label based on new nutrition and public health research, the most recent dietary recommendations from expert groups, and input from four Advance Notices of Proposed Rule Making and various citizens' petitions. Among the changes being considered for the proposed rules are: modifications to the required nutrients, based on the latest nutrition science; updated serving size requirements and labeling requirements for certain package sizes; and a refreshed design.

2. Will you be asking for comment on the proposed changes?

Yes, the two proposed rules are available for public comment for 90 days, and the agency looks forward to receiving comments.

3. Has the Nutrition Facts label changed since 1993?

While the Nutrition Facts label has been an important tool to help people make better food choices over the past 20 years, the only major change has been the requirement, effective in 2006, that trans fat be declared.

4. Are consumers using the label? Do we know what parts of the label they use most often?

Data from FDA's Health and Diet Surveys in 2002 and 2008 show that more and more consumers are using the Nutrition Facts label. For example, the percentage of respondents reporting that they "often" read a food label the first time they purchase a food product rose from 44 percent in 2002 to 54 percent in 2008, and, among these consumers, two-thirds reported using the label to see how high or low the food was in components such as calories, sodium, vitamins, or fat. More than half said they used labels to get a general idea of the nutritional content of the product.

5. How has the label influenced people's eating habits, especially given the obesity epidemic?

The Nutrition Facts label provides information that addresses a number of nutritional concerns, including obesity. However, obesity is not the only important nutritional problem among the U.S. population. While concerns in recent years have largely shifted away from nutritional deficiencies, some population subgroups may still consume inadequate amounts of certain nutrients such as calcium and iron. Also, many nutrients are associated with chronic disease risk such as heart disease. The Nutrition Facts label can help address these nutritional concerns by providing information that consumers can use to make healthy choices.

As for the obesity epidemic, there are many contributing factors, such as exercise and eating behaviors, which are not addressed by the nutrition label. The Nutrition Facts label is one tool to help consumers make informed food choices and maintain healthy dietary practices, but these other factors must be addressed as well.

Also, the label may encourage manufacturers to reformulate existing products and offer new products with a healthier nutrition profile. The food industry has introduced thousands of new product choices with fewer calories, reduced fat, sodium and sugar, and more whole grains since the Nutrition Facts Label requirement was implemented. Following the requirement that trans fat be declared on the label, manufacturers worked to significantly decrease the trans fat content of food products.

Restaurant Foods

6. Because consumers are eating outside the home more and more, shouldn't this nutrition information be found not just on food packages in stores but in restaurants?

Section 4205 of the Affordable Care Act, signed into law on March 23, 2010, directs the FDA to establish labeling requirements for restaurants, similar retail food establishments and vending machines. The FDA issued proposed regulations on April 6, 2011, but they have not yet been finalized.

Sodium

7. Why are you proposing a daily value of 2,300 mg for sodium but asking for comment on a much lower daily value of 1,500 mg?

Although sodium is an essential nutrient in the diet, increases in sodium can increase blood pressure. The FDA is proposing to set a daily value of 2,300 mg for sodium, which is based on the tolerable upper intake level for sodium established in 2005 by the Institute of Medicine (IOM) and current sodium recommendations from other consensus reports. The Daily Value on the current label is 2,400 mg, so the proposed change would not be significant. A Daily Value of 2,300 mg, however, is much lower than the average daily consumption in the United States of about 3,400 mg/day.

Some evidence, however, points to the need for a lower daily value. For example, the 2010 Dietary Guidelines for

Americans recommended a reduction in sodium intake to less than 2,300 mg/day and a further reduction to 1,500 mg/day among groups that are at increased risk of the blood pressure-raising effects of sodium (individuals ages 51 or older, African Americans, and individuals with high blood pressure, chronic kidney disease, or diabetes). These groups account for about half the U.S. population. But a recent IOM report on sodium issued in 2013 concluded that evidence from studies on direct health outcomes is inconsistent and insufficient to conclude that lowering sodium intakes below 2,300 mg/day will increase or decrease the risk of cardiovascular disease outcomes or mortality in the general U.S. population or in identified subgroups. Thus, FDA is proposing a daily value of 2,300 mg but is asking for comment on whether a daily value of 1,500 mg would be more appropriate and alternative approaches for selecting a dietary value for sodium.

Meanwhile, because approximately 75 percent of the sodium consumed by the U.S. population is from sodium added to food during processing, FDA is separately developing a long-term strategy to reduce the sodium content of the food supply to make it easier for people to consume less sodium.

Added Sugars

8. Why are you proposing to require declaration of "added sugars?"

The current label requires declaration of "Sugars." The proposed rule would require declaration of "Added sugars" as well, indented under "Sugars," to help consumers understand how much sugar is naturally occurring and how much has been added to the product. This proposal takes into account new data and information, including recommendations from federal agencies and information from other expert groups, citizen petitions, and public comments. For example, the Dietary Guidelines for Americans recommend reducing caloric intake from added sugars and solid fats because eating these can cause people to eat less of nutrient-rich foods and can also increase how many calories they take in overall. Added sugars provide no additional nutrient value, and are often referred to as "empty calories." Expert groups such as the American Heart Association, the American Academy of Pediatrics, the Institute of Medicine and the World Health Organization also recommend decreasing intake of added sugars.

9. How much added sugars do Americans consume?

On average, Americans get 16 percent of their total calories from added sugars. The major sources of added sugars in the diet (with the highest sources listed first) are soda, energy and sports drinks, grain based desserts, sugar-sweetened fruit drinks, dairy-based desserts and candy.

10. To what level should consumers limit their intake of added sugars?

The government has no specific recommendation for added sugars. Including added sugars on the new Nutrition Facts label would allow consumers who want to limit their added sugar intake to compare various brands of similar products.

Nutrients of Public Health Significance

11. What are nutrients of public health significance?

These are nutrients that, when lacking, are associated with the risk of chronic disease. Essentially, they are nutrients Americans don't eat enough of. The FDA believes these should be declared on the label so that people can see how much of these important nutrients are in the products. The FDA examined data from the National Health and Nutrition Examination Survey to determine which essential vitamins and minerals should be included as nutrients of public health significance. The FDA has proposed that the nutrients of public health significance should include calcium, vitamin D, potassium, and iron. Calcium and iron already are required; vitamin D and potassium are being proposed to be added to the list of mandatory nutrients.

12. Why are Vitamin D and potassium being proposed to be added to the Nutrition Facts label?

Vitamin D is important for its role in bone health, and some population groups are not getting enough of it. Adequate potassium intake is beneficial in lowering blood pressure and intakes of this nutrient also are low among some population groups.

13. Why are you proposing to no longer require vitamins A and C?

Current data indicate that vitamin A and C deficiencies in the general population are not common. These vitamins would still be allowed to be declared on labels on a voluntary basis.

Format Changes

14. What changes are you proposing to make to the design of the Nutrition Facts label and why?

We are not proposing to change the "iconic" look of the label but are proposing several changes to improve the format. These proposed changes include:

- Highlighting the caloric content of foods by increasing the type size and placing in bold type the number of calories and servings per container.

- Shifting information on Percent Daily Value to the left of the label. The Percent Daily Value is intended to help consumers place nutrient information in the context of a total daily diet.
- Declaring the actual amount, in addition to Percent Daily Value, of mandatory vitamins and minerals and, when declared, voluntary vitamins and minerals.
- Changing "Amount Per Serving" to "Amount per ___," with the blank filled in with the serving size in common household measures (e.g., Amount per 2/3 cup).
- Replacing the listing of "Total Carbohydrate" with "Total Carbs" and indenting "Added Sugars" directly beneath the listing for "Sugars."
- Right-justifying the actual amounts of the serving size information.
- Removing the existing footnote and using that area to better explain the Percent Daily Value. This part of the nutrition label is often misunderstood by consumers. We will be conducting an experimental study to help determine information that should be in the footnote to increase consumers' understanding of the Percent Daily Value.

Serving Sizes

15. Would serving sizes on the label be smaller because of the obesity epidemic?

Not necessarily. Some serving sizes would potentially increase and others would potentially decrease. The Nutrition Labeling and Education Act requires the serving sizes to be based on amounts of food and drink that people typically eat, not on how much they should eat. FDA established the current serving size requirements in 1993 based primarily on data from food consumption surveys. More recent food consumption data show that 27 out of 158 (17 percent) of the reference amounts customarily consumed (RACC) used to calculate serving sizes should be changed. This would mean that manufacturers would potentially have to change the serving sizes listed on their labels.

16. How much time would manufacturers have to make these proposed changes?

We are proposing that manufacturers have just over two years (two years after the effective date) to comply with any final requirements.

Imports

17. Would the proposed new requirements apply to imported food?

Yes, foods imported to the United States would need to meet any final requirements.

Critical Thinking

1. Section 4206 of the Affordable Care Act, signed into law on March 23, 2010, directs the FDA to establish labeling requirements for restaurants. Describe the effect this labeling requirement is having on restaurants in your community. If you notice no effect, explain why.
2. Develop a lesson plan for the community explaining to the proposed food labels.
3. Explain how the proposed food labels can be used when providing nutrition education for the following: weight loss programs, cardiovascular disease risk reduction initiatives, diabetic diet instruction, and educational classes specific to the geriatric population.

Create Central

www.mhhe.com/createcentral

Internet References

Food and Drug Administration (FDA)
www.fda.gov

Grocery Manufacturers Association (GMA)
www.gmaonline.org

Article

Prepared by: Janet Colson, *Middle Tennessee State University*

Is the Popular Paleo Diet a Bunch of Baloney?

The Paleo diet might be more successful in generating profit for its proponents than producing health for its followers.

JILL RICHARDSON

Learning Outcomes

After reading this article, you will be able to:

- Describe which foods are allowed on the paleo diet and claims of proponents for the diet.
- Explain why Jill Richardson thinks that the paleo diet "might be more successful in generating profit for its proponents than producing health for its followers."

A decade ago, we went crazy for Atkins. Now, a new grain-free, low-carb diet is sweeping the nation. The so-called "Paleolithic" diet—or "paleo" for short—instructs dieters to eat like their Stone Age ancestors ate. The premise of the diet is simple: your body evolved to eat a radically different diet than what most Americans eat today. Go back to that original diet, and you'll lose weight and eliminate a host of diseases.

Have our bodies evolved to only consume foods found in a hunter-gatherer diet and not from agriculture? And, does the paleo diet, as outlined by the bestselling books by Loren Cordain and Robb Wolf, accurately capture what our cave-dwelling ancestors ate?

The Paleolithic era is defined as the "Old Stone Age." Roughly speaking, it includes everything from the oldest use of stone tools by human ancestors in Africa up to the dawn of agriculture a mere 10,000 years ago. About 1.8 million years ago, our ancestors experienced a massive increase in brain size. The date humans acquired controlled use of fire is debated, but it likely occurred by about 300,000 years ago at the latest. And, at some point during this long period, our ancestors left Africa and spread throughout the world.

Needless to say, it's impossible to accurately lump together the diet of every single human ancestor or even just the *Homo sapiens* who lived in this period. "The truth of the matter is there is no paleo diet," summarizes Katharine Milton, a professor in the Department of Environmental Science, Policy, and Management at UC-Berkeley. "The only thing you can do is generalize very broadly and you can say beyond a shadow of a doubt that paleo peoples were eating wild plant and animal foods because there was no agriculture and there were no domesticated animals." A piece in *Nature* backs her up, showing how difficult it is to reconstruct human diets of the distant past through a variety of means.

Proponents of the paleo diet attempt to distill it into an easy diet plan nonetheless. They tell dieters to eat grassfed meat, seafood, fruits and vegetables, eggs, nuts and seeds, and "healthful" oils (defined as coconut, olive, macadamia nut, avocado, flaxseed, and walnut oils). The list of prohibited foods includes what Cordain calls "Neolithic and industrial-era foods:" all grains, legumes (including peanuts), dairy, refined sugar, potatoes, processed foods, salt, alcohol, and refined vegetable oils.

According to Cordain, "The crucial aspect is to not precisely mimic the exact foods our hunter-gatherer ancestors ate, as this would be impractical or impossible, but rather to mimic the food groups they ate (fresh fruits, vegetables, meat, seafood, poultry, nuts) with commercially available foods from the supermarket." According to him, "nearly 71 percent of the calories in the typical Western diet come from refined sugars, vegetable oils, cereal grains and dairy products—typically via processed foods. Our hunter-gatherer ancestors from any location on the planet or any time period rarely or never consumed these foods."

How does he know? Logic, he answers. It's pretty easy to figure out what kinds of food you can't get when you've got no agriculture and little more than stone tools to work with. But, he notes, there are other techniques one can use, including "ethnographic data from historically studied hunter-gatherers," studying the chemicals in fossilized remains of human ancestors, and finding remains of butchered animal bones or even fossilized human feces.

No matter what, there are several aspects of this diet that deserve praise. Cutting down on sugar, salt, alcohol, and processed foods is a healthy move. So is switching to pasture-raised meat, if you eat animal products. And the oils recommended each provide healthy ratios of omega-6 to omega-3 fatty acids, thus addressing a common problem in the American diet. The diet also preaches variety, telling dieters to switch up what they eat every day, instead of relying on the same handful of foods. These are all concepts that are broadly recommended by many nutrition experts—and they can be adopted without turning back the clock 10,000 years to before the dawn of agriculture.

Let's look at the actual food eaten by a hunter-gatherer societies in the recent past and then examine the elements of the popularized paleo diet one by one. In San Diego County and south of the border into Mexico, the Kumeyaay were hunter-gatherers until recent times and their diet is well recorded. Some foods and traditions are even maintained today. Their dietary staple was the acorn, which they gathered in the fall and stored. Once dried, around February, the acorns were ground into flour, leached to remove the bitter tannins, and eaten as a staple food called *shawii.* In addition to acorns, they ate wild game (deer, bighorn sheep, and rabbits), fish, seeds, seaweed, prickly pear cactus, greens, and wild fruit.

Much of their food was seasonal. During the winter rainy season, they could count on greens like miner's lettuce. Around March and April, they harvested yucca and agave. Over the summer, they gathered seeds, including chia seeds and a wild grain, juniper and manzanita berries, mesquite beans (a legume), and pine nuts. Fruits included berries, prickly pear fruit, palm fruit, and some stone fruits. They dug edible roots, tubers, and corms from wild plants as well. And they had a source of salt, which they included in their diets.

The Kumeyaay were hardly vegetarians, but they did obtain protein from plant sources as well as animals, including from both grains and legumes. They did eat an enormous variety of foods throughout the year, but during some periods they might have been limited to a rather narrow range of foods simply because nothing else was available. Some of their foods are delicious, but you might not wish to eat some unless your only other choice was starvation. And, it's likely that sometimes, that was the choice they were making.

One example does not make a rule, but the Kumeyaay diet blows through several claims made by paleo experts like Cordain. They ate salt, they ate grains, and they ate legumes. Logic tells us that our ancestors absolutely ate grains and legumes elsewhere in the world too. How do we know that? Because our ancestors ultimately domesticated grains and legumes and cultivated them as food on farms. What are the odds that an ancient people found an entirely inedible seed and began planting it and selecting it for desirable traits, trusting that eventually, perhaps in decades or centuries, it would evolve into an edible grain or bean?

It's true that grains and legumes can be inedible in their natural forms. Acorns are too. But the Kumeyaay solved this problem through technology. For acorns, they found a way to remove the bitter tannins before consuming them. For grains, they toasted them over a fire and then ground them into a flour which was eaten as a dish called "pinole." South of the border in Mexico, indigenous peoples there figured out how to make niacin in corn bioavailable by treating corn with lime in a process known as nixtamal. This allowed them to constitute complete protein with grains and beans and to avoid the disease pellagra that is caused by niacin deficiency.

"All humans do is transform their foods," says Milton, commenting on the human ability to turn inedible substances into healthy foods with technology. "That's what being a human is. People only evolve in response to selective pressures. Many different very important foods are not digestible and humans transform them through culture."

Cordain dismisses grains, calling them "nutritionally inferior foods compared to fresh fruits, vegetables, meat, poultry, fish and seafood." He adds that, "most grains in the U.S. are consumed as fiber-depleted refined grains, and as such represent one of the greatest dietary contributors to the ubiquitous high glycemic load in the U.S. diet, which underlies numerous health issues including obesity and the metabolic syndrome."

True—but why not simply tell people to eat whole grains instead of refined ones?

Cordain adds a concern about gluten-containing grains (wheat, rye and barley) because they cannot be eaten by the small percent of the U.S. population that suffers from celiac disease or the slightly larger group of Americans with gluten allergies or sensitivities. Well, it makes sense that those with celiac disease or allergies should avoid gluten, but why does that mean we all should?

How about dairy? In his book *The Paleo Diet Revised,* Cordain explains the dairy prohibition, saying, "Paleolithic people ate no dairy foods. Imagine how difficult it would be to milk a wild animal, even if you could somehow manage to catch one." Good point, but early humans did consume dairy in the same way all mammals do. Human infants drank breast milk. Humans did evolve to consume and digest dairy as infants.

After weaning, Paleolithic humans had no reason to continue producing lactase, the enzyme needed to digest lactose. But sometime after the emergence of agriculture, after humans domesticated livestock, some humans were born with a genetic mutation allowing them to continue producing lactase after weaning, into adulthood.

Milton calls this "a classic case of how human culture modifies their environment and then humans adapt to their own changes in the environment." First, humans domesticated livestock, and then any individuals with the genetic mutation allowing them to digest dairy as adults had an advantage over those who did not.

She notes that whereas some societies with livestock evolved adult lactase secretion, others used technology instead of genes to consume dairy products. "They figured out a way to get the lactose to be eaten by bacteria or drained out—maybe they made a yogurt or something like that—and then they eat the material that remains and it isn't full of lactose anymore."

Cordain acknowledges that some 35 percent of the world's population can digest lactose into adulthood, but points to dairy as the cause of cancer risks, insulin resistance, and acne. A recent study did find a link between high-fat dairy and mortality from breast cancer, but it recommends replacing high-fat dairy products with lowfat or nonfat ones, not cutting dairy out entirely.

What about the paleo diet's claim that one must eat meat? In his book *The Paleo Solution,* Robb Wolf writes, "Your protein source needs to have the following criteria:

1. It needs a face.
2. It needs a soul.
3. You need to kill it, and bring its essence into your being.
4. Really."

Cordain gives vegetarians the bad news a bit more gently, but the data he cites does not back up his assertions. In fact, one study he names backs up the health benefits of a vegetarian diet.

"Ancestral hunter-gatherer diets were never vegetarian," Cordain notes—perhaps correctly. But he goes on to claim, "If they were, these diets would have been rapidly culled by natural selection because they are eventually lethal. Humans require vitamin B12 which is not found in plants, but only in animal foods."

It's true that humans require vitamin B12, which is only found in animal foods—but vegetarians do eat animal foods in the form of dairy and eggs. It's vegans who eschew all animal foods, not vegetarians.

Cordain cites two studies that found that vegetarian diets are not more healthful than omnivorous ones. The first was an Oxford University study published in 1999. Cordain quotes the study's abstract, which reads, "There were no significant differences between vegetarians and nonvegetarians in mortality from cerebrovascular disease, stomach cancer, colorectal cancer, lung cancer, breast cancer, prostate cancer, or all other causes combined."

First of all, this means that vegetarians are no healthier than meat-eaters, but it also means that they are no less healthy.

However, Cordain neglects to mention the sentences that precede what he quotes. These read, "Mortality from ischemic heart disease was 24% lower in vegetarians than in nonvegetarians. . . . Further categorization of diets showed that, in comparison with regular meat eaters, mortality from ischemic heart disease was 20% lower in occasional meat eaters, 34% lower in people who ate fish but not meat, 34% lower in lactoovovegetarians, and 26% lower in vegans."

In other words, Cordain is selectively quoting this study's findings to give a false impression of the results. The study found that vegetarians are 24 percent less likely to die of heart disease than their meat-eating counterparts, and no more or less likely to die of anything else.

A second, more recent study he cites also found no differences in mortality between vegetarians and meat-eaters. Again, he quotes from it selectively, noting that "Within the study, mortality from circulatory diseases and all causes is not significantly different between vegetarians and meat-eaters," leaving off the rest of the sentence: "but the study is not large enough to exclude small or moderate differences for specific causes of death, and more research on this topic is required."

Yet Cordain says, "In fact, if the truth be known, your lifelong dietary deprivations will not prolong your lifespan but rather will produce multiple nutrient deficiencies that are associated with numerous health problems and illnesses. If you have forced plant-based diets upon your children, or unborn fetus they will also suffer."

Long story short, while many aspects of the paleo diet are uncontroversial and beneficial, like increasing fresh fruit and vegetable consumption, switching to pasture-raised meat, and cutting out processed foods, the overall premise of the diet as well as some of its key components appear based on pseudoscience and unsubstantiated claims. But, you might notice that many of the most popular, well-known paleo diet Websites sell books, diet plans and memberships. It appears that this diet might be more successful in generating profit for its proponents than producing health for its followers.

Critical Thinking

1. What was the Paleolithic era and what type foods were consumed in that time?
2. How does the current paleo diet compare to the ancient diet consumed in the Paleolithic era?
3. What do you consider the strongest benefit of the paleo diet? What is the greatest weakness of the diet?
4. Do you agree or disagree with the accusation that the paleo diet "might be more successful in generating profit for its proponents than producing health for its followers"? Justify your opinion.

Create Central

www.mhhe.com/createcentral

Internet References

How to Really Eat Like a Hunter-Gatherer: Why the Paleo Diet Is Half-Baked [Interactive & Infographic]
www.scientificamerican.com/article.cfm?id=why-paleo-diet-half-baked-how-hunter-gatherer-really-eat

Paleo Diet
http://thepaleodiet.com

Paleo Diet Kickstart Plan
http://health.usnews.com/best-diet/paleo-diet

Jill Richardson is the founder of the blog *La Vida Locavore* and a member of the Organic Consumers Association policy advisory board. She is the author of *Recipe for America: Why Our Food System Is Broken and What We Can Do to Fix It.*

Unit 7

UNIT

Prepared by: Janet Colson, *Middle Tennessee State University*

Food Safety and Technology

Foodborne illness constitutes an important public health problem in the United States. The U.S. Centers for Disease Control has reported 76 million cases of foodborne illness each year, out of which 5,000 end in death. The annual cost of losses in productivity ranges from $20 to $40 billion. Foodborne disease results primarily from microbial contamination (bacteria, viruses, and protozoa) and naturally occurring toxins, environmental contaminants, pesticide residues, and food additives.

The Food and Drug Administration (FDA) controls and regulates procedures dealing with food safety, including food service and production. The FDA has established rules (Hazard Analysis and Critical Control Points) to improve the control of food safety practices and to monitor the production of seafood, meat, and poultry.

Surveys show that over 95% of the time people do not follow proper sanitation methods when working with food at home. Thus our best defense is to incorporate safe food-handling practices at home. The U.S. government launched the Food Safety Initiative program to minimize foodborne disease and to educate the public about safe handling practices. An emphasis on improving food safety practices at home is also seen in the *Dietary Guidelines for American, 2010.* The subcommittees of the USDA and HHS recommend creating and offering food safety education programs for children in schools and preschools, along with improving education efforts with adults.

Agricultural trade between nations has led to a truly globalized food supply. This globalization meets the demand of wealthy nations for year-round access to foods grown in tropical environments and strengthens the economies of poorer, underdeveloped countries. One detriment of the global food supply is the translocation of biological contaminants via food. Estimations speculate that less than one percent of foods imported into the United States are inspected each year. Although U.S. demand for a variety of foods has driven the worldwide food trade, our nation has not established an effective method to regulate the safety of foods shipped in from other countries. The current regulatory agency for U.S. food, the Food and Drug Administration, is faced with many challenges of trying to regulate the U.S. food and pharmaceutical industries, much less the newly introduced challenges of the safety of food imports.

Imported foods are not the only concern for biological contaminants. Changes in food production and farming in the United States have led to an increase in the spread of bacterial contamination of our foods. Many conventional poultry and livestock farms raise their animals in crowded, unsanitary conditions. The crowded conditions make the spread of bacteria very likely; therefore, conventional farmers must inoculate their animals with antibiotics to prevent bacteria from spreading throughout the entire stock. An example of poor regulation of foods grown in the United States is the dramatic increase in *Salmonella* and *Campylobacter* bacteria in chickens over the past few years. Possible explanations for the increase in these two microorganisms could be due to the U.S. Department of Agriculture having no standards for *Campylobacter* and testing for *Salmonella* in a very small proportion of animals.

Concern for food safety also applies to the beverages that we drink. An estimated 19.5 million illnesses occur each year in the United States due to microorganisms in our water. The harmful effects may originate from viruses, bacteria, and protozoa or potential health consequences of chemical compounds and contaminants in our drinking water. Recent reports of high levels of arsenic and lead in juice have consumers concerned about the safety of drinking juice, especially by children. Although there is a federally enforced limit on the amount of arsenic and lead in drinking water, no limits exist for juices. Chronic low level consumption of arsenic has been linked to slower cognitive development, various cancers, high blood pressure, diabetes, and infertility.

Advances in food technology are leading to radically different methods of producing and preserving food. Principles of genetic engineering, vertical farms, lab grown meats, bacteriophages, and nanotechnology provide ways to increase production with less burden, enhance food safety, and keep foods fresh longer. Advancing technology in food preservation, most notably high pressure processing, is stretching the concept of longer shelf life. The use of water-absorbing ingredients and edible polymers are also being used to create convenience foods that will not be soggy in the years that the food is on the shelf. These principles of food technology are shaping the future of food.

A controversial topic that is covered in this unit is the concept of growing meat for human consumption in a lab. Harvesting meat tissue grown in petri dishes to be grilled, sautéed, or broiled along with your favorite sauce, is an ingenious idea to some yet bizarre to others. Several labs are working to perfect techniques to grow beef, chicken, and lamb tissue in a chemistry lab. The concept would significantly impact agriculture and food supply.

Genetically modifying our food crops is a controversial topic. The topic has gained much attention from people who perceive the possible threats of genetically altered crops. The positions of people who oppose the practice are fueled by the actions of large agricultural companies that have genetically altered seeds to be resistant to herbicides, which allows for easier and heavy use of the herbicide on the crops. However, there are benefits to using genetically modified crops. Genetically modified crops can be used to increase the world's food supply to meet the demand of its growing population and increase the nutrient density of crops to provide the key nutrients missing in underdeveloped countries' food supply.

The articles in this unit will be useful as a supplement to food safety sections of general nutrition courses. These article topics add a slightly different view of the future of food, food safety, and food technology that are not publicized as often.

Article

Prepared by: Janet Colson, *Middle Tennessee State University*

The Future of Food: Five Frontiers

How nanotechnology, vertical farms, and lab-grown meat may change the way you eat.

ELIZABETH WEINGARTEN

Learning Outcomes

After reading this article, you will be able to:

- Describe new developments that some predict will influence the future of our food supply.
- Explain which of the predictions presented in the article has the greatest likelihood of becoming reality.

Generations of kids have grown up forbidden to taste chocolate cake batter. The rationale for this quasi-torture: fear of salmonella poisoning.

And at the current rate of food technology, the kids of 2040 may be eating healthier cookie dough, too—gooey hunks infused with nano-sized nutrients, with chocolate chips engineered to be less fattening.

But future children may never know what salmonella is: A Dutch company is currently developing a consumer spray to kill the bacteria on contact. Salmonelex may sit next to Windex on future kitchen counters.

But most of the latest advancements in food technology go beyond dessert. Rather, scientists are motivated by an impending agricultural crisis: The world population will likely hit 9 billion by 2050, while climate change may render current agricultural systems and seeds inadequate. To stave off an agricultural doomsday, researchers are developing new techniques to transform our unsustainable practices.

For the month of June, Future Tense—a partnership of *Slate,* the New America Foundation, and Arizona State University—will look at the future of food in both the developed and developing world. We'll explore how we grow food, package it, genetically engineer it, and cook it at home.

To kick things off, here are five of the exciting food frontiers, *Bon appetit.*

1. Coding Corn

Some of the first genetically modified commercial crops in the '90s were tweaked to be tolerant to herbicides and resistant to plant diseases caused by viruses. Scientists built these superfoods by introducing certain genes into the plant's DNA.

Today, most genetically modified foods on the market are commodity crops used for animal feed or processed ingredients, like corn, soybeans, and sugar beets. Typically, they aren't manipulated to be more nutritious for human consumers. But that may soon change. A DuPont-owned company is currently marketing a "high oleic" heart-healthier soybean—meaning its oil has 20 percent less saturated fat than normal commodity soybean oil. Monsanto is also developing omega-3 enriched soybeans.

Researchers are working to enhance the nutrients in staple crops like sweet potatoes and cassava, which provide some populations in developing countires with the majority of their daily calories. That's a problem because though sweet potatoes, for example, are nutritious, they alone don't contain all the nutrients necessary for a balanced diet.

And for a couple of years, another corporation has been seeking FDA approval for genetically engineered salmon, dubbed AquAdvantage, that matures to its full size in half the time. But the process has been mired in controversy, particularly over concerns about the environment.

Gregory Jaffe, the director of the Biotechnology Project at the Center for Science in the Public Interest, says that there are other concerns about GM foods in general. For example, genetic modification could introduce a new gene that produces an allergen in a food, posing consumer health risks. Scientists also have to worry about introducing a new gene and, in the process, inadvertently activating an existing gene in the plant that could produce a harmful substance in the edible part.

2. Tiny Titans

Nanoparticles aren't new: The minuscule units appear naturally in some foods. But in the past decade, researchers have begun trying to use the particles to alter the taste and texture of food. Nanotechnology could be particularly useful for concocting diet-friendly foods: The particles can enhance the flavor and consistency of products without adding calories, sugar, or fat.

The Project on Emerging Nanotechnologies' comprehensive database of nano-products in the United States lists only four in the food and beverage category. Canola Active Oil uses nanoparticles to inhibit "the transportation of cholesterol from the digestive system into the bloodstream." Another product, Nanoceuticals' chocolate-flavored SlimShake, promises "enhanced flavor without the need for excess sugar."

But some scientists worry that nanoparticles in food could pose a danger to human health, and that companies are releasing products without adequate safety testing. Todd Kuiken at the Project on Emerging Nanotechnologies, which is affiliated with the nonpartisan Woodrow Wilson Center and advocates for the advancement of nanotechnology, says he hasn't heard of much current research "on actual food products—what happens when [nanoparticles] get into the body, blood stream, and brain." The FDA says it's funding some research into the safety of nanotech. But the paucity of testing means that right now, no one can be certain that ingesting these tiny particles won't come with big health consequences.

3. Lettuce Skyscrapers

Columbia University professor Dickson Despommier says Babylonians, with their hanging gardens, were first to pioneer the idea of vertical farms. But it was Despommier's 2010 book *The Vertical Farm*—and website, launched in 2004—that inspired the modern movement. Despommier defines a vertical farm as a building that's at least two stories with crops growing inside—stacked greenhouses, if you will. Back in 2010, there were none. Today, seven have sprouted around the world in places like South Korea, Japan, the Netherlands and Chicago.

Horizontal farmland can't grow enough food to sustain the swelling population, Despommier says. Not only do vertical farms do more with less land; they also allow food producers to grow crops in cities next to consumers, eliminating transportation costs. Cultivating food indoors with hydroponics (a system of growing plants without soil) uses 60 percent to 70 percent less water than traditional farming, and indoor crops aren't susceptible to drought, pests, diseases or floods.

PlantLab, based in the Netherlands, is a vertical farm that goes beyond Despommier. Rather than sunlight, it uses red, blue, and far-red LED lights to grow plants. But PlantLab isn't a food producer (though the researchers there do sometimes eat the tomatoes they grow). Rather, they glean information from the plants they grow to create growing recipes for food production companies. These formulas specify the temperature, humidity, carbon dioxide, airflow, nutrients, water, and LED light necessary to grow a crop most efficiently. Gertjan Meeuws, the managing partner of PlantLab, told me he's currently developing recipes of more than 40 crops for about 20 companies—most of which have traditional greenhouses. He guesses that in five to 10 years, retail houses like Wal-Mart will be producing their own vegetables and herbs.

But unlike outdoor farmers, vertical cultivators don't get government subsidies or tax breaks. "Indoor farmers aren't looked at as serious yet by the United States government—there are no major incentive programs to make vertical farming part of the landscape," Despommier says, stressing the vast size and influence of the American farm lobby. That means "the U.S. government will not be a big player in establishing vertical farming in the U.S.—but city governments might. If you talk to the mayor of Chicago or Philadelphia, you'll learn that they're passionate about this idea."

4. Lab Burgers

Dutch scientist Willem van Eelen imagined creating animal meat—or muscle tissue—in a laboratory back in the 1940s. Decades later, Mark Post, a stem cell scientist at the Netherlands' Maastricht University, is currently growing meat by capturing stem cells from cow muscles. His goal: to create a hamburger by November. But it's slow work, as he's forming the patty piece by piece. He's produced about 500 slivers of muscle tissue and estimates he needs 3,000. Once he's finished, Post estimates the hamburger will cost about 250,000 euros.

When will products from Post be on supermarket shelves? With sufficient funding, Post says, "we can probably make it happen in the order of 10 to 15 years." But, he says, "If the research continues to be funded the way it's funded now, it's never going to happen."

Another obstacle: Right now, cell division outside the body is induced with fetal bovine serum—liquid produced from the fetal blood of a dead cow. Not exactly PETA-friendly. Post tells me he would like to create a solution to replace the fluid. Alternative liquids that induce division in certain cells do exist—but so far, Post hasn't found them to work as well with skeletal muscle cells. Creating a replacement will be tough, he says, since fetal bovine serum contains about 10,000 individual proteins. But it's doable. The bottom line: You won't be chowing down on an in-vitro steak any time soon.

5. Salmonella-Fighting Soldiers

Bacteriophages (also referred to as "phages") are viruses that infect and kill bacteria. At Micreos, a company based in the Netherlands, researchers have created a phage spray to target particular bacteria that cause food-borne illnesses, like listeria and salmonella. (If you're keeping track at home—that's the third food technology incubated in the Netherlands.) The technology arose from research into antibiotic alternatives that began at the National Institute of Health in 1993. Micreos, a spinoff from the NIH project, was the first company to introduce phage spray technology—but others are entering the field, too. Recently, the FDA approved an American company's E. coli spray. Right now, its main customers are large scale food producers. But Micreos plans to release a consumer spray in the next year, CEO Mark Offerhaus told me. The industrial spray costs a penny per pound of meat, and Offerhaus guesses that the consumer spray will run about $10 per bottle.

Martin Loesser, a professor of food microbiology at the Institute of Food Science and Nutrition at the Federal Institute of Technology Zurich, has been researching the consumer safety effects of phage technology for 25 years. Though early critics of phage treatments worried that since phages contain proteins they could cause allergic reactions, Loesser dismisses this risk. He's confident because he can identify the proteins that comprise each phage through genetic sequencing and then test those proteins against a database of all known allergenic proteins—like those from wheat, soy, peanuts, and milk. He hasn't found a similarity between a phage protein and a known allergen yet. "The amount of protein that's in [these treatments] is still so low that even if that was allergenic, I doubt that this would cause any kind of reaction," he says.

A Nano-Grain of Salt

Pondering the future of food has long captivated the imaginations of science fiction writers and policymakers. But these visionaries are often way off the mark. Take the food pill. Matt Novak, writer of the Paleofuture blog for *Smithsonian* magazine, recently traced the pill's origins, finding that the premise—encapsulating a meal's worth of calories synthetically—harkens back to the 1893 World's Fair in Chicago. As part of an essay project to promote the fair, suffragette Mary Elizabeth Lease predicted that Americans would be eating synthetic food essences by 1993, freeing women from their kitchen shackles.

The food-pill prediction appeared again in various newspapers, magazines, TV shows (like *The Jetsons*) and in the 1933 Chicago World's Fair. We now know that cramming a meal into a pill isn't scientifically possible. Turns out that consuming 2,000 calories—what the average person needs daily—would mean swallowing about half a pound of pills per day.

Lease's prediction now sounds both quaint and sweeping: Cooks of the future, she wrote, "will take, in condensed form from the rich loam of the earth, the life force or germs now found in the heart of the corn, in the kernel of wheat, and in the luscious juices of the fruits. A small phial of this life from the fertile bosom of Mother Earth will furnish men with substance for days. And thus the problems of cooks and cooking will be solved."

Her prose offers an important reminder: Be wary of any scientist who suggests her technology is a food future panacea. Predicting which technology will radically change the food landscape is tough. For now, we'll have to be content with the promise of licking a safer cake batter spoon.

Critical Thinking

1. Describe how viruses that kill bacteria can be used to curtail outbreaks that cause food borne illness.
2. Critique the theory of providing a nutritious meal in pill form.
3. Define commodity crops.
4. Describe current research being conducted by corporations to develop genetically modified soybeans and salmon.
5. Summarize the concept and the benefits of vertical farms.

Create Central

www.mhhe.com/createcentral

Internet References

Future Tense—Center for Science and the Imagination
http://csi.asu.edu/category/future-tense

Institute of Food Technology
www.ift.org

Monsanto
www.monsanto.com

Project on Emerging Nanotechnologies
www.nanotechproject.org

Society for Science and the Public
www.societyforscience.org

Article

Prepared by: Janet Colson, *Middle Tennessee State University*

Engineering the Future of Food

Tomorrow's genetically modified food and farmed fish will be more sustainable and far healthier than much of what we eat today—if we can overcome our fears and embrace it. Here's how one foodie learned to stop worrying and love "Frankenfood."

Josh Schonwald

Learning Outcomes

After reading this article, you will be able to:

- Discuss the advantages of genetically modified crops.
- Define the potential "input traits" and "output traits" of genetically modified foods.

The Plant Transformation Facility at the University of California, Davis, has been the scene of more than 15,000 "transgenic events," which is the term molecular biologists use when they blast DNA from one life form into another. In room 192 of Robbins Hall, a brick building not far from the student union, thousands of microscopic plantlets grow in Petri dishes bathed in pink and fluorescent blue light.

Here, molecular biologists can mix what were previously sexually incompatible species together using a gas-pump-like tool called the Helium Particle Delivery System. Using bullets (literally) made out of gold, they fire genes from one species into another in a bombardment chamber. The Davis lab has given birth to grapes spiked with jellyfish, tomatoes spiked with carp, transgenic squash, transgenic carrots, transgenic tomatoes.

Another important site in genetic engineering history, an innocuous office building about a ten-minute drive from Robbins Hall, is the birthplace of the most audacious plant in the history of high-tech plants. Among biotech people and anti-bio-tech people, this plant, a tomato, needs no introduction. The so-called Flavr Savr was supposed to be the game changer—longer shelf life, better yield, better taste. Calgene, the company that created the Flavr Savr, claimed it could bring "backyard flavor" to the supermarket tomato.

Achieving "backyard flavor" in an industrial-scale, California-grown tomato has long been one of the holy grails of the $4 billion-plus tomato industry. During the pre-tomato launch hype-a-thon, the president of Calgene claimed that genetic engineering could not only bring us the tomato of our childhood dreams, but also remake the taste of the tomato, tailored to our every desire: "Eventually we're going to design acidic tomatoes for the New Jersey palate and sweet tomatoes for the Chicago palate."

The Flavr Savr turned out to be the Edsel of the produce world, a spectacular failure not just for Calgene, but for the whole biotech industry. This purportedly longer-shelf-life tomato became the lightning rod for much of the anti-genetically modified organism (GMO) movement. People learned about other transgenic crops—a potato with a chicken gene, tobacco with a firefly gene, and, perhaps most notoriously, a tomato with an Arctic flounder gene, which provided an image for a Greenpeace anti-GMO campaign. Nongovernmental organizations cried foul. Consumers were alarmed. It was an op-ed about the Flavr Savr where the term *Frankenfood* first appeared. As for the tomato's taste, most reports said that, far from achieving backyard flavor, it was not that great.

By 1997, supermarkets stopped stocking the bioengineered tomato. The Flavr Savr was a financial disaster for Calgene.

But that was almost fifteen years ago.

One fall day, across campus from the Helium Particle Delivery System, I went to visit Kent Bradford, the director of UC Davis's Seed Biotechnology Center and presumably among the best-positioned people at Davis to answer my burning question: Whatever happened *after* the Flavr Savr?

The Culinary Potential of Frankenfood

Genetic engineering obviously didn't stop with the Flavr Savr debacle; the use of GMOs has exploded. Many genetically engineered foods can be found throughout our food supply. Genetically modified soybeans and canola dominate the market, which means that most processed food—everything from your spaghetti to your Snickers bar—has GM ingredients. More than 90 percent of American cotton and 80 percent of corn crops come from GM seed. All of these crops, though, are what are called "commodity crops." They're not what you pick up at your local greengrocer. They're industrial crops, secondary ingredients. Not what interested me.

What I wanted to know is what was happening with the quest to achieve "backyard flavor"? And what I couldn't get out of my head was this claim that tomatoes could be engineered for precise tastes—"acidic tomatoes for the New Jersey palate and sweet tomatoes for the Chicago palate."

"The process is costly and time-consuming, which partly explains why biotech crop development is largely in the hands of the agribusiness giants."

What was going on? Did they just stop working on "sweet tomatoes for the Chicago palate"? Wouldn't the Flavr Savr creators be intent on redemption, going back to the bench to try again? Or did everything just stop?

Strangely, Bradford, a plant geneticist who has been at UC Davis since the early 1980s, shared my curiosity about the post-Flavr Savr world—he just had a different way of explaining it.

"Yes. Where are all these output traits?" he said. (Input traits are breederspeak for what's so often critical to agriculture—disease resistance, insect resistance, adaptability to particular environments. An output trait is breeder parlance for what I was looking for—traits that improve taste and texture, traits that could change the dining experience of the future.)

Bradford had observed that, almost twenty years after the biotech revolution began, there were few signs of any "Second Generation" crops. The First Generation was the commodity crops: soybean, maize, cotton, canola, sugar beets. Most expected that, after the first wave of crops proved their worth, the next wave would be more consumer focused—better tomatoes, tastier lettuce. But biotech specialty crops (that's the crop scientist term for produce) hadn't appeared. In fact, a GMO specialty crop hadn't been commercialized since 1998. Even Bradford, a longtime biotech believer, considered, "Maybe the genes weren't working?"

A few years ago, Bradford and his collaborator Jamie Miller set out to find out "what was going on" with bioengineered specialty crops. They surveyed the leading plant science journals and tracked GM crop field trials—all subject to government regulation—from 2003 to 2008. Searching for citations related to specialty crops, they found that research not only had never stopped but was thriving.

"There was research on 46 different species," says Bradford. "More than 300 traits were being tested." A lot of it was on input traits (disease, weed resistance), but breeders had also experimented with output traits. "It was happening at the research level, but it just didn't move to the next step. It just stopped there."

There was an obvious explanation, Bradford says, sighing. "It was regulatory."

Post Flavr Savr, in response to growing consumer concerns about transgenic breeding, a regulatory process was created that treated genetically modified foods differently from conventionally bred crops. If you have iceberg lettuce, using classic plant-breeding techniques (crossing, back-crossing), the assumption is that the resulting lettuce is safe. There's no requirement for pretesting. You just introduce the product into the market. But with GMOs, Bradford says, the attitude was that "it's guilty until proven innocent."

A genetically engineered crop must pass review by the U.S. Department of Agriculture, the Environmental Protection Agency, and the Food and Drug Administration before it is commercialized. The cost could range from $50,000 to tens of millions of dollars to win regulatory approval. For every "transgenic event," the genetic engineer must show exactly what genes went into the plant and how they function, and then prove how the plant makeup has been altered. That research is costly. So is plant storage. Once a transgenic creation is spawned at the Plant Transformation Facility, it is whisked to the UC Davis Controlled Environment Facility, where it will stay in a tightly secured warehouse. Or it will be airmailed to some other place, where it'll live out its life in another intensely biosecure environment.

The process is costly and time-consuming, which partly explains why biotech crop development is largely in the hands of the agribusiness giants—the Monsantos, Syngentas, and Bayer CropSciences of the world—who have the resources to undertake the process. With such high approval costs, big companies have favored commodity crops with market potential for hundreds of millions of dollars in sales, not tens of millions.

We talked about the reasons for what Bradford calls "the bottleneck" for the biotech specialty crops. It was NGOs such as Greenpeace and the Union of Concerned Scientists that were the bogeymen, in his view. Big Organic, a $20 billion industry, had a vested interested in stopping GMOs. Back in 2000, when the USDA was developing the National Organic Program standards, the first draft did not prohibit genetically modified foods, but then activists launched an anti-GMO campaign, flooding the USDA with a tidal wave of letters—275,026, to be exact. The USDA then determined that genetically modified organisms would not be included under the standard for organic produce. Being deemed un-kosher in the organic world is a hard stigma to overcome.

The anti-GMO movement hasn't lost momentum; the Non-GMO Project has become the fastest-growing food eco-label in North America, with sales eclipsing $1 billion in 2011. As for Europe: After a 12-year moratorium on GMO crops, the European Union greenlighted a GMO potato—but not for human consumption. It would be used to produce higher levels of starch, which is helpful for industries like paper manufacturing. In short, the European market is still overwhelmingly closed for genetically modified foodstuffs.

What If the World Embraced Agricultural Biotechnology?

According to the World Health Organization, 250 million children worldwide, mostly in the developing world, have diets lacking in vitamin A. Between 250,000 and 500,000 of these children go blind every year. Yet, there is a crop, developed more than 13 years ago, that is fortified with vitamin A compounds. If children unable to get vitamin A from other protein sources simply eat this crop, they will not go blind and die. It is named "golden rice" because of its yellowish hue, and every health organization in the world has declared it to be safe to eat.

But golden rice was not bred through traditional means; it was bred in a lab. So golden rice is, by its opponents' definition, Frankenfood, and therefore, like many other GMO crops, it's been ferociously opposed.

Now let's say that golden rice does get approved (as some predict it will in 2013), and let's say it saves millions of children from starvation and blindness in Asia. Or let's say bioengineered crops slow down the creation of algal dead zones in the Gulf of Mexico. Or a low-fat, anti-cancer potato becomes a smash hit at McDonald's. Consumer worries about GMOs evaporate, becoming as anachronistic as fears of microwave ovens causing cancer. The regulatory barriers are gone; transgenic plants are treated the same as any other. The Monsanto juggernaut is over; small, boutique companies and open-source plant breeders in the comfort of a Brooklyn loft have a chance to contribute to the vegetable economy. Then what happens?

- **Food will look different.** There will almost surely be more varieties. Austrian heirloom lettuce varieties like Forellenschluss and heirloom tomatoes like the Brandywines and Cherokee Purples could become readily available. So many vegetables today aren't commercially viable because of disease vulnerabilities or production inefficiencies. But in a genetically engineered future, all the flaws that make them ill-suited for commercialization become mere speed bumps.

  "You could have disease immunity almost immediately." says Bradford. "And it would be very easy to take care of these other variables. Instead of taking a decade to ready a crop for commercialization, it will take a matter of months."

  It's possible that colors would change. You could find pink lettuce and blue arugula—maybe with a green orange slice for St. Patrick's Day. Color becomes malleable because it's often a single trait.
- **Food will taste different.** It is also likely, some geneticists say, that in 2035 some lettuces won't taste anything like lettuce. The notion of tomatoes with customized flavor was a reckless ambition in the 1990s when the Flavr Savr debuted; modifying taste is among the most challenging tasks for plant geneticists. You can silence a gene in the potato genome, tuning down the bitterness or acidic quality, but it's still a fractional impact on taste.

  Taste is complex. A tomato, for instance, has between five and twenty compounds that influence flavor. Changing flavor requires not one gene, but packages of genes, and the genes must be placed precisely. Then there is texture, inextricably linked to flavor. Modifying taste eludes technologists today, but in the next ten years, that could change, as bioengineers will be able to choose from a genetic cassette—stacks of genes that together confer desired traits. With a few mouse clicks, geneticists say, they could choose from a range of flavors, textures, and colors.

  "Think of it like Photoshop," says C. S. Prakash, director of the Center for Plant Biotechnology Research at Tuskegee University. "At some point that won't be a far-fetched metaphor." It will be technologically possible, therefore, to create a Caesar salad without the Caesar dressing; the flavor of the Caesar could be bred into the lettuce.

  Textures would also be far easier to change. You could bite into an apple that has the consistency of a banana. In a biotech-friendly future, fruits and vegetables would merely be another frontier for adventurous and often mind-bending culinary pioneers.
- **We'll see produce that doesn't spoil.** In a biotech future, the sell-by dates will be different; instead of rushing to eat your lettuce in a week, loose leaf lettuce could languish, unsealed, for a month or more. One of the huge problems in the produce industry is perishability, with close to one-third of all fresh fruits and vegetables produced lost to over ripening or damage during shipment. But bioengineers are already making progress in changing the post-harvest behavior of plants. By having an enzyme shut off, an apple has been modified so that it won't turn brown after it is sliced, and a banana has been engineered to ripen more slowly.

  Although small organic farmers are often the most hostile to technologized solutions and may be the least likely group to adopt high-tech crops, it's possible that GMOs could change the farmers' markets in places like Chicago or Buffalo.

  "In New York and Illinois, it's pretty hard to grow a lot of crops because they're going to freeze," explains Dennis Miller, a food scientist at Cornell University. "But you could engineer in frost tolerance. You could extend the growing season and bring in more exotic crops into new regions. I don't know if we'll be growing bananas in upstate New York, but it would expand the options for locally grown fruits and vegetables."

"With a few mouse clicks, geneticists say, they could choose from a range of flavors, textures, and colors."

How Frankenfood Will Improve Health

Most breeders expect that the biggest change for consumers would be something that's already familiar to any Whole Foods shopper. We already have calcium-fortified orange juice and herbal tea enhanced with antioxidants, but in an agbiotech-friendly world, the produce section would likely be overflowing with health enhancements. Orange potatoes enhanced with beta-carotene, calcium-enhanced carrots, and crops with enhanced antioxidants are already in the pipeline. By the 2030s, vegetables and fruits will be vitamin, nutrient, and beneficial-gene-delivery vehicles.

To illustrate how this would play out, Prakash points to the work of Cynthia Kenyon, a University of California—San Francisco molecular biologist, who extended the life span of a ground worm by six times by changing a gene called "def 2."

While this is in the realm of basic science, Prakash also suggests that, if something like a "fountain of youth" gene is found to benefit humans, it could be bred into vegetables. By combining genetics and plant science, a whole new realm of products would likely appear.

Some geneticists envision a future in which crop development would become a highly collaborative process: Nutritionists, geneticists, physicians, chefs, and marketers would work to develop new fruits and vegetables aimed at various consumer wants.

Another Kind of Foodie Hero

A scientist in a white lab coat doesn't conjure the same feelings as a micro-farmer in a straw hat. Growing fish in a warehouse isn't quite as stirring as pulling them out of a choppy Alaskan sea. A meat-spawning bioreactor doesn't have the same allure as a dew-covered Virginia pasture.

But it's time to broaden the foodie pantheon.

Let's continue to celebrate our heirloom-fava-bean growers and our grass-fed-goat herders. Let's carefully scrutinize the claims of nutritional science and keep a wary eye on new technologies, especially those with panacea-like claims from multinational corporations with monopolistic aims and a history of DDT and Agent Orange production. But let's not be so black-and-white; let's not be reflexively and categorically opposed to any and all technological solutions. Savoring the slowest food and foraging for wild asparagus shouldn't be viewed as at odds with championing lab-engineered vitamin A–enhanced rice that could save children from blindness.

Pairing a locally grown, seasonal mesclun mix from an organic micro-farm with cobia, a saltwater fish grown in an industrial-sized warehouse, is not an incompatible, ethically confused choice.

I make this point because of the rising tide of food-specific neo-Luddism in America. While well intentioned and often beneficial in its impact, this foodie fundamentalism is unfortunately often associated with a dangerous antiscientism. If we're going to meet the enormous challenges of feeding the world's still-growing population, we are going to need all the ingenuity we can bring to bear.

My modest hope: Let's keep an open mind. Let's consider even the fringy, sometimes yucky, maybe kooky ideas. Let's not miss opportunities to build a long-term sustainable future for our planet.

Critical Thinking

1. Define the potential "input traits" and "output traits" of genetically modified foods.
2. Outline the history of GM foods.
3. Explain why biotech crop development occurs primarily in large agribusiness corporations. Evaluate why opponents of large agribusiness corporations view this as negative.
4. Evaluate the potential benefits of GM foods.

Create Central

www.mhhe.com/createcentral

Internet References

FDA's Role in Regulating Safety of GE Foods.
www.fda.gov/ForConsumers/ConsumerUpdates/ucm352067.htm

Monsanto
www.monsanto.com

Project on Emerging Nanotechnologies
www.nanotechproject.org

Society for Science and the Public
www.societyforscience.org

World Future Society
www.wfs.org/futurist

Josh Schonwald is the author of *The Taste of Tomorrow: Dispatches From the Future of Food* (Harper, 2012).

Article

Prepared by: Janet Colson, *Middle Tennessee State University*

Who Should You Believe When It Comes to the Safety of Genetically Engineered Foods?

Conflicting studies and tons of controversy surrounding GE foods are muddying up the water.

JILL RICHARDSON

Learning Outcomes

After reading this article, you will be able to:

- Explain why corn is genetically engineered.
- Compare the design and results of the GE corn study conducted by Séralin to the study conducted by Monsanto.
- List the seven GE crops grown in the United States.

Controversy and genetic engineering go together like peanut butter and jelly, so naturally, there's another brouhaha over genetically engineered (GE) crops in the news. Back in September 2012, a French study led by Gilles-Eric Séralini found that rats fed Monsanto's GE corn were more likely to develop tumors than rats fed non-GE corn. The study was published in the journal *Food and Chemical Toxicology,* the same journal that routinely publishes Monsanto's own studies finding that its GE corn is safe to feed to rats. Now, over two years later, the journal retracted the Séralini study.

So what's going on? Does GE corn give rats tumors? How about people? And how do Americans, the vast majority of whom are not scientists, know what is safe to eat? Here's a look at what the Séralini study found, why it should not have been retracted, and how to tell the difference between valid and bogus claims about GE food.

Both Monsanto and Séralini's feeding studies follow the same general model. Get a large group of a type of rats called Sprague-Dawley and divide them into groups. Feed some groups GE corn and feed the others non-GE corn. Occasionally test their blood and urine, and watch to see if any get sick and die. At the end of the study, euthanize the remaining rats and dissect them to check their organs. Pretty simple, right?

Here are the differences. Monsanto studied its rats for only 90 days, but Séralini studied the rats for two years. Monsanto used twice as many rats—20 male rats and 20 female rats in each group—as Séralini.

Then there's the corn used. Both studied a variety of Roundup Ready corn called NK603. (Roundup Ready means that the corn resists Monsanto's herbicide Roundup, so cornfields can be sprayed by Roundup, killing the weeds and leaving the corn alive.) In addition to the Roundup Ready corn that was sprayed by Roundup, as a control they used what's known as a "near isoline." A near isoline means corn that is genetically identical to the Roundup Ready corn, with the exception of the Roundup Ready gene. The near isoline corn was grown in the same location at the same time as the Roundup Ready corn, so they would be as similar as possible.

But each study added some additional groups. Séralini examined groups fed Roundup Ready corn that was never sprayed by Roundup. He also studied rats fed a control diet but given water spiked with Roundup herbicide. The extra groups would help find out if any impacts of the Roundup Ready corn were attributable to the Roundup and not to the corn itself.

Monsanto, for its part, added extra groups called "reference controls" that obscured its data. Rats fed reference control diets were fed various kinds of non-GE corn grown in different locations.

Whenever Monsanto found a statistically significant difference between the Roundup Ready rats and the control rats, they could often dismiss the differences by saying that the results of the Roundup Ready rats were within the normal range for the reference control rats. Michael Hansen, senior scientist at Consumers Union, compares this to a pharmaceutical company testing a drug. If the group taking the drug gains 10 pounds and the control group doesn't, it's not okay for the pharmaceutical company to brush that off because a 10 pound weight gain is a relatively normal occurrence within the wider human population.

Monsanto, of course, concluded that its Roundup Ready corn is perfectly safe to eat. Séralini did not, because more rats fed GE corn developed tumors than rats fed non-GE corn. What accounted for the different results?

Perhaps it's because Séralini's study continued for two years, whereas Monsanto ended its study after 90 days. Imagine a study of the health of a human population. You'd find more disease among a study that continued to age 80 than you would in a study that ended at age 30.

There's also the different sizes of the study groups. Monsanto studied 20 rats per sex per group, and Séralini studied only 10. However, Monsanto only gathered and analyzed blood and urine from 10 rats per sex per group. So, in essence, the study groups were the same size for many of the measurements taken.

Séralini's study is not conclusive. As Hansen and others point out, the number of rats in each group is too small. "However," Hansen adds, "Both the French Food Safety Agency (ANSES) and the European Food Safety Authority (EFSA) have agreed with Dr. Séralini that such long-term safety assessment should be done on GE foods." The European Commission announced on June 28, 2013, that it would spend 3 million euros to do just that.

So why did the journal retract the study? In its statement, *Food and Chemical Toxicology* noted that the study was neither fraudulent nor did it intentionally misrepresent the data. However, there were concerns with the size of the study groups and the strain of rats used. "Ultimately," the press release concluded, "the results presented (while not incorrect) are inconclusive, and therefore do not reach the threshold of publication for *Food and Chemical Toxicology*."

"This really is a scandal," Hansen says when asked about the retraction. He points to the journal's own policy for *what merits a retraction:* "Infringements of professional ethical codes, such as multiple submission, bogus claims of authorship, plagiarism, fraudulent use of data or the like. Occasionally a retraction will be used to correct errors in submission or publication."

The reasons given for retracting the Séralini study do not meet those criteria.

Why is it okay for Monsanto to use Sprague-Dawley rats—which it does in numerous feeding studies published in the same journal—but not Séralini? Hansen points to a *Chinese study* the journal just published that used the same strain of rats in a two-year feeding study of GE rice. The study concluded that the GE rice "exerts no unintended adverse effects on rats."

Likewise, Hansen notes Monsanto's studies based its conclusion that its GE corn is safe on blood and urine from only 10 rats. "If you're going to say that 10 is too small a number to conclude that there's a health problem, how can you turn around and include a study that concludes there's no problem?" he asks.

If inconclusiveness is a fatal flaw in a study, an awful lot of other studies ought to be retracted, too.

"It's a double standard," Hansen says. "Any study that concludes a problem with genetic engineering is gone through with a fine-tooth comb and they try to rip it up but the same is not done" for studies with conclusions favorable to genetic engineering. "This is a form of scientific censorship. When you retract a paper, it means it no longer appears in that journal so it's no longer in the public domain."

Séralini study notwithstanding, how do we know what to believe about GE crops? In addition to any good science out there, there are ideologues and kooks on both sides of the debate.

To start, a 2011 article found that professional associations with the biotech industry impact study outcomes. The study examined a total of 94 different journal articles published on the nutritional and health impacts of GE food and feed. Of those studies, 41 had at least one author with a professional tie to the biotech industry. All 41 had outcomes favorable to biotech. The remaining 53 papers, in which none of the authors had professional ties to the biotech industry, were split: 39 in favor of biotech, 12 against, and 2 neutral.

In other words, any time a study has at least one author with a professional tie to the biotech industry, you don't even have to read the study to know the conclusion. It concluded that GE crops are a-okay.

You might conclude that the best way to go is simply to find independent research on GE crops. That's a great idea. Unfortunately, the biotech companies use their intellectual property rights to restrict independent research on their products. Even scientists see this as a problem: in 2009, 26 university entomologists wrote to the EPA protesting scientists' inability to conduct independent research.

Even the FDA does not test these crops for safety. In fact, Hansen points out, they only require biotech companies like Monsanto to perform voluntary "safety consultations" on their crops. After Monsanto does its own safety check, the FDA sends back a letter confirming that Monsanto found its own product to be safe. Since we already know that 100 percent of nutrition and health studies in which one or more authors were affiliated with the biotech industry, it's a foregone conclusion that 100 percent of Monsanto's voluntary "safety consultations" found that Monsanto's products were perfectly safe.

A Norwegian study examined the differences in opinions on GE crops among different groups of scientists. It found that ecologists were more likely to have a moderately negative attitude to GE crops and worry about the uncertainty and ignorance involved when human beings tinker with plant genes, whereas molecular biologists—particularly those who worked for the biotech industry or those funded by industry—had a strongly favorable view of GE crops and felt that the crops are useful and "do not represent any unique risks." The only molecular biologists who sided with the ecologists were those working in foundations, with public funding, studying the risks of GE crops.

The paper notes that "industry funding might impose limits on scientists' possibilities to reflect on the social dimension of their work or at least that the recruitment process is biased and thereby indirectly influences the reflection that will take place." In other words, as noted before, independent research is key.

The authors suggest a solution may be more interdisciplinary training for scientists or even dialogue between scientists of different disciplines. However, "open-minded dialogue might be difficult to facilitate, as there seems to be a lack of trust between the different groups."

Unfortunately, in the end, it's hard for most of us to figure out whether the headlines we read about GE foods are true or not. Look for independent research that is not conducted by scientists employed by the biotech industry, and consider the perspectives of scientists from a variety of scientific disciplines, not just molecular biology. Consider the research of social scientists like economists and anthropologists as well.

If that's not enough to make you feel good about eating GE foods, the only option is to try to avoid them. So far, only a few GE crops are grown and sold, but they are found in an awful lot of our food: corn, soy, cotton, canola, sugar beet, alfalfa, and papaya. Since they aren't labeled, the easiest way to avoid them is to buy organic.

Hopefully, a few years from now, the European Commission's long-term rat feeding study will shed more light on this issue—although by then, odds are the United States will have legalized a whole bunch of new GE crops for us to worry about.

Critical Thinking

1. Explain why the *Food and Chemical Toxicology* journal retracted Séralin's study and discuss what happened to the study after retraction.
2. Write an essay on the impact that banning GE corn in the state of Iowa will have on the United States.

Create Central

www.mhhe.com/createcentral

Internet References

Food and Drug Administration
www.fda.org

Monsanto
www.monsanto.com

National Environmental Health Association
www.neha.org/index.shtml

Jill Richardson is the founder of the blog *La Vida Locavore* and a member of the Organic Consumers Association policy advisory board. She is the author of *Recipe for America: Why Our Food System Is Broken and What We Can Do to Fix It.*

Article Prepared by: Janet Colson, *Middle Tennessee State University*

The Organic Foods Debate: Are They Healthier Than Conventional?

Many consumers believe organics are healthier than conventional options, as studies show some organics contain more nutrients and significantly less pesticide residues that research suggests may be harmful to your health.

JUDITH C. THALHEIMER

Learning Outcomes

After reading this article, you will be able to:

- Explain why consumers buy organic foods.
- Compare the nutrition and health qualities of organic foods to foods that are grown conventionally.

"Should I buy organic?" As dietitians, you've probably heard this question from clients time and again. Given the higher cost of organic foods and new questions being raised regarding their health benefits, clients are right to ask.

Despite these new questions, however, demand for organic products is growing. According to the Organic Trade Association's (OTA) 2012 Organic Industry Survey, sales of food and nonfood organic products grew by 9.5% in 2011 to reach $31.5 billion.[1] Of the 81% of families that said they bought organic food products, as part of the OTA's newly released 2013 US Families' Organic Attitudes and Beliefs Study, 48% said their primary motivation was the belief that organic products are a healthier choice for themselves and their children.[2] But are organic foods, in fact, more healthful than conventional foods?

Finding the Truth

A meta-analysis conducted by Stanford University researchers and published in the September 2012 issue of *Annals of Internal Medicine* touched off a media firestorm when it concluded that "the published literature lacks strong evidence that organic foods are significantly more nutritious than conventional foods."[3] With the exception of higher phosphorus levels in organic produce and limited evidence suggesting higher omega-3 fatty acids in organic milk, no significant difference was found between the nutrient levels in organic and conventional foods.[3]

Similarly, a 2007 meta-analysis by the British Nutrition Foundation found no overall differences in the nutrient profiles of organic and conventional foods. However, there was evidence of higher levels of vitamin C in some organically grown produce, such as potatoes and dark, leafy greens.[4]

Mary Ann Moylan, RD, LDN, CDE, an in-store dietitian for Ahold USA's Giant Superstore supermarket in Willow Grove, Pennsylvania, has seen firsthand the impact of the media surrounding the Stanford study. "More customers are asking me about the benefits of organic foods," she says. "They want to know what I think. As a registered dietitian, I need to be able to answer these questions in an informed and evidenced-based way."

Comparative analysis of plant nutrients is complicated. A plant's nutrient profile depends on the plant species or variety, weather during that particular growing season, soil makeup, and other conditions. In studies that compare the same varieties of fruits and vegetables grown in similar locations, organic food contains higher levels of some nutrients about 60% of the time, according to Charles Benbrook, PhD, a research professor at Washington State University's Center for Sustaining Agriculture and Natural Resources.[5]

While the Stanford analysis averaged crops from multiple years into a single data point, a 2011 review that looked at separate years as separate data points to account for the effects of weather came to a very different conclusion.[6] The 2011 review, a meta-analysis conducted by scientists at Newcastle University in England, concluded that organic produce has a 12% higher content of secondary metabolites and a 6% higher vitamin C content than corresponding conventional samples.[6] Secondary metabolites are phytochemicals that increase a plant's ability to survive in its environment. Since organic plants are forced to defend themselves against disease and pests without the aid of manmade chemicals, they may develop more of these natural defenses.

The Newcastle researchers posited that the defense-related secondary metabolites in fruits and vegetables are the reason higher intake is linked to reduced risk of cancer and cardiovascular disease. While it's possible that higher levels of beneficial phytochemicals and vitamin C make organic foods better for our long-term health outcomes than conventional products, there have been no large studies in humans to address this issue.[6]

What Is Organic?

When examining the value of organic foods, it's important to understand the definition of organic. In the United States, organic is a labeling term defined by the USDA. To be considered organic, a product must meet federal standards for production, processing, and certification under the Organic Food Production Act of 1990. The National Organic Program oversees these standards, which have been in full effect since October 2002.

According to the USDA, organic products have "been produced through approved methods that integrate cultural, biological, and mechanical practices that foster cycling of resources, promote ecological balance, and conserve biodiversity."[7] The national organic standards forbid the use of synthetic fertilizers and pesticides, sewage sludge, irradiation, and genetic engineering to grow fruits, nuts, vegetables, and grains. Organic meat and poultry can't be irradiated. The animals must have access to the outdoors, and they can't be given any growth hormones, antibiotics, or other drugs. All feed must be 100% organic, with no animal by-products.[8]

"The most important aspect of this conversation is that organic produce is about much more than nutrients; it's about the way crops are grown," says Sharon Palmer, RD, author of The Plant-Powered Diet. "Organic produce generally has lower levels of pesticide residues, which is one of the main reasons people are attracted to them. In addition, organic production is more sustainable; it uses less energy, produces fewer greenhouse gas emissions, and creates healthier soils. If anything, this widely publicized [Stanford] study highlights what's really important about organic food production; it's not just the nutrients."

Reasons for Buying Organic

The 2010 Nielsen Global Online Survey found that worldwide people buy organic foods for more than just their perceived vitamin or phytochemical content. North America was the "region most likely to buy organics to avoid toxins (71%), promote environmentally friendly organic farms (59%), help small farmers (58%), avoid genetically modified products (45%), do the right thing (38%), and vote against modern farming methods (23%)."[9]

Moylan says her customers choose organic foods for a variety of reasons: "Some prefer the taste of organic produce or milk. Others are interested in protecting the environment or want to support sustainable agriculture. Food safety and the use of chemicals in food manufacturing are common concerns. I see a particular interest from pregnant women and people with young children."

Evidence for some of the benefits of organic foods can be found in the Stanford study. The researchers reported evidence of pesticide residues in 38% of conventional foods and 7% of organics. In absolute terms, organic fruits and vegetables had a 30% lower risk of pesticide contamination than conventional produce.[3]

While farmers can't apply synthetic pesticides to organic produce, there can be what the USDA calls "inadvertent or indirect contact from neighboring conventional farms or shared handling facilities" as long as the level of prohibited pesticides remains below 5% of the accepted tolerance levels.[10] In the 2013 US Families' Organic Attitudes and Beliefs Study, 30% of families cited limiting exposure to pesticides as a reason they buy organic foods.[2]

In the Stanford study, pesticide levels in conventional foods generally fell within the Environmental Protection Agency's (EPA) acceptable limits.[3] Despite the EPA's control of residue levels, concerns still exist about the safety of ingesting pesticides, especially in adults with chronic health conditions, children, and pregnant women. Studies have shown that eating organic foods reduces pesticide exposure. A 2003 study by Curl and colleagues found that children aged 2 to 5 who ate conventional foods had six times more urinary organophosphorus pesticide metabolites than children who ate organic foods.[11] Three studies funded by the National Institute of Environmental Health Sciences and the EPA found that women with higher pesticide exposure during pregnancy had children with lower IQ scores.[12]

Moreover, the detrimental environmental impact of pesticide use should be taken into account. Air- or water-borne pesticides can deplete the ozone, harm or kill nontarget species and beneficial soil organisms, contaminate drinking water, or adversely effect marine life.

Twenty-nine percent of families who buy organic foods are concerned about hormone and antibiotic use in conventional foods.[2] The increase in antibiotic-resistant bacterial infections in humans primarily is a result of unnecessary antibiotic use in both humans and animals. On conventional farms, low levels of antibiotics routinely are used in healthy animals to speed up growth and discourage the development or spread of bacterial disease. In 2011, about 80% of all reported antibiotic sales in the United States were for use in livestock (29.9 million lbs for animals vs. 7.7 million for humans).[13]

The Stanford study found that, while bacterial contamination was common in chicken and pork regardless of farming method, conventional chicken and pork had a 33% higher risk of contamination with bacteria that was resistant to three or more antibiotics than organic products. There was no difference in the risk of E coli contamination between organic and conventional produce.[3]

The 2011 report by the National Antimicrobial Resistance Monitoring System found that more than 27% of all bacteria isolated from chicken showed resistance to five or more classes of antibiotics. Researchers also found 10 different serotypes of bacteria resistant to six or more classes of antibiotics in ground turkey. Fifty-five percent of Salmonella isolated from retail poultry was drug resistant, up from 50% in 2010.[14] In 2012, the FDA restricted the use of the cephalosporin class of antibiotics in animals in response to rising resistant strains of bacteria.[15]

Advising Clients

When answering clients' questions about organic foods, dietetics professionals clearly must take into account a definition of healthy that goes beyond nutrient content. "I think it's important for RDs to discuss the whole situation about organics, not just nutrients. We should feel informed and empowered to discuss the entire food system in our conversations with people," Palmer says. "Dietitians should be the experts in areas such as food sustainability and production. Otherwise people will turn to less informed people for information about organics." For evidence-based information on organics, Palmer recommends the Hunger and Environmental Nutrition Dietetic Practice Group of the Academy of Nutrition and Dietetics (the Academy).

It's important to recognize that organic products may be hard to find in some areas. The good news for those seeking organic products is that they're more available now than ever. In 2010, natural retailers sold 39% of all organic foods, and 54% was sold by mass-market retailers such as mainstream supermarkets, club/warehouse stores, and mass merchandisers.[16] Many mainstream retailers today offer their own line of natural and organic foods, use shelf tags to promote natural and organic choices throughout the store, or devote a section of the store to these products. Moylan sees the impact of this trend firsthand. "The customers I counsel at Giant are pleasantly surprised to see how many items throughout the supermarket have those purple 'organic' food tags, and grouping items in our Nature's Promise Marketplace has been a big help to customers looking for those options. Having programs like these in mainstream markets is really broadening options for the average shopper."

The growing availability of organic products is fueled by studies showing that organic buyers are spending more per shopping trip and are shopping more frequently than those who never purchase organic food. Organic buyers spend more because organics can cost 20% to 100% more than their conventionally produced counterparts. Many factors lead to the higher cost: Growing crops without herbicides and pesticides causes more losses from crop damage and incurs higher labor costs for weeding and pest control; animals raised to produce organic meats must be fed more expensive organic feed; and there's a fee for organic certification.[17]

If price is a concern, Vandana Sheth RDN, CDE, a spokesperson for the Academy, recommends choosing fruits and vegetables that provide the most potential health benefit for the money. "The Environmental Working Group tests more than 10,000 pesticides in fruits and vegetables and develops a Dirty Dozen list," she says. "Conventionally grown versions of these fruits and vegetables have been found to have higher levels of pesticide residue." The group also publishes The Clean 15, a list of the 15 conventionally grown fruits and vegetables found to have the least pesticide residues[18] (see Table 1). The FDA recommends washing all fresh produce, organic as well as conventional, for food safety reasons and to reduce or eliminate pesticide and fungicide residues.[19]

Moylan counsels customers on a budget seeking organic choices to begin with foods they eat most often or in the greatest quantities. "Choosing organic produce in season is a great way to stretch your organic foods budget too," Moylan says. "They're more likely to be locally grown and cost less to transport, leading to lower prices in the store."

Table 1 Produce with the Most and Least Pesticides[18]

Dirty Dozen	Clean 15
Apples	Asparagus
Celery	Avocados
Cherry tomatoes	Cabbage
Cucumbers	Cantaloupe
Grapes	Sweet corn
Hot peppers	Eggplant
Nectarines (imported)	Grapefruit
Peaches	Kiwi
Potatoes	Mangos
Spinach	Mushrooms
Strawberries	Onions
Sweet bell peppers	Papayas
	Pineapples
	Sweet peas (frozen)
	Sweet potatoes

**According to the Environmental Working Group, kale/collard greens and summer squash "do not meet traditional Dirty Dozen criteria but were commonly contaminated with pesticides exceptionally toxic to the nervous system."*

Palmer suggests looking outside traditional stores and making wise choices. "There are more affordable ways to eat organic, such as using your farmers market and community-supported agriculture programs to purchase foods that may be grown in an organic fashion but not necessarily with the certification. Don't waste money on purchasing organic junk food [eg, cookies, chips, candy]. I see that as a waste of food dollars. You also can find less expensive organic foods at stores that specialize in it rather than stores that have a small selection," she says. Buying in bulk and what's on sale, using coupons, and purchasing the growing number of private label brands are other money-saving ways to buy organic.[20]

What Really Matters

Whether people buy organic or conventional, it's the nutritional quality of the overall diet that matters. "The key is to enjoy a wide variety of foods, including fruits, vegetables, whole grains, lean protein, nuts, seeds, and beans," Sheth says. "I advocate that people meet their fruit and vegetable servings as their primary goal," Palmer adds, regardless of whether that produce is organically grown.

In November 2012, the American Academy of Pediatrics (AAP) published a clinical report on the health and environmental advantages and disadvantages of organic foods. The report concluded with advice for pediatricians, which nutrition professionals can use as a guide as well. In summary, the AAP recommended encouraging a health-promoting diet; answering questions about organics using the latest scientific evidence regarding nutrition, cost issues, and the environmental impact; and directing clients who express concern about the potential health impact of pesticide residues in food to resources such as the Environmental Working Group's "Shoppers Guide to Pesticides."[21]

"Choosing to buy organic foods is a personal decision," Sheth says. "At this point, there's no conclusive scientific evidence that shows that organically produced foods are healthier. Similarly, taste and appearance of organic or conventionally grown foods don't show a significant difference. If your goal is to limit your exposure to pesticides, antibiotics, and hormones or if you have concerns about environmental impact, look for the organic label on foods."

7 Ways to Reduce Pesticide Residues

The FDA offers the following tips to reduce or eliminate any pesticide residues and bacteria that may be present on conventional or organic produce and meats[1,2]:

- **Wash your hands for 20 seconds** with warm water and soap before and after preparing fresh produce to prevent the spread of bacteria.
- **Cut away any damaged or bruised areas** before preparing or eating.
- **Wash produce** with large amounts of cold or warm running tap water and scrub with a brush when appropriate. There's no need to use soap or a produce wash.
- **Wash produce before you peel it** so dirt and bacteria aren't transferred from the knife onto the fruit or vegetable.
- **Dry produce with a clean cloth** or paper towel to further reduce bacteria that may be present.
- **Throw away the outer leaves** of leafy vegetables such as lettuce and cabbage.
- **Trim the fat from meat** and the fat and skin from poultry and fish. Residues of some pesticides concentrate in animal fat.

Sidebar References

1. 7 tips for cleaning fruits, vegetables. US Food and Drug Administration website. http://www.fda.gov/ForConsumers/ConsumerUpdates/ucm256215.htm. Updated April 12, 2013. Accessed April 25, 2013.
2. Pesticide Q & A. US Food and Drug Administration website. http://www.fda.gov/Food/FoodborneIllness-Contaminants/Pesticides/ucm114958.htm. Updated February 20, 2013. Accessed April 23, 2013.

Main Article References

1. Consumer-driven US organic market surpasses $31 billion in 2011. Organic Trade Association website. http://www.organicnewsroom.com/2012/04/us_consumerdriven_organic_mark.html. April 2012. Accessed April 18, 2013.
2. Eight in ten US parents report they purchase organic products. Organic Trade Association website. http://www.organicnewsroom.com/2013/04/eight_in_ten_us_parents_report.html. April 4, 2013. Accessed April 17, 2013.
3. Smith-Spangler C, Brandeau ML, Hunter GE, et al. Are organic foods safer or healthier than conventional alternatives? A systematic review. ***Ann Intern Med.*** 2012;157(5):348–366.
4. Is organic food really more nutritious? Tufts University Health & Nutrition Letter website. http://www.tuftshealthletter.com/ShowArticle.aspx?rowId=368. September 2007. Accessed April 19, 2013.
5. Schardt D. Going organic: what's the payoff? Center for Science in the Public Interest website. http://www.cspinet.org/nah/articles/going-organic.html. October 2012.
6. Brandt K, Leifert C, Sanderson R, Seal CJ. Agroecosystem management and nutritional quality of plant foods: the case of organic fruits and vegetables. ***Crit Rev Plant Sci.*** 2011;30(1–2):177–197.
7. What is organic? United States Department of Agriculture website. http://www.ams.usda.gov/AMSv1.0/nop. Updated May 3, 2013. Accessed April 18, 2013.
8. Organic standards. United States Department of Agriculture website. http://www.ams.usda.gov/AMSv1.0/ams.fetchTemplateData.do?template=TemplateN&navID=Organic-StandardsLinkNOPFAQsHome&rightNav1=OrganicStandardsLinkNOPFAQsHome&topNav=&leftNav=&page=NOPOrganicStandards&resultType=&acct=nopgeninfo. Updated April 4, 2013. Accessed April 18, 2013.
9. Global trends in healthy eating. Nielsen website. http://www.nielsen.com/us/en/newswire/2010/global-trends-in-healthy-eating.html. Updated August 30, 2010. Accessed April 21, 2013.
10. USDA National Organic Program, USDA Science and Technology Programs. 2010–2011 Pilot Study: Pesticide Residue Testing of Organic Produce. United States Department of Agriculture website. http://www.ams.usda.gov/AMSv1.0/getfile?dDocName=STELPRDC5101234. November 2012.
11. Curl CL, Fenske RA, Elgethun K. Organophosphorus pesticide exposure of urban and suburban preschool children with organic and conventional diets. ***Environ Health Perspect.*** 2003;111(3):377–382.
12. Parker-Pope T. Pesticide exposure in womb affects IQ. The New York Times website. http://well.blogs.nytimes.com/2011/04/21/pesticide-exposure-in-womb-affects-i-q. April 21, 2011. Accessed April 23, 2013.
13. Record-high antibiotic sales for meat and poultry production. The Pew Charitable Trusts website. http://www.pewhealth.org/other-resource/record-high-antibiotic-sales-for-meat-and-poultry-production-85899449119. February 6, 2013.
14. National Antimicrobial Resistance Monitoring System. 2011 retail meat report. US Food and Drug Administration website. http://www.fda.gov/downloads/AnimalVeterinary/SafetyHealth/AntimicrobialResistance/NationalAntimicrobialResistanceMonitoringSystem/UCM334834.pdf.
15. Cephalosporin order of prohibition goes into effect. US Food and Drug Administration website. http://www.fda.gov/AnimalVeterinary/NewsEvents/CVMUpdates/ucm299054.htm. April 6, 2012.
16. Industry statistics and projected growth. Organic Trade Association website. http://www.ota.com/organic/mt/business.html. June 2011. Accessed April 18, 2013.
17. 10 reasons organic food is so expensive. FOX News website. http://www.foxnews.com/leisure/2012/03/11/10-reasons-organic-food-is-so-expensive/-ixzz2RbCdXLXr. March 11, 2012. Accessed April 23, 2013.

18. EWG's 2013 shopper's guide to pesticides in produce. Environmental Working Group website. http://www.ewg.org/foodnews/summary.php. Accessed April 22, 2013.
19. Pesticide Q & A. US Food and Drug Administration website. http://www.fda.gov/Food/FoodborneIllnessContaminants/Pesticides/ucm114958.htm. Updated February 20, 2013. Accessed April 23, 2013.
20. Buying organic is easier and more affordable than ever before. Organic: It's Worth It website. http://www.organicitsworthit.org/get/buying-organic-easier-and-more-affordable-ever.
21. Forman J, Silverstein J; Committee on Nutrition; Council on Environmental Health; American Academy of Pediatrics. Organic foods: health and environmental advantages and disadvantages. ***Pediatrics.*** 2012;130(5):e1406–e1415.

Critical Thinking

1. Why do consumers choose organic foods over conventionally grown ones?
2. What are the differences between the nutritional quality of organic foods and conventionally grown foods?
3. What populations benefit from eating organic foods?
4. What advice should dietitians give to consumers about use of organic foods in meal planning?

Create Central

www.mhhe.com/createcentral

Internet References

Food and Drug Administration
www.FDA.gov

National Organic Program
www.ams.usda.gov/AMSv1.0/nop

Organic Trade Association
www.ota.com/index.html

Judith C. Thalheimer, RD, LDN, is a freelance nutrition writer and community educator living outside Philadelphia.

Article

Prepared by: Janet Colson, *Middle Tennessee State University*

Food That Lasts Forever

Want to shop once a month? New techniques can keep meals fresh longer—much longer

DEBORAH BLUM

Learning Outcomes

After reading this article, you will be able to:

- Describe the advances in food technology that help extend the shelf-life of foods.
- Explain how high pressure processing is used in foods processing.

In his basement office at the University of Wisconsin, Rich Hartel lines up the failures. The 10-year-old jar of marshmallow crème in which the corn syrup settled into a thick amber pool at the bottom. The two-year-old petrified Peeps. "I have some one-year-old Twinkies at the back of my cabinet," offers Hartel, a professor of food science. Contrary to popular belief that they're immortal, Twinkies are designed for no more than a four-week shelf life, and they tend to become more chewy than soft after the first week. The fact is that most desserts—barring, famously (or infamously), fruitcake—devolve into a sticky wad of starch in a depressingly short time.

At least for now. Scientists like Hartel are working to change that, with some startling recent success. A new generation of food-preservation technologies is starting to transform how long we can keep food tasting fresh, exponentially increasing its life span. NASA recently reported that it has come up with bread pudding that can last a solid four years. Over at the Pentagon, there's pound cake that stays springy for up to five years. And that's just the desserts. Long-lasting entrées and side dishes are being concocted, with enormous implications: in the future we may have to go to the grocery store only once a month and will rarely, if ever, need to throw out food because it has gone bad. Further, if fruits and vegetables can be better preserved, food scientists hope they will become less expensive and more available for people on limited budgets.

Without new and more sophisticated methods of preservation, we could fall short of feeding a global population expected to top 7 billion this year.

Consumers are already taking advantage. Tuna in those vacuum-sealed pouches that started popping up in stores a few years ago tastes fresher than canned tuna and has a similar shelf life, about 2 ½ years. Foodmakers had conquered one part of the equation. Spam is famously imperishable—but palate-wise, it's practically in a category of its own and not a likely standard bearer for fresh-tasting, everyday meals. Though Spam is sold with an expiration date two years in the future, Phil Minerich, vice president of research at Hormel, says that actually underestimates its durability. "We really put that on there to help the consumer move it through," he says. "We don't want it to be sitting on the shelf for 12, 15 years." But, he adds, a well-sealed can of Spam would remain edible that long, if not longer.

The new food preservationists aren't just after longevity; they're reaching for a different standard of edibility. "In the last decade, there's been an evolution in the way we think of long-lasting foods," says Lauren Oleksyk, leader of the food-processing, engineering and technology team at the U.S. Department of Defense Combat Feeding Directorate.

"We're not just talking about long-term space missions," says John Floros of Penn State. "We're talking about survival here on earth."

Much of the new technology stems from the military's need for long-lasting food for troops, packaged as MREs (meals, ready to eat)—rations that have never been famous for tasting good. In 2002, Oleksyk and her colleagues introduced their first alternative option, an "indestructible" sandwich: a bread envelope stuffed with pepperoni or barbecued chicken, designed to last three to five years without refrigeration at standard room temperature.

There are three big challenges to making food with a long life span, and a sandwich presents all of them: controlling moisture, controlling atmosphere and controlling microorganisms, from bacteria to mold. (Many traditional food-preservation techniques, such as drying and salting, work because they kill microorganisms or limit their growth.)

Oleksyk's team members needed to keep liquids from the sandwich filling from seeping into the bread, so they mixed water-absorbing ingredients including glycerol and sorbitol into the filling. They also increased the use of fine, edible polymer films, which are undetectable in the mouth. (Hartel notes that in desserts, chocolate is often used as a moisture barrier. His favorite example is the Twix, designed so that chocolate separates the dry cookie from the moist peanut butter or caramel inside.)

The supersandwich also limits exposure to oxygen, which accelerates chemical changes in food, by tucking packets of oxygen-scavenging chemicals in the outer wrapping. And the packaging is as impervious as possible, with layers of heat-resistant polypropylene and metal foil.

But the most important advance may be innovative ways of controlling bacteria, like a newly refined method of high-pressure processing (HPP), which greatly improves taste. The old method of sterilization requires 30 minutes of 250°F (121°C) heat, and as any cook knows, every hot minute changes the food. With HPP, food is sealed in a plastic pouch, placed in a chamber and subjected to 87,000 lb. of pressure per sq. in., effectively killing any bacteria. The makers of some commercially available lunch meats, like Hormel's Natural Choice line, already rely on high-pressure processing rather than chemical preservatives. Companies that handle delicate seafood products like raw oysters are also adopting the approach. Oleksyk says the technique may soon allow the military to offer sandwiches stuffed with ingredients like tuna salad and mayonnaise.

Will consumers bite? Better taste and texture are critical for makers to change the way people think about preserved foods.

"It's night and day compared to the old heating process," Oleksyk says. "The foods taste like they're freshly prepared." The Defense Department hopes to introduce packaged HPP fruit that will retain its crispness for at least three years in a way that cannot be achieved by canning. Oleksyk's goal is to eventually create meals that can last up to 10 years. That would mean—especially if combat rations continue to be delivered on the standard three-to-five-year schedule—that there would never be a point when the food didn't taste fresh, she says. "They wouldn't have any idea how old it actually was."

Oleksyk admits that these are still mostly dreams of the future, but researchers at NASA have also been pushing the boundaries of old-time heat treatment. A report published in December in the *Journal of Food Science* offered a detailed portrait of the outer limits of shelf stability for heat-treated, or thermostabilized, foods. The report was based on a three-year study of 13 foods, including vegetable side dishes (carrot coins, three-bean salad), pork chops, vegetable omelettes and apricot cobbler. Once processed and packaged, the foods were stored at Johnson Space Center and taste-tested on a regular basis over the three years. They remained edible for a surprising length of time, although they had clearly aged, turning darker and changing in texture. "We tested a tuna-fish casserole," says lead author Michele Perchonok, a food scientist at the center's Habitability and Environmental Factors Division. "The pasta got soft, but the tuna held up very well."

Shelf Lives in the Balance

- **Bread:** Fresh bread quickly gets moldy when unrefrigerated
- **Twinkies:** Rumors of their immortality are greatly exaggerated
- **Canned Peas:** It's best to throw out canned goods after about a year
- **Tuna:** Vacuum packaging means even more salad days
- **Pork Chops:** Thermostabilizing grilled chops gives a boost to longevity
- **Spam:** No everyday food lasts longer than this icon (yet)

"It's night and day compared to the old heating process. The foods taste like they're freshly prepared," says the U.S. Defense Department's Lauren Oleksyk.

The best results consistently came from meat products, she says. For instance, extrapolating from its three-year study, the agency calculated that grilled pork chops could remain edible for nearly seven years and tuna or salmon for close to eight years (far longer than desserts, which had shelf lives of 1¼ to five years). She attributes the durability of meats mostly to their tough protein fibers.

Ultimately, long-lasting foods could have global impact. We rely on shelf-stable foods after disasters and when electricity fails. After Hurricane Katrina in 2005, many Gulf Coast residents subsisted on MREs provided by the military; these and similar products feed victims of everything from earthquakes and blizzards to drought. What's more, frozen- and chilled-food sections are expensive for grocers. In a future when energy supplies may be increasingly limited, researchers suggest, investment in food preservation looks like a smart move.

That's one of the main messages in a recent analysis titled "Feeding the World Today and Tomorrow" from the Chicago-based Institute of Food Technologists. The lead author, John Floros, head of the food-science department at Penn State University, says that without good food preservation, we could fall short of meeting the needs of a global population expected to top 7 billion this year. The problem, he says, is that we lose too much food to rot and decay. In developing countries without sophisticated food-distribution and cooling systems, the loss is consistently 30 percent a year and in some places as high as 70 percent. He expects such challenges to increase, along with uncertainties in food production related to projected global climate change. Floros works with NASA on its food-stability projects, but "we're not just talking about long-term space missions," he says flatly. "We're talking about survival here on earth."

Critical Thinking

1. Identify the three big challenges of producing food with a long shelf life.
2. Describe methods used as moisture barriers in food processing
3. Define high pressure processing (HHP). List three examples of foods preserved by (HHP).

Create Central

www.mhhe.com/createcentral

Internet References

Institute of Food Technology
www.IFT.org

National Institute of Food and Agriculture
www.csrees.usda.gov

Society for Science and the Public
www.societyforscience.org

Deborah Blum is a science writer and the author of *The Poisoner's Handbook.*

Article

Prepared by: Janet Colson, *Middle Tennessee State University*

FDA Taking Closer Look at "Antibacterial" Soap

Learning Outcomes

After reading this article, you will be able to:

- Compare the germ-killing effectiveness of over-the-counter antibacterial soap to regular soap and water.
- Describe what makes soap "antibacterial."

When you're buying soaps and body washes, do you reach for the bar or bottle labeled "antibacterial"? Are you thinking that these products, in addition to keeping you clean, will reduce your risk of getting sick or passing on germs to others?

Not necessarily, according to experts at the Food and Drug Administration (FDA).

Every day, consumers use antibacterial soaps and body washes at home, work, school, and in other public settings. Especially because so many consumers use them, FDA believes that there should be clearly demonstrated benefits to balance any potential risks.

In fact, there currently is no evidence that over-the-counter (OTC) antibacterial soap products are any more effective at preventing illness than washing with plain soap and water, says Colleen Rogers, PhD, a lead microbiologist at FDA.

Moreover, antibacterial soap products contain chemical ingredients, such as triclosan and triclocarban, which may carry unnecessary risks given that their benefits are unproven.

"New data suggest that the risks associated with long-term, daily use of antibacterial soaps may outweigh the benefits," Rogers says. There are indications that certain ingredients in these soaps may contribute to bacterial resistance to antibiotics, and may have unanticipated hormonal effects that are of concern to FDA.

In light of these data, the agency issued a proposed rule on December 16, 2013 that would require manufacturers to provide more substantial data to demonstrate the safety and effectiveness of antibacterial soaps. The proposed rule covers only those consumer antibacterial soaps and body washes that are used with water. It does not apply to hand sanitizers, hand wipes, or antibacterial soaps that are used in health care settings such as hospitals.

According to Rogers, the laboratory tests that have historically been used to evaluate the effectiveness of antibacterial soaps do not directly test the effect of a product on infection rates. That would change with FDA's current proposal, which would require studies that directly test the ability of an antibacterial soap to provide a clinical benefit over washing with non-antibacterial soap, Rogers says.

A large number of liquid soaps labeled "antibacterial" contain triclosan, an ingredient of concern to many environmental and industry groups.

What Makes a Soap "Antibacterial?"

Antibacterial soaps (sometimes called antimicrobial or antiseptic soaps) contain certain chemical ingredients that plain soaps do not. These ingredients are added to many consumer products in an effort to reduce or prevent bacterial contamination.

A large number of liquid soaps labeled "antibacterial" contain triclosan, an ingredient of concern to many environmental and industry groups. Animal studies have shown that triclosan may alter the way hormones work in the body. While data showing effects in animals don't always predict effects in humans, these studies are of concern to FDA as well, and warrant further investigation to better understand how they might affect humans.

In addition, laboratory studies have raised the possibility that triclosan contributes to making bacteria resistant to antibiotics. Such resistance can have a significant impact on the effectiveness of medical treatments.

Moreover, recent data suggest that exposure to these active ingredients is higher than previously thought, raising concerns about the potential risks associated with their use regularly and over time.

A Chance to Weigh In

FDA encourages consumers, clinicians, environmental groups, scientists, industry representatives and others to discuss and weigh in on the proposed rule and the data it discusses. The comment period extends for 180 days.

In the meantime, FDA is emphasizing that hand washing is one of the most important steps people can take to avoid getting sick and to prevent spreading germs to others. Another good source for tips and information about benefits of appropriate hand washing is the Centers for Disease Control and Prevention (CDC). Consumers can go to www.cdc.gov/handwashing.

How do you tell if a product is antibacterial?

- Most antibacterial products have the word "antibacterial" on the label.
- A Drug Facts label on a soap or body wash is a sure sign a product contains antibacterial ingredients. Cosmetics must list the ingredients, but are not required to carry a Drug Facts Label.

FDA and EPA Working in Tandem on Triclosan

FDA and the Environmental Protection Agency (EPA) have been closely collaborating on science and regulatory issues related to triclosan. This joint effort will help to ensure government-wide consistency in the regulation of the chemical.

The two agencies are reviewing the effects of triclosan from two different perspectives.

EPA regulates the use of triclosan as a pesticide, and is in the process of updating its assessment of the effects of triclosan when it is used in pesticides. FDA's focus is on the effects of triclosan when it is used by consumers on a regular basis in hand soaps and body washes. By sharing information, the two agencies will be better able to measure the exposure and effects of triclosan and how these differing uses of triclosan may affect human health.

For more information on EPA's most recent assessment of triclosan, see: www.epa.gov/pesticides/reregistration/triclosan/triclosan-questions.htm

EPA re-evaluates each pesticide active ingredient every 15 years. EPA's Preliminary Work Plan for the triclosan risk assessment, can be found in docket EPA-HQ-OPP-2012-0811 at www.regulations.gov.

Critical Thinking

1. Compare the prices of a bottle of liquid antibacterial soap to a regular bar of soap.
2. Discuss why the FDA is concerned about the long-term use of antibacterial soaps.

Create Central

www.mhhe.com/createcentral

Internet References

Food and Drug Administration
www.fda.org

Food Safety.gov
www.foodsafety.gov

Article Prepared by: Janet Colson, *Middle Tennessee State University*

Antibiotic Resistance

Wasting a Precious Life Saver

David Schardt

Learning Outcomes

After reading this article, you will be able to:

- Define antibiotic resistant.
- Trace the route of antibiotic-resistant bacteria from a farm animal to the consumer.
- Explain the impact that antibiotic-resistant livestock and poultry have on the health status of the public.

The Director-General of the World Health Organization was blunt. The world is facing "an end to modern medicine as we know it," Margaret Chan warned last year. Strep throats could once again kill people, and hip replacements, organ transplants, and cancer chemotherapy "would become far more difficult or even too dangerous to undertake."

That's because we're losing our first-line antimicrobial drugs to antibiotic resistance, Chan noted. As for new antibiotics to replace them, Chan wasn't optimistic: "The pipeline is virtually dry. The cupboard is nearly bare."

Happy Halloween

On the evening before Halloween in 2011, Danielle Wadsworth, a healthy 31-year-old insurance agent, shared a dinner of beef tacos with friends at her home in Lewiston, Maine.

"Then, seemingly out of nowhere, I started feeling like I had the flu," she told the Web site keepantibioticsworking.com. By the next day, "I just wanted to be left alone."

But Wadsworth got worse. When her persistent bloody diarrhea wouldn't stop, she went to the emergency room, where intravenous fluids brought temporary relief. But when the bloody diarrhea returned, she ended up back in the hospital.

For the next four days, as she suffered intense pain and alternating pangs of hunger and thirst, Wadsworth was treated with morphine every few hours while her doctors tried to figure out what was wrong.

"I love life, but was beginning to wonder if fighting was worth it," she recalled. "It never crossed my mind that it could be something I'd eaten."

Nor did that occur to the hospital staff until the stool cultures came back positive for *Salmonella typhimurium,* one of the leading causes of food poisoning in the United States.

Wadsworth was one of 20 known victims infected with a new strain of *S. typhimurium,* one that was resistant to at least eight antibiotics, including streptomycin and tetracycline. The Centers for Disease Control and Prevention (CDC) eventually traced the resistant *S. typhimurium* to contaminated ground beef sold by a supermarket chain, but the CDC couldn't identify the meat supplier because the chain hadn't kept good records.

Fortunately, the bug was still susceptible to the antibiotic ciprofloxacin. Cipro helped cure Wadsworth's infection, but it couldn't heal the anxiety that she says she still feels about what can happen from eating tainted food.

Or what could happen to her loved ones. "I am the legal guardian for my grandfather. Considering that I cook for him, I hate to even think about the outcome had he eaten the same meat that made me sick."

Bugs Galore

The seven-state outbreak that sickened Danielle Wadsworth was one of 55 food poisoning outbreaks since 1973 that were caused by antibiotic-resistant bacteria, according to a new report by the Center for Science in the Public Interest (publisher of *Nutrition Action Healthletter*).[1]

More than two-thirds of the bacteria fingered in those outbreaks were resistant to antibiotics that the World Health Organization considers "critically important" for treating humans or that the Food and Drug Administration (FDA) regards as "highly important."

Of the 55 outbreaks, 14 involved dairy foods (usually raw milk or raw-milk cheese), while 10 came from ground beef, 7 from poultry, 4 from produce, 2 from seafood, 1 each from pork and eggs, and 3 from multiple ingredients. (In 13 of the outbreaks, no specific food could be identified.) Antibiotic-resistant *Salmonella typhimurium,* the bug that made Danielle Wadsworth so sick, was the bacterium found most often.

Course of *most* Resistance

"There's this huge population of antibiotic resistance genes in bacteria in nature and nobody quite knows why they're there," says microbiologist Julian Davies of the University of British Columbia in Vancouver. "You can even find them in caves where no human has ever been."

"What we do know," explains Lance Price, an environmental health scientist at George Washington University in Washington, D.C., "is that when you use antibiotics, it's very clear and undisputable that you promote the development of drug-resistant bacteria. It's one of the strongest evolutionary forces in nature."

Handle with Care

If you cook meat, poultry, and fish thoroughly, you'll kill any harmful bacteria they may contain. Beyond that, here's some good advice about how to help prevent the spread of antibiotic-resistant bacteria:

- **Don't expect antibiotics to treat** colds, flu, most coughs, bronchitis, sore throats not caused by strep, or runny noses. They're caused by viruses, which antibiotics don't kill.
- **Don't stop taking prescribed antibiotics** early because you start feeling better.
- **Alcohol-based hand sanitizers** like Purell don't increase antibiotic resistance. The jury is still out on whether antibacterial soaps and dish detergents that contain triclosan do.

Sources: CDC, CSPI.

Antibiotics stop bacteria by killing them or halting their growth. Resistant bacteria have genes that enable them to survive certain antibiotics by neutralizing the drugs, by pumping the drugs out of their cells, or by altering the cell structure that the antibiotic attacks so that it's no longer vulnerable.

To make matters worse, bacteria can swap their resistance genes with each other, so that the instructions for resistance are passed on to other bacteria that have yet to be exposed to the antibiotic.

Every time an antibiotic is used, susceptible bacteria are killed, paving the way for resistant bugs to grow and multiply.

The consequences can be deadly.

"People sickened by antibiotic-resistant bacteria are more likely to have longer and more expensive hospital stays, and may be more likely to die as a result of the infection," Price notes. And these aren't obscure bacteria, he adds. "They're the same kind of *E. coli,* for instance, that cause urinary tract infections and sepsis, or blood infections."

When the first-choice antibiotics are useless, physicians have to resort to drugs that may be less effective, more toxic, and more expensive, according to the CDC.

Unfortunately, much of the damage to the effectiveness of antibiotics has already occurred.

"There's no doubt that antibiotic resistance is now widespread throughout the world," says Davies.

A major cause: the chronic misuse of antibiotics in hospitals, physicians' offices, and homes. Some doctors, for example, still prescribe—and some patients still demand—antibiotics to treat colds or the flu, even though both are caused by viruses, not bacteria. (Antibiotics don't attack viruses.)

"Humans are to blame in large part for creating this huge problem," says George Zhanel, a microbiologist at the University of Manitoba and director of the Canadian Antimicrobial Resistance Alliance.

But reducing the inappropriate use of antibiotics in human medicine alone won't be enough, concluded a 2003 report from the National Academy of Sciences.[2] "Substantial efforts must be made to decrease inappropriate overuse of antimicrobials in animals and agriculture as well."

That's because three-quarters of the antibiotics that are used in the United States are given to animals, not people.

Antibiotics to Grow On

Most meat and poultry farms rely on antibiotics to treat sick animals and to prevent healthy animals from becoming sick. Modern facilities crowd many animals together, which makes it easier for disease to spread throughout the herds or flocks. (Antibiotics are also widely used in fish farming.)

"The antibiotics approved by the FDA for use in animals represent nearly every class of antibiotic important for treating humans," says Price.

Much of the antibiotics that are given to animals, however, are not to treat or prevent disease, but to stimulate growth.

In the 1950s, scientists discovered that animals fed small, "sub-therapeutic" doses of antibiotics grew more quickly on the same amount of food. And farmers need no prescription for those low doses.

"It's a big economic advantage because the animals are larger and healthier, and their time to slaughter is shorter," explains Zhanel. "The drawback is that this use of antibiotics selects out antibiotic-resistant bacteria for survival."

For example, fluoroquinolone antibiotics (which include the Cipro that helped Danielle Wadsworth) can kill a wide range of disease-causing bacteria. After the FDA approved their use in poultry in 1995, resistance to fluoroquinolones among *Campylobacter* bacteria on chickens tested at slaughter houses and supermarkets rose so sharply that in 2000, the FDA reversed its decision and tried to ban the use of fluoroquinolones in poultry. (The ban was delayed for five years while Bayer, which manufactures fluoroquinolones, fought it unsuccessfully in court.)

Resistant Bacteria Spread

Antibiotic-resistant bacteria usually reside in an animal's intestines and are excreted in its waste. From there, they can be spread by polluted water, farm workers, the wind, birds, and even flies.

In North Carolina, for example, swine waste is commonly stored in open pits before being sprayed onto nearby fields. "Many of these waste pits are located in flood plains and can overflow, while the fields sprayed with waste can contaminate groundwater," says epidemiologist Steve Wing of the University of North Carolina.

"This clearly is a potential source for human exposure to antibiotic-resistant bacteria."

Bugs on Food

Some antibiotic-resistant bacteria wind up on the meat and poultry in the refrigerator case at the supermarket.

"Our food supply is tainted with disease-causing bacteria that are often resistant to many different antibiotics," says George Washington University's Lance Price, who serves on a U.S. Department of Agriculture advisory panel on food safety.

The National Antimicrobial Resistance Monitoring System (NARMS), which consists of the FDA, the CDC, and about a dozen state public-health laboratories, buys chicken, ground turkey, ground beef, and pork chops at retail stores nationwide every year and tests them for antibiotic-resistant bacteria. It has no trouble finding them.

In 2011, the latest year available, NARMS detected *Salmonella* in 12 percent of the chicken samples that it tested. About three-quarters of the bugs were resistant to at least one antibiotic, and more than a quarter were resistant to at least five classes of antibiotics. That's eight times the level of multiple resistance found in 2002.[3]

Salmonella also turned up in 12 percent of the ground turkey samples. About three-quarters of the bacteria were resistant to at least one antibiotic, and 19 percent—double the percentage found in 2002—were resistant to at least five classes of antibiotics.

E. coli was detected in two-thirds of the beef and around 40 percent of the pork samples. Roughly half of the *E. coli* on pork and a fifth of the *E. coli* on beef were resistant to at least one antibiotic. About 1 percent of the *E. coli* on each meat was resistant to at least five classes of antibiotics. For beef, that's triple the percentage found in 2002, and for pork, it's one-third the level.

"The evidence is unequivocal that drug-resistant pathogens have contaminated meat and other animal foods and infected people with drug-resistant infections," says Price. "What we don't know is the full extent of it."

How to Decode the Claims

Want to find meat and poultry grown without antibiotics? It's tricky.

- **What these terms on food labels mean:**
  Antibiotic free: Term not permitted by the U.S. Department of Agriculture because *all* foods should be free of antibiotic residues.

  No antibiotics administered or **Raised without antibiotics:** Animal never received antibiotics. Not independently verified, so claim depends on the honesty of the company making it.

  USDA Certified Organic or **American Grassfed Certified:** Use of antibiotics prohibited. Verified by independent audits.

  Certified Humane or **Animal Welfare Approved:** Antibiotics permitted only to treat sick animals. Verified by independent audits.

- **Companies that told us that they use or sell meat from animals that were *never* treated with antibiotics:**
  Supermarkets: Whole Foods

  Restaurants: Chipotle Mexican Grill

  Brands: Applegate, Bell & Evans, Coleman Natural Foods, Murray's Chicken, Niman Ranch, Heritage Acres, Laura's Lean Beef, Harvestland

- **Companies that told us that they use or sell meat from animals that were treated with antibiotics *only* if they were sick:**
  Restaurants: Burger King, In-N-Out Burger, Panera (only items marked on the menu)

  Brands: Perdue

To find stores, farmers' markets, farms, and restaurants near you that sell meat and poultry raised without the routine use of antibiotics, go to realtimefarms.com/fixantibiotics. The information is "crowd sourced," which means that anyone can add to it. So be sure to verify with the company before you buy.

Sources: 2012 survey by Rep. Louise Slaughter of New York, companies.

Ending Drug Abuse

How practical would it be to end the routine use of antibiotics to promote growth in animals that are raised for food? Very practical, says Price, because it's already been done.

In the late 1990s, Denmark, the world's largest exporter of pork, banned the use of antibiotics on farms except to treat sick animals.

"Nothing bad happened as a result," Price notes. Ending the use of antibiotics for growth promotion caused no sustained harm to animal survival, production rates, or feed efficiency, a World Health Organization expert panel found.[4]

"And these are industrial farms," adds Price. "They're cleaner, the density of animals is lower, and the quality of life is a little better than in the U.S., but these are still highly efficient industrial farms."

Most importantly, ending the routine use of antibiotics helped slash rates of resistance.

According to the Danish Veterinary and Food Administration, the percentage of *Campylobacter* bacteria in pigs that was resistant to antibiotics like erythromycin dropped from 80 percent before the ban to less than 20 percent. And the percentage of vancomycin-resistant *E. coli* in broiler chickens plummeted from 75 percent to less than 5 percent.[5]

The ban also led to a decline in resistant bacteria isolated from the intestines of healthy Danes.

What to Do

How can you lower your odds of getting food poisoning from resistant bacteria?

It may help to buy meat or poultry that comes from animals that were never given antibiotics (see "How to Decode the Claims"). According to a 2012 Stanford University meta-analysis, conventionally produced chicken and pork were 33 percent more likely than organic chicken and pork to be contaminated with bacteria that were resistant to at least three antibiotics.[6]

But that won't guarantee that you—or your child or parent—won't get a bout of antibiotic-resistant food poisoning like the one that hit Danielle Wadsworth.

"As a society, we have to say that antibiotics are too valuable for treating sick people and that we cannot afford to squander them as production tools for raising animals," says Price.

"We're talking about the future of medicine. We don't have new drugs coming up through the pipeline. And even if we did, if we abuse them the same way, they're going to be useless again very quickly."

Notes

1. www.cspinet.org/foodsafety.
2. www.nap.edu/openbook.php?isbn=030908864X
3. www.fda.gov/AnimalVeterinary/SafetyHealth/AntimicrobialResistance/NationalAntimicrobialResistanceMonitoringSystem/ucm334828.htm.
4. www.who.int/gfn/en/Expertsreportgrowthpromoter denmark.pdf.
5. democrats.energycommerce.house.gov/index.php?q=hearing/hearing-on-antibiotic-resistance-and-the-use-of-antibiotics-in-animal-agriculture-subcommitt.
6. *Ann. Intern. Med. 157:* 348, 2012.

Critical Thinking

1. What is meant by antibiotic-resistant bacteria and how do these type of bacteria develop?
2. Why are antibiotics given to animals?
3. Explain what the Director-General of the World Health Organization meant when she said that "the world is facing *an end to modern medicine as we know it.*"
4. What claims on a food label assure consumers that the product was raised without using any antibiotics?
5. What does the claim "raised without antibiotics" mean?

Create Central

www.mhhe.com/createcentral

Internet References

Center for Health in the Public Interest
www.cspinet.org

Keep Antibiotics Working
www.keepantibioticsworking.com

Food and Drug Administration
www.FDA.gov

National Organic Program
www.ams.usda.gov/AMSv1.0/nop

United States Department of Agriculture
www.usda.gov

Article

Prepared by: Janet Colson, *Middle Tennessee State University*

Arsenic in Your Juice

How much is too much? Federal limits don't exist.

CONSUMER REPORTS

Learning Outcomes

After reading the article, you will be able to:

- Identify the natural and man-made sources of lead and arsenic exposure.
- Describe how the FDA regulates arsenic and lead in U.S. food and beverages.

Arsenic has long been recognized as a poison and a contaminant in drinking water, but now concerns are growing about arsenic in foods, especially in fruit juices that are a mainstay for children.

Controversy over arsenic in apple juice made headlines as the school year began when Mehmet Oz, M.D., host of "The Dr. Oz Show," told viewers that tests he'd commissioned found 10 of three dozen apple-juice samples with total arsenic levels exceeding 10 parts per billion (ppb). There's no federal arsenic threshold for juice or most foods, though the limit for bottled and public water is 10 ppb. The Food and Drug Administration, trying to reassure consumers about the safety of apple juice, claimed that most arsenic in juices and other foods is of the organic type that is "essentially harmless."

But an investigation by *Consumer Reports* shows otherwise. Our study, including tests of apple and grape juice, a scientific analysis of federal health data, a consumer poll, and interviews with doctors and other experts, finds the following:

- Roughly 10 percent of our juice samples, from five brands, had total arsenic levels that exceeded federal drinking-water standards. Most of that arsenic was inorganic arsenic, a known carcinogen.

In our tests, apple and grape juice had arsenic and lead at varying levels.

- One in four samples had lead levels higher than the FDA's bottled-water limit of 5 ppb. As with arsenic, no federal limit exists for lead in juice.
- Apple and grape juice constitute a significant source of dietary exposure to arsenic, according to our analysis of federal health data from 2003 through 2008.
- Children drink a lot of juice. Thirty-five percent of children 5 and younger drink juice in quantities exceeding pediatricians' recommendations, our poll of parents shows.
- Mounting scientific evidence suggests that chronic exposure to arsenic and lead even at levels below water standards can result in serious health problems.
- Inorganic arsenic has been detected at disturbing levels in other foods, too, which suggests that more must be done to reduce overall dietary exposure.

Our findings have prompted Consumers Union, the advocacy arm of *Consumer Reports*, to urge the FDA to set arsenic and lead standards for apple and grape juice. Our scientists believe that juice should at least meet the 5 ppb lead limit for bottled water. They recommend an even lower arsenic limit for juice: 3 ppb.

"People sometimes say, 'If arsenic exposure is so bad, why don't you see more people sick or dying from it?' But the many diseases likely to be increased by exposure even at relatively low levels are so common already that its effects are overlooked simply because no one has looked carefully for the connection," says Joshua Hamilton, Ph.D., a toxicologist specializing in arsenic research and the chief academic and scientific officer at the Marine Biological Laboratory in Woods Hole, Mass.

As our investigation found, when scientists and doctors do look, the connections they've found underscore the need to protect public health by reducing Americans' exposure to this potent toxin.

Many Sources of Exposure

Arsenic is a naturally occurring element that can contaminate groundwater used for drinking and irrigation in areas where it's abundant, such as parts of New England, the Midwest, and the Southwest.

But the public's exposure to arsenic extends beyond those areas because since 1910, the United States has used roughly 1.6 million tons of it for agricultural and other industrial uses.

About half of that cumulative total has been used since only the mid-1960s. Lead-arsenate insecticides were widely used in cotton fields, orchards, and vineyards until their use was banned in the 1980s. But residues in the soil can still contaminate crops.

For decades, arsenic was also used in a preservative for pressure-treated lumber commonly used for decks and playground equipment. In 2003 that use was banned, (as was most residential use) but the wood can contribute to arsenic in groundwater when it's recycled as mulch.

Other sources of exposure include coal-fired power plants and smelters that heat arsenic-containing ores to process copper or lead. Today the quantity of arsenic released into the environment in the U.S. by human activities is three times more than that released from natural sources, says the federal Agency for Toxic Substances and Disease Registry.

The form of arsenic in the examples above is inorganic arsenic. It's a carcinogen known to cause bladder, lung, and skin cancer in people and to increase risks of cardiovascular disease, immunodeficiencies, and type 2 diabetes.

The other form that arsenic takes is organic arsenic, created when arsenic binds to molecules containing carbon. Fish can contain an organic form of arsenic called arsenobetaine, generally considered nontoxic to humans. But questions have been raised about the human health effects of other types of organic arsenic in foods, including juice.

Use of organic arsenic in agricultural products has also caused concern. For instance, the EPA in 2006 took steps to stop the use of herbicides containing organic arsenic because of their potential to turn into inorganic arsenic in soil and contaminate drinking water. And in 2011, working with the FDA, drug company Alpharma agreed to suspend the sale of Roxarsone, a poultry-feed additive, because it contained an organic form of arsenic that could convert into inorganic arsenic inside the bird, potentially contaminating the meat. Or it could contaminate soil when chicken droppings are used as fertilizer. Other arsenic feed additives are still being used.

What Our Tests Found

We went shopping in Connecticut, New Jersey, and New York in August and September, buying 28 apple juices and three grape juices. Our samples came from ready-to-drink bottles, juice boxes, and cans of concentrate. For most juices, we bought three different lot numbers to assess variability. (For some juices, we couldn't find three lots, so we tested one or two.) In all, we tested 88 samples.

Five samples of apple juice and four of grape juice had total arsenic levels exceeding the 10 ppb federal limit for bottled and drinking water. Levels in the apple juices ranged from 1.1 to 13.9 ppb, and grape-juice levels were even higher, 5.9 to 24.7 ppb. Most of the total arsenic in our samples was inorganic, our tests showed.

As for lead, about one fourth of all juice samples had levels at or above the 5-ppb limit for bottled water. The top lead level for apple juice was 13.6 ppb; for grape juice, 15.9 ppb.

The following brands had at least one sample of apple juice that exceeded 10 ppb: Apple & Eve, Great Value (Walmart), and Mott's. For grape juice, at least one sample from Walgreens and Welch's exceeded that threshold. And these brands had one or more samples of apple juice that exceeded 5 ppb of lead: America's Choice (A&P), Gerber, Gold Emblem (CVS), Great Value, Joe's Kids (Trader Joe's), Minute Maid, Seneca, and Walgreens. At least one sample of grape juice exceeding 5 ppb of lead came from Gold Emblem, Walgreens, and Welch's. Our findings provide a spot check of a number of local juice aisles, but they can't be used to draw general conclusions about arsenic or lead levels in any particular brand. Even within a single tested brand, levels of arsenic and lead sometimes varied widely.

Arsenic-tainted soil in U.S. orchards is a likely source of contamination for apples, and finding lead with arsenic in juices that we tested is not surprising. Even with a ban on lead-arsenate insecticides, "we are finding problems with some

How to Reduce Your Family's Risk

Test your water. If your home or a home you're considering buying isn't on a public water system, have the home's water tested for arsenic and lead. To find a certified lab, contact your local health department or call the federal Safe Drinking Water Hotline at 800-426-4791. To find contact information for your public water system, go to cfpub.epo.gov/safewater/ccr/index.cfm.

Limit children's juice consumption. Nutrition guidelines set by the American Academy of Pediatrics can help. The academy recommends that infants younger than 6 months shouldn't drink juice; children up to 6 years old should consume no more than four to six ounces a day and older children, no more than 8 to 12 ounces a day. Diluting juice with water can help meet those goals.

Consider your food. Buying certified organic chicken makes sense because organic standards don't allow the use of chicken feed containing arsenic. But for juice and other foods, it's not so certain. Organic standards prohibit the use of synthetic fertilizers and most pesticides, but organic juices still may contain arsenic if they're made from fruit grown in soil where arsenical insecticides were used.

Need a home-treatment system? Contact NSF International at www.nsf.org/certified/DwTu or 800-673-8010 for info on systems certified to lower arsenic levels to no more than 10 ppb. The University of Georgia Cooperative Extension discusses treatment technologies at aesl.ces.uga.edu/publications/watercirc. (Click on "Removal of Arsenic from Household Water.")

If you're concerned, get tested. Ask your doctor for a urine test for you or your child to determine arsenic levels. Don't eat seafood for 48 to 72 hours before being tested to avoid misleadingly high levels from "fish arsenic." For a medical toxicologist in your area who can interpret results, call the American Association of Poison Control Centers at 800-222-1222.

Washington state apples, not because of irresponsible farming practices now but because lead-arsenate pesticides that were used here decades ago remain in the soil," says Denise Wilson, Ph.D., an associate professor at the University of Washington who has tested apple juices and discovered elevated arsenic levels even in brands labeled organic.

Over the years, a shift has occurred in how juice sold in America is produced. To make apple juice, manufacturers often blend water with apple-juice concentrate from multiple sources. For the past decade, most concentrate has come from China. Concerns have been raised about the possible continuing use of arsenical pesticides there, and several Chinese provinces that are primary apple-growing regions are known to have high arsenic concentrations in groundwater.

A much bigger test than ours would be needed to establish any correlation between elevated arsenic or lead levels and the juice concentrate's country of origin. Samples we tested included some made from concentrate from multiple countries including Argentina, China, New Zealand, South Africa, and Turkey; others came from a single country. A few samples solely from the United States had elevated levels of lead or arsenic, and others did not. The same was true for samples containing only Chinese concentrate.

The FDA has been collecting its own data to see whether it should set guidelines to continue to ensure the safety of apple juice, a spokeswoman told us.

The Juice Products Association said, "We are committed to providing nutritious and safe fruit juices to consumers and will comply with limits established by the agency."

Answering a Crucial Question

We also wanted to know whether people who drink juice end up being exposed to more arsenic than those who don't.

So we commissioned an analysis of data from the National Health and Nutrition Examination Survey (NHANES), conducted annually by the National Center for Health Statistics. Information is collected on the health and nutrition of a nationally representative sample of the U.S. population, based on interviews and physical exams that may include a blood or urine test. Officials and researchers often use the data to determine risk factors for major diseases and develop public health policy. In fact, data on lead in the blood of NHANES participants were instrumental in developing policies that have successfully resulted in lead being removed from gasoline.

Our analysis was led by Richard Stahlhut, M.D., M.P.H., an environmental health researcher at the University of Rochester with expertise in NHANES data, working with Consumer Reports statisticians. Ana Navas-Acien, M.D., Ph.D., a physician—epidemiologist at Johns Hopkins University's Bloomberg School of Public Health, also provided guidance. She was the lead author of a 2008 study in the *Journal of the American Medical Association* that first linked low-level arsenic exposure with the prevalence of type 2 diabetes in the U.S.

Over time, people who ingest even low arsenic levels can become sick.

Stahlhut reviewed NHANES data from 2003 through 2008 from participants tested for total urinary arsenic who reported their food and drink consumption for 24 hours the day before their NHANES visit. Because most ingested arsenic is excreted in urine, the best measure of recent exposure is a urine test.

Following Navas-Acien's advice, we excluded from our NHANES analysis anyone with results showing detectable levels of arsenobetaine, the organic arsenic in seafood. That made the results we analyzed more likely to represent inorganic arsenic, of greatest concern in terms of potential health risks.

The resulting analysis of almost 3,000 study participants found that those reporting apple-juice consumption had on average 19 percent greater levels of total urinary arsenic than those subjects who did not, and those who reported drinking grape juice had 20 percent higher levels. The results might understate the correlation between juice consumption and urinary arsenic levels because NHANES urinary data exclude children younger than 6, who tend to be big juice drinkers.

"The current analysis suggests that these juices may be an important contributor to dietary arsenic exposure," says Keeve Nachman, Ph.D., a risk scientist at the Center for a Livable Future and the Bloomberg School of Public Health, both at Johns Hopkins University. "It would be prudent to pursue measures to understand and limit young children's exposures to arsenic in juice."

Robert Wright, M.D., M.P.H., associate professor of pediatrics and environmental health at Harvard University who specializes in research on the effect of heavy-metals exposure in children, says that findings from our juice tests and database analysis concern him: "Because of their small size, a child drinking a box of juice would consume a larger per-body-weight dose of arsenic than an adult drinking the exact same box of juice. Those brands with elevated arsenic should investigate the source and eliminate it."

A Chronic Problem

Arsenic has been notoriously used as a poison since ancient times. A fatal poisoning would require a single dose of inorganic arsenic about the weight of a postage stamp. But chronic toxicity can result from long-term exposure to much lower levels in food, and even to water that meets the 10-ppb drinking-water limit.

A 2004 study of children in Bangladesh suggested diminished intelligence based on test scores in children exposed to arsenic in drinking water at levels above 5 ppb, says study author Joseph Graziano, Ph.D., a professor of environmental health sciences and pharmacology at Columbia University. He's now conducting similar research with children living in New Hampshire and Maine, where arsenic levels of 10 to 100 ppb are commonly found in well water, to determine whether better nutrition in the United States affects the results.

People with private wells may face greater risks than those on public systems because they're responsible for testing and treating their own water. In Maine, where almost half the population relies on private wells, the USGS found arsenic levels in well water as high as 3,100 ppb.

And a study published in 2011 in the International Journal of Environmental Research and Public Health examined the long-term effects of low-level exposure on more than 300 rural Texans whose groundwater was estimated to have arsenic at median levels below the federal drinking-water standard. It found that exposure was related to poor scores in language, memory, and other brain functions.

Warning Signs

Chronic arsenic exposure can initially cause gastrointestinal problems and skin discoloration or lesions. Exposure over time, which the World Health Organization says could be five to 20 years, could increase the risk of various cancers and high blood pressure, diabetes, and reproductive problems.

Signs of chronic low-level arsenic exposure can be mistaken for other ailments such as chronic fatigue syndrome. Usually the connection to arsenic exposure is not made immediately, as Sharyn Duffy of Geneseo, N.Y., discovered. She visited a doctor in 2007 about pain and skin changes on the sole of her left foot. She was referred to a podiatrist and eventually received a diagnosis of hyperkeratosis, in which lesions develop or thick skin forms on the palms or soles of the feet. It can be among the

Our Test Findings of Apple and Grape Juice

There's no federal limit for arsenic or lead in juice. In our tests, 25 percent of samples exceeded the 5-ppb lead limit for bottled water, and 10 percent exceeded the 10-ppb limit for arsenic in drinking water. Most arsenic we detected was inorganic. Our tests don't offer conclusions about overall levels in any juice type or brand. We tested three lots of most juices. Smaller containers are noted. For more details see www.ConsumerReports.org/juicebox.

Juice (in alphabetical order)	Total arsenic[1] (ppb)	Lead (ppb)
365 Everyday Value Organic 100 percent Apple Juice (Whole Foods)[2]	7.0 to 7.1	3.5 to 3.8
America's Choice 100 percent Apple Juice (A&P)	1.4 to 4.4	0.5 to 5.6
Apple & Eve 100 percent Apple Juice (6.75-ounce juice boxes)	5.0 to 10.5	1.9 to 3.4
Gerber 100 percent Apple Juice (4-ounce bottles)	5.8 to 9.7	3.4 to 13.6
Gerber Organic 100 percent Apple Juice (4-ounce bottles)	5.5 to 5.7	2.2 to 2.3
Gold Emblem 100 percent Apple Juice (CVS)	3.1 to 9.4	2.9 to 5.6
Gold Emblem 100 percent Grape Juice (CVS)	5.9 to 7.5	6.5 to 8.6
Great Value 100 percent Apple Juice (Walmart)	10.1 to 13.9	3.7 to 5.1
Great Value 100 percent Apple Juice (Walmart, 10-ounce bottles)[3]	5.5	3.4
Great Value 100 percent Apple Juice with fiber Not from Concentrate (Walmart)	2.9 to 3.9	0.1 to 0.2
Joe's Kids 100 percent Apple Juice (Trader Joe's, 6.75-ounce Juice boxes)	4.1 to 5.7	5.3 to 9.7
Juicy Juice 100 percent Apple Juice Non Frozen Concentrate[4]	1.9 to 4.2	1.4 to 2.2
Juicy Juice 100 percent Apple Juice	1.7 to 3.0	0.8 to 2.3
Juicy Juice 100 percent Apple Juice (10-ounce bottles)	1.7 to 1.9	1.1 to 3.5
Juicy Juice 100 percent Apple Juice (6.75-ounce juice boxes)	1.3 to 2.8	1.4 to 2.8
Lucky Leaf 100 percent Apple Juice[2]	2.3 to 3.2	0.8 to 1.2
Minute Maid 100 percent Apple Juice (10-ounce bottles)	6.2 to 6.7	4.2 to 6.5
Minute Maid 100 percent Apple Juice (juice box packaged for McDonald's)	2.0 to 5.6	0.8 to 5.3
Mott's Original 100 percent Apple Juice	4.0 to 7.9	2.1 to 3.8
Mott's Original 100 percent Apple Juice (4.23-ounce juice boxes)	4.0 to 10.2	0.6 to 0.7
Mott's Original 100 percent Apple Juice (6.75-ounce juice boxes)	2.1 to 2.8	0.6 to 1.3
Nature's Own 100 percent Apple Juice[2]	2.3 to 2.4	0.9 each
Old Orchard 100 percent Apple Juice Frozen Concentrate[4]	1.6 to 4.8	0.6 to 1.3
Red Jacket Orchards 100 percent Fuji Apple Juice	1.3 to 1.8	0.1 to 0.2
Rite Aid Pantry 100 percent Apple Juice	1.1 to 6.4	0.4 to 2.6
Seneca 100 percent Apple Juice Frozen Concentrate[4]	2.3 to 4.4	0.9 to 5.5
Tropicana 100 percent Apple Juice (15.2-ounce bottles)	1.5 to 2.1	0.5 to 1.0
Walgreens 100 percent Apple Juice	4.0 to 6.8	2.3 to 6.9
Walgreens 100 percent Grape Juice	9.7 to 24.7	10.1 to 15.9
Welch's 100 percent Apple Juice Pourable Concentrate[4]	1.1 to 4.1	0.6 to 1.3
Welch's 100 percent Grape Juice	7.1 to 12.4	3.5 to 9.2

[1] Includes organic and inorganic arsenic.
[2] Two lots tested.
[3] One lot tested.
[4] Reconstituted; assumes no arsenic or lead from added water.

earliest symptoms of chronic arsenic poisoning. But she says it was roughly two years before she was finally referred to a neurologist, who suggested testing for arsenic. She had double the typical levels.

"Testing for arsenic isn't part of a routine checkup," says Duffy, a retiree. "When you come in with symptoms like I had, ordering that kind of test probably wouldn't even occur to most doctors."

Michael Harbut, M.D., chief of the environmental cancer program at Karmanos Institute in Detroit, says, "Given what we know about the wide range of arsenic exposure sources we have in this country, I suspect there is an awful lot of chronic, low-level arsenic poisoning going on that's never properly diagnosed."

Emerging research suggests that when arsenic exposure occurs in the womb or in early childhood, it not only increases cancer risks later in life but also can cause lasting harm to children's developing brains and endocrine and immune systems, leading to other diseases, too.

Case in point: From 1958 through 1970, residents of Antofagasta, Chile, were exposed to naturally occurring arsenic in drinking water that peaked at almost 1,000 ppb before an arsenic removal plant was installed. Studies led by researchers at the University of California at Berkeley found that people born during that period who had probable exposure in the womb and during early childhood had a lung-cancer death rate six times higher than those in their age group elsewhere in Chile. Their rate of death in their 30s and 40s from another form of lung disease was almost 50 times higher than for people without that arsenic exposure.

"Recent studies have shown that early-childhood exposure to arsenic carries the most serious long-term risk," says Joshua Hamilton of the Marine Biological Laboratory. "So even though reducing arsenic exposure is important for everyone, we need to pay special attention to protecting pregnant moms, babies, and young kids."

Other Dietary Exposures

In addition to juice, foods including chicken, rice, and even baby food have been found to contain arsenic—sometimes at higher levels than the amounts found in juice. Brian Jackson, Ph.D., an analytical chemist and research associate professor at Dartmouth College, presented his findings at a June 2011 scientific conference in Aberdeen, Scotland. He reported finding up to 23 ppb of arsenic in lab tests of name-brand jars of baby food, with inorganic arsenic representing 70 to 90 percent of those total amounts.

Similar results turned up in a 2004 study conducted by FDA scientists in Cincinnati, who found arsenic levels of up to 24 ppb in baby food, with sweet potatoes, carrots, green beans, and peaches containing only the inorganic form. A United Kingdom study published in 2008 found that the levels of inorganic arsenic in 20-ounce packets of dried infant rice cereals ranged from 60 to 160 ppb. Rice-based infant cereals are often the first solid food that babies eat.

How Much Juice Do Children Drink?

Too many children drink too much juice, according to our poll of parents. One in four toddlers 2 and younger and 45 percent of children ages 3 to 5 drink 7 or more ounces of juice a day.

The American Academy of Pediatrics cautions that to help prevent obesity and tooth decay, children younger than 6 should drink no more than 6 ounces a day, about the size of a juice box. (Infants younger than 6 months shouldn't drink any.) The possible presence of arsenic or lead in juices is all the more reason to stick with those nutrition-based limits.

Our findings are from 555 telephone interviews in October with parents, who were asked about children's juice consumption the previous day. Totals don't equal 100 percent because some said they didn't know how much juice their kids drank.

Amount of juice consumed	Children 2 and under	Children 3 to 5	Total children 5 or younger
None	40 percent	22 percent	31 percent
1 to 6 oz.	28	26	27
7 to 12 oz.	18	29	23
16 oz. or more	8	16	12

Consumers Union wants federal limits for arsenic and lead in juice.

Rice frequently contains high levels of inorganic arsenic because it is among plants that are unusually efficient at taking up arsenic from the soil and incorporating it in the grains people eat. Moreover, much of the rice produced in the U.S. is grown in Arkansas, Louisiana, Mississippi, Missouri, and Texas, on land formerly used to grow cotton, where arsenical pesticides were used for decades.

"Initially, in some regions rice planted there produced little grain due to these arsenical pesticides, but farmers then bred a type of rice specifically designed to produce high yields on the contaminated soil," says Andrew Meharg, professor of biogeochemistry at the University of Aberdeen, in Scotland. Meharg studies human exposures to arsenic in the environment. His research over the past six years has shown that U.S. rice has among the highest average inorganic arsenic levels in the world—almost three times higher than levels in Basmati rice imported from low-arsenic areas of Nepal, India, and Pakistan. Rice from Egypt has the lowest levels of all.

Infant rice cereal for the U.S. market is generally made from U.S. rice, Meharg says, but labeling usually doesn't specify country of origin. He says exposure to arsenic through infant rice cereals could be reduced greatly if cereal makers used techniques that don't require growing rice in water-flooded paddies or if they obtained rice from low-arsenic areas. His 2007 study found that median arsenic levels in California rice were 41 percent lower than levels in rice from the south-central U.S.

Setting a Standard

Evidence of arsenic's ability to cause cancer and other life-threatening illnesses has surged because some of the diseases linked to it have latency periods of several decades. Only recently have scientists been able to more fully measure the effects in populations that were exposed to elevated levels of arsenic in drinking water many years ago.

The Environmental Protection Agency periodically revises its assessment of the toxicity of various chemicals to offer guidance on drinking-water standards. Based on such a review, the agency changed the water standard for arsenic to 10 ppb, effective in 2006, from the 50-ppb limit it set in 1975. The EPA had proposed a 5-ppb limit in 2000, so the current limit is a compromise that came only after years of haggling over the costs of removing arsenic. Since 2006, New Jersey has had a 5-ppb threshold, advising residents that water with arsenic levels above that shouldn't be used for drinking or cooking.

For known human carcinogens such as inorganic arsenic, the EPA assumes there's actually no "safe" level of exposure, so it normally sets exposure limits that include a margin of safety to ideally allow for only one additional case of cancer in a million people, or at worst, no more than one in 10,000. For water with 10 ppb of arsenic, the excess cancer risk is one in 500.

Debate over that standard is likely to begin anew. The agency's latest draft report, from February 2010, proposes that the number used to calculate the cancer risk posed by ingesting inorganic arsenic be increased 17-fold to reflect arsenic's role in causing bladder and lung cancer. The proposal "suggests that arsenic's carcinogenic properties have been underestimated for a long time and that the federal drinking-water standard is underprotective based on current science," says Keeve Nachman, the Johns Hopkins scientist.

Each year the FDA tests a variety of foods and beverages for arsenic and other contaminants. It also started a program in 2005 to test for specific toxins such as arsenic and lead in domestic and imported products. As of late November, that program had published results for 160 samples of apple juice and concentrate. And the agency can alert inspectors at U.S. ports to conduct increased surveillance for products suspected to pose risks. Currently there's an alert for increased surveillance of apple concentrate from China and six other countries "where we have a suspicion there may be high levels of arsenic in their products," says FDA spokeswoman Stephanie Yao. But in fiscal 2010, the agency conducted physical inspections of only 2 percent of imported food shipments.

Consumers Union urges federal officials to set a standard for total arsenic in apple and grape juice. Our research suggests that the standard should be 3 ppb. Concerning lead, juice should at least meet the bottled-water standard of 5 ppb. Such standards would better protect children, who are most vulnerable to the effects of arsenic and lead. And they're achievable levels: 41 percent of the samples we tested met both thresholds.

Moreover, the EPA should impose stricter drinking-water standards for arsenic, Consumers Union believes. (The drinking-water threshold for lead is 15 ppb, which acknowledges that many older homes have water pipes or solder with lead.) Officials should also ban arsenic in pesticides, animal-feed additives, and fertilizers.

As our tests show, sources of lead haven't been eliminated, but dramatic progress has been made: Since the 1970s, average blood lead levels in children younger than 6 have dropped by about 90 percent, thanks to a federal ban on lead in house paint and gas. The U.S. should be equally aggressive with arsenic, suggests Joseph Graziano at Columbia University. "We tackled every source, from gasoline to paint to solder in food cans," he says, "and we should be just as vigilant in preventing arsenic from entering our food and water because the consequences of exposure are enormous for adults as well as children."

Critical Thinking

1. Identify the natural and man-made sources of exposure to lead and arsenic.
2. Differentiate between organic and inorganic arsenic.
3. Describe how the FDA regulates arsenic and lead in U.S. food and beverages.
4. Identify potential signs of chronic low-level exposure to arsenic.

Create Central

www.mhhe.com/createcentral

Internet References

Arsenic in Drinking Water—Enviornmental Protetive Agency (EPA)
http://water.epa.gov/lawsregs/rulesregs/sdwa/arsenic

FDA Center for Food Safety and Applied Nutrition
www.fda.gov/food/foodsafety/default.htm

Food Safety Project (FSP)
www.extension.iastate.edu/foodsafety

National Institute of Food and Agriculture
www.csrees.usda.gov

USDA Food Safety and Inspection Service (FSIS)
www.fsis.usda.gov

Article

Prepared by: Janet Colson, *Middle Tennessee State University*

Food Fears

Which Ones *Should* You Worry About?

DAVID SCHARDT

Learning Outcome

After reading this article, you will be able to:

- Determine which of the following poses the greatest health risk: farmed salmon, bagged salads greens, meat "glue," microwave popcorn, bean sprouts, rice, or non-stick skillets.

Don't eat this, don't do that. Every week, it seems, someone announces that this or that food or cooking technique is harmful. Here's a guide to which fears you should—and which ones you needn't—be concerned about.

Farmed Salmon Is Contaminated

"We found that farmed salmon contained seven to 10 times higher levels of PCBs, dioxins, and pesticides than wild salmon," said David Carpenter of the State University of New York at Albany nine years ago, after he and colleagues analyzed 700 farmed and wild salmon samples that had been bought in 2002.

Farmed salmon absorb PCBs and other industrial chemicals from the fishmeal and fish oil they're fed. In Carpenter's study, salmon farmed in Canada, Chile, Norway, and Scotland had 20 to 50 parts per billion (ppb) of PCBs, compared with 1 to 17 ppb in wild salmon. (Most of the farmed salmon sold in the U.S. comes from Canada and Chile. It's typically called Atlantic salmon, even if it's raised in the Pacific Ocean.)

Using Environmental Protection Agency guidelines, Carpenter advised consumers to eat farmed salmon no more than once a month (see *Nutrition Action,* June 2004).

Are the fish cleaner now? No one has tested enough salmon to know. "I'm not aware of other studies that have systematically analyzed farmed salmon for contaminants since our work," says Carpenter, who is now director of his university's Institute for Health and the Environment.

"Unfortunately, we really don't have hard information to show that commercial interests have done much to clean up farmed salmon," he adds.

Environmental organizations oppose most salmon farming. The Monterey Bay Aquarium, for example, warns that large amounts of wild fish are needed to feed farmed salmon and that waste from farmed salmon pollutes the oceans.

The Bottom Line

Until more studies are done, err on the side of caution and don't eat farmed salmon more than once a month.

Unwashed Bagged Greens Aren't Safe

U.S. companies recalled bagged salad greens at least eight times in 2012, usually because of contamination with *Listeria* bacteria.

Luckily, there were no reported illnesses from the contamination. *Listeria,* which can multiply at refrigerator temperatures, can cause miscarriages in pregnant women and potentially deadly blood poisoning or meningitis in older adults and those with compromised immune systems.

So should you wash bagged greens that say "washed" on the label? "No. Rewashing bagged salad greens that were washed before being packaged is very unlikely to create a safer salad," says Food and Drug Administration produce-safety expert Michelle Smith. "Once disease-causing bacteria become attached to leafy greens, it's difficult to remove them by rinsing with water."

In fact, "the greater likelihood is that you'll make a safe product unsafe because of cross-contamination with bacteria from your fingers, cutting boards, countertops, or the sink," adds Smith.

If the bag doesn't say "washed," though, you *do* need to wash the greens thoroughly.

What about slimy leaves?

"Spoilage is not just a quality issue," says Smith. "It can also be a food-safety issue. Once spoilage organisms start to attack, a vegetable or fruit becomes more susceptible to pathogens because its skin or surface begins to break down, allowing easier entry of pathogens." And once inside the plants' cells, the germs can chow down . . . and flourish.

The Bottom Line

Don't rewash bagged washed greens. As for spoilage, "I would look carefully at the leaves from the top of the bag as I pull them out," says Smith. "If they are starting to spoil, I would discard the entire bag. If the bulk of the lettuce appears sound and there are a few spoiled leaves at the bottom of the bag, I might use what's at the top and discard the slimy leaves and any leaves they may have touched."

Microwave Popcorn Ruins Lungs

"Popcorn lung" is an irreversible scarring of the smallest airways in the lungs. It's caused by inhaling vapors of a buttery-tasting chemical that some manufacturers may be adding to their microwave popcorn.

Diacetyl is a natural compound found in cheese, butter, yogurt, and wine. It's not harmful when swallowed, but it can damage the lungs if large amounts are inhaled. Nearly all "popcorn lung" victims worked in popcorn or flavoring manufacturing facilities, where they breathed in the chemical every day. The most severe cases needed lung transplants.

Several consumers also claim to have the disease, including a middle-aged man in Colorado who inhaled the buttery steam from the two bags of popcorn he microwaved every day for 10 years "because it smells good." His $7 million award is being appealed by the supermarket chain that sold him the popcorn.

"Generally, flavor manufacturers have reduced the amount of diacetyl they use, and, in some instances, diacetyl has been replaced with other, similar flavoring substances," says John Hallagan of the Flavor and Extract Manufacturers Association.

How can you tell if your favorite microwave popcorn contains diacetyl? You can't.

"FDA food-labeling regulations don't require the specific declaration of individual flavoring substances," notes Hallagan, "so butter-flavored microwave popcorn labels will simply list them as 'natural,' 'artificial,' or 'natural and artificial' flavors."

The Bottom Line

If you eat butter-flavored microwave popcorn and want to lower any potential risk of inhaling flavoring compounds, says Kathleen Kreiss of the Centers for Disease Control and Prevention (CDC), "allow the bag to cool before you open it, and use a kitchen exhaust hood if you have one."

Meat Glue Is Dangerous

If you've attended a wedding reception or conference where every piece of beef looked exactly the same, you've probably ingested one of two enzymes that some call "meat glue."

Transglutaminase, which is produced by bacteria, and beef fibrin, which is extracted from cow's blood, can seamlessly bind one piece of meat to another to make small pieces look like steak. The enzymes have been used for years to minimize waste and turn out uniform portions. What's wrong with that?

The enzymes themselves are harmless. What's dicey is the fate of any disease-causing bacteria that might be on the outside of meat that ends up "glued" in the inside.

Normally, bacteria on the surface of steaks and roasts are killed when the meat is seared, roasted, or grilled. "But using meat glue can move that surface inside, where it might not be cooked thoroughly enough to kill bacteria," says Sarah Klein, an attorney and food-safety advocate at the Center for Science in the Public Interest, *Nutrition Action*'s publisher.

Meat-glue manufacturers claim that no food-poisoning outbreaks have been blamed on rare or undercooked glued meat. "Foodborne outbreaks have been linked to eating steak," counters Klein, "but the victims usually don't know if what they were eating was fabricated with the enzymes."

You're most likely to find transglutaminase and beef fibrin in food served at events like conferences and weddings, at casinos, on cruise ships, and by some high-end chefs. You probably won't run into them at the supermarket.

The Bottom Line

Klein's advice: "If you're eating at a wedding, conference, or other function, it's safest to order your beef medium or well done."

Raw Bean Sprouts are Likely to Make You Sick

The Kroger supermarket chain announced in October that it would no longer sell raw bean sprouts because they are too often contaminated with disease-causing bacteria. Wal-Mart stopped selling sprouts two years ago.

"There have been at least 35 outbreaks from contaminated sprouts since the mid-1990s," says the Food and Drug Administration's Michelle Smith. The primary culprits: *Salmonella* and *E. coli.*

Unsprouted seeds can be contaminated by dirty water, animals, or improperly composted manure in the field or during distribution or storage. A single *Salmonella* bacterium on a seed can easily grow to an infectious dose during the two to seven days it takes for the seed to sprout, notes the FDA.

"Rinsing the sprouts can remove dirt and some bacteria, but not the bacteria that have become firmly attached," says Smith. "In the nutrient-rich, wet environment that sprouts are grown in, bacteria can enter root hairs and other plant structures where they can't be washed off." The only way to kill any bacteria that may be present is to stir-fry, boil, or thoroughly cook sprouts in some other way.

The Bottom Line

If you eat sprouts, make sure they're thoroughly cooked, not added at the end for crunch.

Arsenic in Rice Causes Cancer

Last September, *Consumer Reports* magazine found "troubling" levels of inorganic arsenic in almost every rice-containing food it tested.

Arsenic is found in a wide range of foods, including fruits and vegetables, chicken, and grains. Rice takes up arsenic from soil and water more readily than other grains do.

In the *Consumer Reports* tests, a quarter cup of uncooked white rice ranged from roughly 1 microgram to 7 micrograms of inorganic arsenic, while brown rice ranged from 4 mcg to

10 mcg. (Brown rice tends to have more arsenic than white rice because the metal concentrates in the bran.) Rice cakes ranged from 2 mcg to 8 mcg per serving, while hot and ready-to-eat rice cereals ranged from 2 mcg to 7 mcg.

Arsenic is a known human carcinogen.

"Ingestion of inorganic arsenic in drinking water can cause cancer of the skin, bladder, lung, liver, and kidney," says Allan Smith, director of the Arsenic Health Effects Research Program at the University of California, Berkeley.

That's based on studies in people who were exposed to large amounts of arsenic for many years. In Bangladesh, people who drank tap water that contained 50 to 149 micrograms of arsenic per liter for 20 to 30 years, for example, were 44 percent more likely to die of cancer than those who drank water with less arsenic.[1]

Americans are exposed to much lower levels. How concerned should we be? There isn't enough data to set a limit on inorganic arsenic in food, says the Institute of Medicine of the National Academy of Sciences.

The U.S. Environmental Protection Agency limits the total amount of arsenic in drinking water to 10 micrograms per liter. (A liter is roughly a quart.) But some 2 percent of U.S. drinking water has more than twice that much. (Check with your water utility for arsenic levels in your community's drinking water. To get rid of arsenic at home, you'll need an under-the-sink reverse osmosis filter. A pitcher or faucet filter won't do.)

The Bottom Line

The less arsenic you ingest, the better. *Consumer Reports* recommends that adults eat no more than 1½ to 2 cups of cooked (brown or white) rice a week. (For arsenic levels by brand, see consumerreports.org/cro/magazine/2012/11/arsenic-in-your-food/index.htm.)

You can remove about half the arsenic in your rice by rinsing it, cooking it in six parts water to one part rice until it reaches eating texture, then pouring off the extra water.[2]

---

[1] *Epidemiology 20:* 824, 2009.
[2] *J. Environ. Monitor. 11:* 41, 2009.

Nonstick Cookware Fumes Are Toxic

"Beware: Your Non-Stick Cookware is Heating Up Your Risk of Getting Cancer and Other Health Hazards!" warns Joseph Mercola, who runs the popular Web site mercola.com.

The villain: PFOA, a compound that the U.S. Environmental Protection Agency is studying as a suspected human carcinogen. Some companies use PFOA to help their nonstick coatings spread evenly over the cookware during manufacturing. Most is burned off before the cookware leaves the factory.

"Companies that rely on PFOA were saying that none of it is released during the use of their nonstick cookware," says Kurunthachalam Kannan of the New York State Department of Health. "But PFOA emissions are difficult to measure, and not many facilities have the equipment to do it."

With funding from Consumers Union, Kannan and his coworkers found that new nonstick cookware heated to 356° F to 444° F *did* emit PFOA, both into the air and into water that was being heated in the cookware. But the amounts were "very little," varied dramatically from brand to brand, and declined with each use of some brands. (The study didn't name any of the brands tested.)[1]

"The highest level was around 100 times lower than published animal studies suggest are levels of concern," concluded consumerreports.org.

Some people also worry that nonstick coatings, when heated, can break down and release toxic particles and fumes. But that breakdown occurs only when the cookware is heated beyond normal, to more than 500° F. At that temperature, foods begin to scorch and smoke and plastic handles can start to melt.

As for PFOA, virtually all Americans have it in their bloodstream, but very little likely comes from cookware. The chemical is widely used in stain- and water-resistant coatings for carpets, upholstery, and clothing, and in food packaging and fire-resistant foams and paints.[2]

The Bottom Line

There's no need to throw out your nonstick cookware. Just keep the burner below high.

---

[1] *Environ. Sci. Technol. 41:* 1180, 2007.
[2] *Arch. Intern. Med. 172:* 1397, 2012.

Critical Thinking

1. What advice would you give a friend about using non-stick pans to grill a farmed salmon?
2. When using bagged salad greens, what steps should be taken to assure it is safe to eat?
3. Why do some chain grocery stores not sell bean sprouts? If you choose to eat sprouts, what is the safest way to prepare them?
4. What is diacetyl and what health risks does it pose?
5. What is transglutaminase and what health risks does it pose?
6. Why should we limit the amount of rice we consume?

Create Central

www.mhhe.com/createcentral

Internet References

Center for Health in the Public Interest
www.cspinet.org

Food and Drug Administration
www.FDA.gov

United States Department of Agriculture
www.usda.gov

Article

Prepared by: Janet Colson, *Middle Tennessee State University*

The Side Effect of America's Growing Obsession with Greek Yogurt

These days, Greek yogurt is hugely popular. But it also poses a problem: what to do with that leftover whey?

JILL RICHARDSON

Learning Outcomes

After reading this article, you will be able to:

- List the three components that are derived from fresh milk.
- Outline the steps in making Greek yogurt.

About a year ago, I decided to try and make my own cheese. I opted for an easy one—cream cheese—and chronicled it on my blog. Figuring that I ought to start with high quality ingredients, I got about a gallon of the best non-homogenized organic whole milk I could afford—and set to work. A day later, I had a pint and a half of cream cheese and six and a half pints of whey.

This is similar to the dilemma the Greek yogurt industry now faces. So-called "Greek" yogurt is nothing more than yogurt with the whey removed. (Greeks don't have a monopoly on eating yogurt minus whey, but it would not behoove marketers to change their winning brand based on accuracy at this point.) With two to three ounces of whey for every ounce of Greek yogurt produced, the industry faces a challenge to dispose of all that whey.

Yet, as I learned by necessity following my cheese-making experiment, there are uses for whey. So much so that Joanne Rigutto, a small farmer in Oregon, sometimes makes cheese just to get the whey from the process. Once again, it appears, an industry has succeeded in turning an asset into a waste product.

Rigutto compares it to manure. She produces whey in small quantities as she needs it, just as her horses, goats, and chickens produce just as much manure as she requires to fertilize her soil organically. "I know how much manure I need, so that's how much livestock I have, and that works. If I had too many animals on the farm, then the manure becomes a problem and not an asset." You might not like to think of food product as something comparable to manure, but both are nutrient dense and useful, but toxic when produced in excessive quantities.

To start, what is whey? Milk is an incredibly complex food, but it can be easily separated into three parts.

After it leaves the cow, if you let the milk sit, the cream will rise to the top. You can skim this off to use as cream, or you can turn it into whipped cream or even butter. The fat-free milk that remains, of course, is what we know as skim milk. The dairy industry generally removes the butterfat from the milk via centrifuge and then adds it back in to make 1 percent, 2 percent, and "whole" milk. And while the "whole" milk found in stores contains 3.25 percent butterfat, that's not how it comes out of the cow. Cows vary in the amount of butterfat in their milk, with the favorite industrial breed, the Holstein, producing a lower percentage than some other dairy breeds like Jerseys.

But aside from separating out the butterfat, you can also separate the curds from the whey. Either starting with skim milk or whole milk, add a bit of lemon juice and the milk solids will curdle, separating out from a cloudy liquid called whey. Strain the curdled milk with a cheesecloth to fully separate the curds (the solids) from the whey. This is how you make the paneer cheese found in Indian food.

Separating curds from whey is a key part of making cheese. Paneer is not technically cheese, as no cultures were added and no fermentation takes place. Cheesemaking—and yogurt making—requires heating the milk to a specified temperature, adding cultures, and holding the milk at that temperature for a period of time. To make yogurt, heat the milk to 180°F and then cool it to 115°F before adding the cultures. Some recipes recommend holding it around that temperature for longer periods, but I find that keeping it between 105° and 115° for 4 hours generally does the trick.

For cheese, you add a substance called rennet—an enzyme typically taken from the stomach of a calf, although now vegetarian options are available—to induce curdling. Once the cultures have done their job, most cheeses require straining through a cheesecloth to separate the curds from the whey.

Yogurt's a different story. Even if you never plan to make your own cheese, you can separate the curds from the whey with store-bought yogurt at home. This is all that the product sold as Greek yogurt actually is. Strain any kind of yogurt through a cheesecloth and the whey will drip out, leaving behind what some believe is a creamier and healthier product for you to eat.

The notion that Greek yogurt is healthier than normal yogurt comes from the fact that Greek yogurt is a more concentrated product with the whey removed. Compared to plain yogurt, one cup of Greek yogurt contains more protein, fewer carbs, and less lactose. Therefore, if you don't tolerate lactose well, or if you subscribe to the notion that all carbs are the devil and protein is the most valuable macronutrient around, Greek yogurt is for you.

The runaway marketing success of Greek yogurt has left manufacturers with a problem on their hands: what to do with all of that whey. The very same problem I faced after my first bold steps into the world of cheesemaking.

But whey, while watery, is not the nutritional equivalent of water. Yes, it contains some of the lactose from milk, but it's also rich in calcium and other nutrients, not to mention beneficial microbes. Whey, it turns out, is useful.

For one thing, you can use whey to make your own ricotta cheese. Ricotta is simply the Italian word for "recooked." First, you make cheese or yogurt. Then you take what's leftover—whey—and "recook" it into ricotta. Recipes that specifically call for whey drained from yogurt are available online.

When looking for a way to put my own whey to good use, I turned to a few friends and a few websites for help. One friend gave me a cookbook called Nourishing Traditions by Sally Fallon and Mary Enig, as it contained several recipes calling for whey. Fallon and Enig often recommend soaking grains overnight prior to using them to break down an antinutrient in them called phytic acid. You can help this process along by adding a bit of whey to the soak water. A nice bonus is that whole grains like steel cut oats and brown rice cook faster following soaking. You can add whey when you soak beans too.

Farmer Joanne Rigutto contributed more tips for using whey. When she's in a "cheesy mood," she makes a few pounds of paneer cheese per week, yielding about three quarters of a gallon of whey per pound of cheese. "If I'm eating soup all the time and doing a lot of stews and whatnot," she says, "it will take me anywhere from one big stew to four to five days to use all that up."

She replaces water in her recipes with whey for soups, stews, breads, muffins, cornbread, and more. "If you make pancakes, if you use whey instead of water, it will produce the lightest fluffiest pancakes you've ever had."

"Anywhere you use water," she continues, "it adds a little extra flavor. It adds umami." That's the fifth flavor, named for the Japanese word meaning deliciousness. "You can't really taste that it's whey but it enhances the flavor to everything." Rigutto used to use wine in her cooking, but found she could now use whey instead. "It's cheaper than using wine for one thing, and if you're making cheese, you're gonna have the whey anyway."

She also feeds whey to her animals. "I just started malting barley for beer-making and because I have enough animals right now, I can brew beer all the time and I'll have animal feeds from the spent grains. I'm going to start milking the goats here soon too, which means I'm going to be making cheese on a regular basis." She then mixes the whey with her spent beer grains and feeds it to the chickens and—in small quantities—to the horses. When she gets pigs, they will receive spent grains and whey too.

"When you're making cheese," she summarizes, "You're pulling out the protein mostly. So the whey has all the other good things." Using the whey is "just another way to get the squeal out of the pig."

In other words, if you'd like to help Greek yogurt makers with their pollution problem, a simple way to do so is by depriving them of your business. Opt for regular yogurt instead and using the whey yourself.

(And if you're feeling brave and you try making yogurt at home, here's some advice from my yogurt-making exploits: don't give up if it does not work the first time. Yogurt is very easy to make, but it's also easy to screw up. I've done so by using dead cultures instead of live ones, by attempting to make yogurt in a metal pot that was too conductive and cooked the cultures, and by using a broken thermometer without realizing it wasn't working. But if so long as you use live cultures and keep the milk at the right temperature, it's a cinch.)

Critical Thinking

1. Compare the nutritional quality of skim milk to plain, fat-free Greek yogurt.
2. Describe products that can be made from whey at home and by the food industry.
3. Write an essay on the trends in Greek yogurt consumption by college students.

Create Central

www.mhhe.com/createcentral

Internet References

American Dairy Association and Dairy Council
www.adadc.com

National Yogurt Association
www.aboutyogurt.com

U.S. Department of Agriculture
www.usda.gov

Jill Richardson is the founder of the blog *La Vida Locavore* and a member of the Organic Consumers Association policy advisory board. She is the author of *Recipe for America: Why Our Food System Is Broken and What We Can Do to Fix It.*

Unit 8

UNIT

Prepared by: Janet Colson, *Middle Tennessee State University*

Hunger, Nutrition, and Sustainability

Considering the economic instability over the past few years, more Americans are living at or below the poverty level. The changes in our economy and employment rates have caused many Americans to spend less money on food for themselves and their families. It is possible to consume fresh and nutritious foods on a tight budget, but it is challenging in our current food culture. Several articles in this unit describe some of the challenges that low-income populations face to obtain nutritious foods and what can be done to improve the accessibility of nutritious foods for those that struggle to feed their families.

The international food supply is a complex global process that is influenced by natural and secular phenomena. Unpredictable weather, climate change, government regulation of agriculture, tariffs on trade, trading and speculation of commodity crops, and increased meat consumption have all influenced the world's food supply. Global food prices are directly linked to changes in supply and the price of food. Over the past decade, food prices have increased at dramatic rates, with prices of grains increasing at the highest speed. The sharp increases in food prices lead to political protests in African, South American, and Asian countries. The food crisis has culminated in greater political instability in developing countries that rely on rice and wheat as their main source of calories.

The regulations that helped to stabilize agriculture prices and production after the Great Depression and World War II have diminished or been eliminated. As a result of this deregulation, the price of food has increased and has experienced much great volatility in prices. The populations that feel the most effect of rising food costs are the poorer areas of developing countries.

Nutrient deficiencies magnify the effect of disease, resulting in more severe symptoms and greater complications in countries with developing economies. For example, vitamin A deficiency leads to blindness in about 250,000–300,000 children annually and exacerbates the symptoms of measles. Iron deficiency, which is widespread among pregnant women and those in the child-bearing years in developing countries, increases the risk of death from hemorrhage in their offspring and reduces physical productivity and learning capacity. Finally, iodine deficiency causes brain damage and mental retardation. It is estimated that 1.5 billion people are at risk for iodine deficiency such as goiters or cretinism.

Malnutrition is the main culprit for lowered resistance to disease, infection, and death, especially among children in developing countries. The malnutrition-infection combination results in stunted growth, lowered mental development in children, lowered productivity, and higher incidence of degenerative disease in adulthood. This directly affects the economies of developing countries. Over 1 billion people globally suffer from micronutrient malnutrition frequently called "hidden hunger." In addition, partnerships between the public and private sectors may prove valuable in combating malnutrition. Solutions to these problems such as building sustainable systems through indigenous knowledge and practices that are community based and environmentally friendly with emphasis on biofortification and dietary diversification may combat hunger and nutrient deficiencies in the future.

Malnutrition not only affects children and adults in developing countries, but it is also prevalent in the United States. Thirty million Americans (including 11 million children), experience food insecurity and hunger. In a country where one-fifth of the food is wasted and 130 pounds of food per person is thrown away each year, it is unacceptable that Americans go hungry. Food security is now critical to consumers worldwide.

Sustainable agriculture versus conventional agricultural practices are another topic of concern. Current conventional agricultural techniques depend on nitrogen-based fertilizers for crop production; however, as the use of these chemical fertilizers spreads to other countries, it is posing threats to the health of our ecosystems. Additionally, the high nitrogen content may damage the atmosphere. Even though genetically modifying crops may increase yield and reduce costs to the farmer, controversy exists over the safety of genetic modification.

Our agricultural grain crops are annuals, meaning the plants must be planted each year from seed and the plants are cleared from the fields at the end of the growing season. Plant geneticists are now able to develop perennial grain plants that could have significant ecological, environmental, and health benefits to the world's food supply. But does the modified grain threaten the health of those who consume them?

Many of the articles in this unit focus on food insecurity, hunger, and food/health disparities. This topic was emphasized in this unit because of the growing number of food insecure households in the United States. The topic of hunger has always been a central focus in international nutrition; however, more people in the United States are affected by food insecurity, even with the abundant amount of food that is wasted here. Food assistance programs are needed domestically as well as for the millions of undernourished people living in developing countries.

Article

Prepared by: Janet Colson, *Middle Tennessee State University*

Behind the Label: How Fair Are Organic and Fairtrade Bananas?

The Dominican Republic's organic and Fairtrade boom has helped banana growers, but what about the slum-dwelling Haitian migrant workers? Tom Levitt reports on the plight of the forgotten people in the banana trade.

TOM LEVITT

Learning Outcomes

After reading this article, you will be able to:

- Summarize how price competition from large retail stores impacts the laborers on plantations where organic and fairtrade products are grown.
- Evaluate the effectiveness of the price premium on production of fairtrade agriculture.

Like many young Dominicans, Federico left for the United States when he finished school to look for work, ending up in a Spanish store in New York. After 20 years working seven days a week he grew tired of the long hours and yearned for his homeland and the tropical climate of the Caribbean.

He had heard about the booming banana trade with the export market growing fast, a cheap and plentiful workforce, and land and water in abundance. It seemed like an ideal opportunity, with money to be made for entrepreneurs willing to set up a plantation. Today he is half way towards his dream, 35 hectares of indigenous forest have been cleared with half already planted with banana trees. The other half will be up and running later this year, together with a new building to wash and pack the harvested bananas.

Not far away Jan Luis Moneta is still waiting for his dream: a work visa. He migrated from Haiti, one of the poorest countries in the world, when he was 14 years old. After 30 years working on banana plantations he is still classed as an illegal worker. With his daily wage he cannot afford to live in anything more than a corrugated iron hut, with no water, toilet facilities or electricity.

Jan Luis is just one of many thousands of 'invisible' Haitian migrants working in the banana sector, where they make up an estimated 90 per cent of the total workforce [the government says the figure is 66 per cent]. Union activists told the *Ecologist* that 90–95 per cent of them are working in the country illegally.

Although their stories are wildly different, both Federico and Jan Luis have together helped fuel the Dominican Republic's banana boom. The country is the UK's biggest supplier in value terms, with more than half of all their bananas exported to our shores. The majority of these are Fairtrade and/or organic. Despite the economic downturn, overall Fairtrade sales in the UK grew by 12 per cent in 2011.

But by buying organic and Fairtrade bananas, are consumers in the UK helping to improve conditions for workers and the environment on the ground? And is the switch to organic and Fairtrade providing a template for other banana-producing countries to replicate?

A favourite at breakfast and in packed lunches, the banana's unrivalled popularity has seen major supermarkets such as Tesco and Asda vying to offer the best deal. Between 2002 and 2008, a price war between major supermarkets saw the price of bananas plummet by up to 41 per cent. The price cuts are almost invariably kicked off by Walmart (owner of Asda in the UK) and have continued to this day. At one point in 2009, German discounter Aldi led others down to the UK's lowest price ever, at 37p per kilo, one third the price at the beginning of the decade.

A decision by Sainsburys and Waitrose to only source Fairtrade bananas from 2007 seemed to signal a change or at least a part change. In 2012 the Co-op followed suit. These decisions have contributed to creating a £150 million Fairtrade banana market, accounting for one in every three bananas sold.

The Dominican Republic has been one the main beneficiaries of this boom. Its Fairtrade and organic banana industry has been growing rapidly over the past decade with an estimated 60 per cent of banana production certified organic and a quarter certified Fairtrade.

The principles of organic farming insist on fairness to all workers, while Fairtrade standards are meant to ensure fair payments to banana plantation owners and their workers, with the additional Fairtrade premium being spent on projects to help small producers and plantation workers.

While the health problems normally associated with banana plantations and daily contact with toxic pesticides and fungacides were not apparent in the Dominican Republic, the industry the *Ecologist* saw in the country was still one reliant on a migrant workforce paid poverty wages, living in slums and with no legal status. What's more, in an effort to tackle criticism of its treatment of illegal workers, the Dominican Republic government is now planning to force many of these migrants underpinning the banana industry to leave the country.

The Organic and Fairtrade Boom

The seeds of an organic, and latterly, Fairtrade industry in the Dominican Republic were sown in the 1980s when private foundations from Germany encouraged organic cocoa production. Producers later switched to bananas. Growing consumer demand, together with technical support from multinational marketing companies, helped the banana sector grow considerably from the 1990s onwards.

The organic farms we visited had managed to replace often dangerous chemicals used to protect banana trees with a natural pesticide, a mixture of garlic and rotting vegetables. But the prevalence of black sigatoka (or 'leaf streak'), the fungal disease that wreaks havoc in banana growing countries across the world, is becoming a major problem, with farms regularly reporting losses of up to 30 per cent of their crop. The disease attacks the tree and can cut fruit production by half.

A particularly devastating outbreak in late 2011 wiped out an estimated 40 per cent of production in the main banana growing region. For smaller producers in particular, the growing prevalence of diseases like black sigatoka make it a struggle to meet the low and non-chemical requirement in Fairtrade and organic standards. Larger conventional and organic farms in the country can afford to operate aerial spraying every 20 to 30 days to protect their crops.

Federico runs an organic plantation in the north-west of the Dominican Republic in the province of Monte Cristi. Like many organic farms he hopes to get Fairtrade certification soon too. Along with the neighbouring province of Valverde, this is the heart of the banana-growing industry in the country. One government official we spoke to estimated 90 per cent of employment here is related to bananas.

On his farm, Federico is proud of his chemical-free plantation, even as it expands onto more former forested land. The irony is that forested land can be converted straight into organic production whereas former conventional agricultural land would have to go through a two-year conversion period to remove traces of chemicals in the soils.

He uses a mixture of roots and chicken manure to fertilise the plants, which means he loses out on the unnaturally large bananas of conventional farms. 'My smaller bananas are much healthier and stronger', says Federico. Like all other plantations, every bunch of bananas is protected by a plastic bag, although in his case dipped in a mixture of hot pepper, garlic and soap rather than chemicals.

The use of plastic bags in particular is one of the most wasteful parts of banana production. On both conventional and organic farms, they are used to protect the bananas from overexposure to the sun and thrown out after three months. Disposal of the bags is badly regulated and local roads and rivers throughout the banana growing regions are strewn with plastic waste, white bags from organic plantations and blue chemical coated bags from the conventional ones.

Ironically, if it wasn't for the colour coded plastic bags covering the bunches of bananas, it would be impossible to spot the difference between the organic and conventional farms. They often lie just metres apart (sometimes even on the same farm) and look identical in terms of layout, stretching for tens of acres with no attempt at mixed cropping or diversity to encourage natural wildlife. The monoculture landscape is little different to the oil palm plantations of south-east Asia which have devastated the once biodiversity-rich tropical rainforests of countries like Malaysia and Indonesia.

'This region has lost its biodiversity,' says Fasto Pena, director of Naturaleza, a local environmental group. 'It's equally bad on organic and conventional farms. Plantation owners need to look after the natural environment better so it is still there for us in the future.'

The Forgotten Banana Workers

There is also a less visible side to banana production. As with the majority of banana growing countries, a key component of the growth in the Dominican Republic has been a cheap migrant workforce. When the Haiti earthquake struck in 2010, thousands fled across the border, ending up in the north-west banana-growing states. However, the supply of migrant workers has actually been constant for the past 20 to 30 years. But a better life is unlikely to be found on a banana plantation.

Lying hidden off a main road, around 1,000 Haitian migrants live crowded together in a community of corrugated iron shacks. Most of them are young and male, some have families but no-one has water, toilets or electricity. Some of them have jobs. Some don't. Of the ones that do, nearly all work on banana plantations, including some for a well-known organic plantation.

Most of the workers get 250 to 300 pesos a day when they work (about £4). 'It is barely enough to eat,' a group of young men tell us. 'It allows us one meal a day of beans and rice but is not enough to rent a house or look after a family.'

Nearby, off a main road near the town of Mao in Valverde, in another community of mainly wooden huts, live around 130 Haitian migrants. One of them, a 34-year-old Haitian Sabin James, told us he works on an organic plantation and after 15 years in the country is still trying to get legal status. Even though he gets paid 300 pesos, Sabin can't afford to buy a US$225 (8,800 pesos) passport that would give him access to social security. His company offers help to apply for one but won't help him pay for it. 'They say they are helping us but they know it's no help at all,' says Sabin.

'The companies don't want to know about workers or bother themselves with how much they earn, where they live or what they eat,' says Padre Regino Martinez, co-founder of Asomilin.

His organisation has been helping migrants get passports at a reduced cost of US$140 and overcoming their fears of being deported if they try and apply.

Padre says Dominican workers don't get paid more but were given fixed contracts and the opportunity for promotion to higher paid positions, which Haitians never occupied, leaving them trapped in poverty.

'They don't have enough to cover the costs of living. And have no way of getting a higher salary to rent a home or buy a visa or passport. No power to negotiate with plantation owners. There are plenty of workers who need a job, so they are all too scared to stand up to employers,' says Padre.

Another migrant, Emmantel Audige, was one of a number of workers we met living near the Haitian border and is employed on a Fairtrade certified banana plantation. He told us that he and other migrants had signed a contract for eight hours a day but actually worked six am to five pm without rest or overtime and for wages of no more than the average 250 pesos reported by non-Fairtrade workers. He said he had been in the country for 11 years but was still an illegal worker, with no rights to social security. All migrants can use state hospitals but we were told care was very poor, with long waiting times.

According to the Fairtrade Foundation the premium consumers pay for Fairtrade bananas has been used to help migrants get passports and working visas, however, Emmantel says he has no idea what the premium gets spent on. He and other migrants would like to have access to a healthcare centre to deal with work injuries and for use by their families. After one year workers should also get 14 days paid holiday but Emmantel says he gets none.

Even migrants like Jean Baptiste who has been working in the country in the banana sector for over 30 years—currently six days a week for an organic and Fairtrade certified plantation—are still forced to live in the community of wooden huts with no electricity, water or toilet facilities. Jan gets 280 pesos a day but says a fair wage would be 500 pesos (£8), something that would allow him to continue to live comfortably in the wooden huts with fellow migrants, but not enough to rent a home with water and electricity.

Back on his organic farm, Federico, who hopes to be certified Fairtrade, admits that some of his workers are illegal migrants with no work permits. He uses around 40 workers on day-to-day contracts, although he is not sure about where they live or their living conditions. He says his farm does not have enough money yet to help workers get visas or passports.

The Fairtrade Foundation in the UK acknowledges that migrant workers in Dominican Republic's banana industry need help in getting better housing, access to healthcare and legal status. It says many of the small-scale producers are often disadvantaged themselves and it takes time for them to assume more responsibility for the living conditions of migrant workers.

Trade union groups in the Dominican Republic say Fairtrade standards do not do enough to help migrant workers. 'There is no doubt that they are improving international trade but it isn't helping migrant workers to earn a fair salary,' says Luciano Robles, from the Trade Union Autonomous Federation (CASC). 'International standards need to be adapted to local situations.'

Supermarket Price Wars

The Fairtrade Foundation says calls for using the Fairtrade premium to subsidise migrant workers' wages may undermine the responsibility of farm owners and employers to tackle the 'living wage' issue. It points the blame, in part, at the continual use of bananas in price wars between supermarkets, saying it has devalued the fruit in the eyes of the consumer and left producers with low returns, even in the Fairtrade sector, which has to remain competitive against conventional alternatives. Although the minimum price for Fairtrade bananas has risen slightly in the past two years, the price wars make it harder than ever to improve the conditions of slum-dwelling Haitian migrants.

Campaigners are hoping the new supermarket watchdog, the Groceries Code Adjudicator, will help stop supermarkets pressuring their suppliers. 'Supermarkets are the most powerful actors along supply chains and make vast profits however the unsustainably low prices they pay to suppliers can leave the workers who plant, harvest and pack our food in poverty,' says Banana Link campaigner Anna Cooper.

While campaigners fight for a better standard of living for banana workers, there are fears many of the illegal Haitian migrants could soon be expelled. Tough new rules, which union groups say are politically motivated, state that at least 80 per cent of a firm's employees must be Dominican—a figure at odds with the reality of the migrant-dominated banana industry. Government officials told the *Ecologist* this was to 'regularise' the workforce and ensure Haitians were legal citizens in the country. But it puts the plight of thousands of other illegal migrants in peril.

'Until now the Dominican Republic government has allowed the existence of illegal Haitian workers, knowing the extreme difficulties they face in their own country and which can be partly solved by work here,' says Marike de Pena, from Banelino, a well-known Fairtrade producer group that sells bananas to many UK supermarkets.

She admits some of their small-scale producers may be using illegal workers but says the group wants more Haitian migrants to be able to stay in the country and get better wages and legal status. To that end, the Fairtrade Foundation, together with banana producers, have been lobbying the government to resolve the issue.

For now though, the difficulties for many migrants persist. 'The network of migration, exploitation and violation of rights is mutually beneficial for Haiti and Dominican Republic. There is even money to be made on the border from trafficking people. The institutions issuing visas, the Dominican economy and the banana industry getting cheap labour. Everyone benefits,' union organiser Luciano Robles told the *Ecologist.*

Critical Thinking

1. Describe the working conditions of organic and Fairtrade banana plantations in the Dominican Republic.
2. Evaluate the effectiveness of the price premium on production of Fairtrade agriculture.
3. Summarize how price competition from large retail stores impacts the laborers on plantations where organic and Fairtrade agriculture is grown.

Create Central

www.mhhe.com/createcentral

Internet References

Fair Trade USA
www.fairtradeusa.org

Food and Agriculture Organization of the United Nations (FAO)
www.fao.org

National Institute of Food and Agriculture
www.csrees.usda.gov

Organic Consumers Association
www.organicconsumers.org

World Health Organization (WHO)
www.who.int/en

Article

Prepared by: Janet Colson, *Middle Tennessee State University*

Rising Prices on the Menu

Higher Food Prices May Be Here to Stay

THOMAS HELBLING AND SHAUN ROACHE

Learning Outcomes

After reading this article, you will be able to:

- Summarize the factors that influence the price of foods throughout the world.
- Explain why food prices are volatile and projected to remain higher than in previous years.

Around the world, poor weather has reduced harvests and driven up food prices, fueling inflation risks and hitting the most vulnerable. Floods in Australia, Pakistan, and parts of India have helped push up the cost of food, as have droughts in China, Argentina, and Eastern Europe. Energy prices are again on the rise, with likely knock-on effects for food.

Many countries—especially developing and emerging economies—are struggling with the implications of high food prices, given their effects on poverty, inflation, and, for importing countries, the balance of payments. Higher food prices may also have contributed to social unrest in the Middle East and North Africa.

International food prices were broadly stable through the first half of 2010, but they surged in the second half of 2010, and have continued rising in 2011. The IMF's food price index (see box) is now close to the previous spike in June 2008.

The increase in food prices is, of course, bad news for all consumers. But the poor—as well as consumers in developing and emerging economies in general—are hit harder by higher food costs because food represents a much larger share of their overall spending (IMF, 2011). At the same time, rapidly rising food prices pose important macroeconomic policy challenges for decision makers in emerging and developing economies.

International Food Markets

Food, more than perhaps any other product, is laden with both symbolic and practical value. Concerns about food security, sufficient domestic production, and relative incomes in agriculture mean that food is not traded as readily as manufactured goods, because of protectionist agricultural policies. Despite these trade barriers, some major food items—especially major grains and oilseeds—are traded internationally. In this article we focus on the international prices of such products. Much food is not traded, so international food prices are only one determinant of domestic food inflation.

The world grew accustomed to relatively low international food prices in the 1980s and the 1990s, when prices adjusted for inflation were below those recorded during the Great Depression. But since the turn of the century, food prices have been rising steadily—except for declines during the global financial crisis in late 2008 and early 2009—and this suggests that these increases are a trend and don't just reflect temporary factors.

Expensive Tastes

Perhaps the most important explanation for the trend increase in food prices is that consumers in emerging and developing economies are becoming richer and changing their diet as a result. In particular, consumers in these economies are eating more high-protein foods such as meat, dairy products, edible oils, fruits and vegetables, and seafood. These products are more "income elastic" than staple grains. In other words, as people get richer, they demand more of these high-protein foods, whereas their consumption of grains may grow more slowly or even decline.

This increases the demand for scarce agricultural resources—for example, more land might be devoted to cattle grazing instead of crop planting, while more crops are used for animal feed. Reflecting these changes, emerging and developing economies have accounted for about three-quarters of the total growth in global demand for major crops since the early 2000s.

Food and Fuel

Another influence on the markets for food products over the past decade has been the boom in biofuels. High oil prices and policy support have boosted demand for biofuels, which are used as supplements in transportation fuels, particularly in the advanced economies and also in some emerging economies, including Brazil. This demand, in turn, has buoyed the demand for feedstock crops. In 2010, for example, the production of

Tracking Food

The IMF food price index tracks the spot prices of the 22 most commonly internationally traded agricultural food items.

These include major grains—wheat, rice, and corn; oil seeds—soybeans; edible oils—palm oil; basic meats—beef carcasses; some basic seafood items—fish meal; some tropical fruits—bananas; and sugar.

The index was created to facilitate assessment of food market developments and prospects for the IMF's *World Economic Outlook*. The commodities it follows are those with the largest shares in international trade, and those shares determine the weight of each commodity in the index. These items generally have an international reference price—for example, the price of U.S. corn exports at Gulf of Mexico ports.

corn-based ethanol absorbed some 15 percent of the global corn crop. Other crops whose demand is correlated with that of biofuels are cane sugar, palm kernels, and rapeseed.

In addition to these indirect effects, high oil prices also have a direct effect on the cost of producing food because fuel—including natural gas—is used to produce inputs, such as fertilizers. Fuel is also used in all stages of the agricultural production cycle—from sowing to harvesting to distribution. Food prices are partly dependent on oil prices, and biofuels have likely strengthened this link.

Yielding Crops

With the structural increases in the demand for many crops and other foods, prices can only remain stable over the medium term if there is a matching structural increase in supply. In other words, average prices have to increase to provide the incentives for increased supply. While farmers have responded to the opportunities from rising demand, their response has only been gradual. The interplay between productivity and acreage growth is key to understanding the supply response. Traditionally, rapid productivity growth in agriculture helped drive down food prices. But over the past decade, global productivity growth—as measured by the amount of crop produced per hectare—has fallen for rice and wheat compared with the 1980s and 1990s and has been broadly stagnant for corn and soybeans. Less productivity growth means higher prices, everything else being equal.

With lower yield growth, production increases have had to be achieved by using more land. But increasing the amount of land devoted to producing more of a crop comes at a cost, which is reflected in higher prices. The higher cost is due to two main factors.

First, crops compete for land. Since there are geographical limits to where crops can be produced, higher acreage for one crop often means lower acreage for another. Farmers decide what to plant depending on crops' relative prices. Second, because demand for many crops has been rising at the same time, overall acreage also had to increase. To encourage farmers to plant and harvest more acreage, particularly on marginal land that is less productive, crop prices need to rise.

From a longer-term perspective, the recent decline in yield growth is worrying. It means that continued growth in demand for food will require further increases in acreage. But some of the additional land will be less productive than that now being used, whether due to lack of irrigation in arid areas, poor infrastructure, or simply lower soil fertility. In areas with rapid urbanization, fertile land is being used for purposes other than agriculture. And soil degradation and climate change have hampered yield growth.

Low yield growth and limited land availability amid rapid demand growth in an economy can lead to shifts in international trade patterns. In China, for example, rising demand for animal feed has turned that country into a net importer of corn and soybeans. Because international food markets are still relatively shallow—that is, only a small share of global production is exported, as most production is consumed locally—such developments can have large effects on world prices.

Weathering Production Cuts

The ongoing structural change in international food markets is clearly one factor behind the trend increase in food prices. But trends usually don't result in abrupt price movements. To really understand recent price surges, we have to look at other factors. Indeed, the catalyst of the food price surge since mid-2010 has been a series of weather-related supply shocks. The sequence of events is well known by now.

First, drought and wildfires caused a decline in wheat production in Russia, Ukraine, and Kazakhstan. As a result, the global wheat harvest for the current crop year is now estimated to have declined by over 5 percent. Then, a hot and wet summer led to a lower-than-expected corn harvest in the United States. Finally, starting in fall 2010, one of the strongest La Niña weather episodes in the past 50 years began to hit harvests—including rice—in Asia. The damage to harvests in Asia not only caused rises in the price of international food commodities but also affected local food markets, notably through the negative impact on local fruit and vegetable production.

The global price response to a supply shortfall depends not only on the size of the shortfall but also on other factors. One amplifying factor was the imposition of grain export restrictions in Russia and Ukraine. This helps to keep domestic prices low and stable but leads to higher world prices. A pattern of protectionist trade policy responses to supply shocks have also been observed during past price surges for food commodities, including in the 1973–74 and the 2006–08 booms (see Martin and Anderson, 2011).

Stocking Up

Food prices are also affected by the level of stocks. Many of the major food commodities—as opposed to perishable food—are storable and, when there are harvest shortfalls, stocks can add to supply. The lower stocks are relative to consumption—the so-called stock-use ratio—the more reluctant inventory holders will be to release parts of their stocks at any given price, assuming they are maintaining them partly to protect against future shortages. So the effect of supply shocks on prices goes up as stock-use ratios fall.

Low stock-use ratios have amplified the effects on prices of recent supply disappointments and have contributed to an uptick in food price volatility. Stock levels relative to consumption decreased substantially over the past decade. At the previous food price peak in 2008, they had reached a low comparable to that recorded during the 1973–74 commodity and food price boom. Favorable harvest outcomes in the second half of 2008 and early 2009 allowed for only minor rebuilding of stocks. So when supply shocks started to hit in mid-2010, food markets were still vulnerable.

The effects of supply shocks tend to be short lived. Crop production usually returns to trend quickly as weather normalizes. Indeed, periods with production shortfalls and large price spikes are usually bracketed by long periods of relative price stability (Deaton and Laroque, 1992, among others, have emphasized this pattern). In the absence of further weather disturbances, the recent food price surge can be expected to ease when the new Northern Hemisphere crop season begins later this year. But the upward trend in prices is unlikely to reverse soon because the supply adjustment to the structural increases in demand for major food commodities will take time.

Impact

The surge in international food prices has already caused higher domestic food inflation and headline consumer price inflation as of early 2011 in many economies. Such direct effects are referred to as "first-round," and are part of the normal pass-through of prices. As in 2007–08, these effects have been greater in emerging and developing economies, where the share of food items in the consumer basket is higher than in advanced economies (IMF, 2008).

Just as poorer countries and households spend a higher proportion of their budget on food, so too the actual cost of food makes up a larger proportion of the cost of food products in poor countries than in rich countries, where the cost of labor, transportation, marketing, and packaging add value that are not in the form of calories.

But if international food prices stabilize, the first-round effects fade unless underlying, or core, inflation is affected. Economists call these indirect or "second-round" effects and they occur if the food price increases affected expectations of future inflation. If people expect food to continue to go up in price, they begin to demand higher wages, leading to increased core inflation.

The experience of the past two decades has been that risks of a pass-through from rising food prices to core inflation are low for advanced economies, but are significant for emerging and developing economies.

The main reasons for this difference are twofold (IMF, 2008). First, with the much larger expenditure shares for food and larger cost shares of raw food in the latter group of countries, food price spikes are more likely to unhinge inflation expectations and trigger increases in wage demands. Second, monetary policy credibility in emerging and developing economies remains lower despite recent improvements, implying that economic actors will be less confident in a strong central bank response to emerging inflation pressures and will thus be more likely to adjust their medium-term inflation expectations.

The IMF has traditionally advised countries to accommodate the first-round, direct effects of rising commodity prices on inflation, but to be prepared to tighten monetary policy to avoid second-round effects. At the same time, such policies have to be complemented by measures that strengthen social safety nets and protect the poor from the ravages of rising grocery bills.

Higher Food Prices—Here to Stay?

The world may need to get used to higher food prices. A large part of the recent surge is related to temporary factors, such as the weather. Nevertheless, the main reasons for rising demand for food reflect structural changes in the global economy that will not be reversed.

Over time, supply growth can be expected to respond to higher prices, as it has in previous decades, easing pressures on food markets, but this will take time counted in years rather than months. There is also the prospect that the world may face increasing scarcity in inputs important for food production, including land, water, and energy. Technology and higher yield growth could compensate for such scarcity.

In the meantime, policymakers—particularly in emerging and developing economies—will likely have to continue confronting the challenges posed by food prices that are both higher and more volatile than the world has been used to.

References

Deaton, Angus, and Guy Laroque, 1992, *"On the Behavior of Commodity Prices," Review of Economic Studies,* vol. 59, no. 1, pp. 1–23.

Grilli, Enzo, and Maw Cheng Yang, 1988, *"Primary Commodity Prices, Manufactured Goods Prices, and the Terms of Trade of Developing Countries: What the Long Run Shows," The World Bank Economic Review,* vol. 2, no. 1, pp. 1–47.

International Monetary Fund, 2008, *World Economic Outlook,* Chapter 3, *"Is Inflation Back? Commodity Prices and Inflation"* (Washington, October).

_____, 2011, *World Economic Outlook* (Washington, April).

Martin, Will, and Kym Anderson, 2011, *"Export Restrictions and Price Insulation During Commodity Price Booms"* Revised version of a paper presented at the World Bank-UC Berkeley Conference on Agriculture for Development—Revisited, Berkeley, October 1–2, 2010.

Pfaffenzeller, Stephan, Paul Newbold, and Anthony Rayner, 2007, *"A Short Note on Updating the Grilli and Yang Commodity Price Index," The World Bank Economic Review,* vol. 21, no. 1, pp. 151–63.

Critical Thinking

1. List the factors that impact the price of the global food supply.
2. How has the economic growth in emerging and developing countries impacted the price and supply of food?
3. Explain why growing crops for biofuels impacts the supply and price of food crops.
4. As a consumer, how can you plan your menus to save money?

Create Central

www.mhhe.com/createcentral

Internet References

Fair Trade USA
www.fairtradeusa.org

Food and Agriculture Organization of the United Nations (FAO)
www.fao.org

International Monetary Fund
www.imf.org

National Institute of Food and Agriculture
www.csrees.usda.gov

Thomas Helbling is an Advisor and **Shaun Roache** is an Economist, both in the IMF's Research Department.

Article

Prepared by: Janet Colson, *Middle Tennessee State University*

Taking the SNAP Challenge

SHARON PALMER

Learning Outcomes

After reading this article, you will be able to:

- Outline the history of the Supplemental Nutrition Assistance Program (SNAP) in the United States.
- Explain why it is important for dietitians to understand what SNAP is and keep current on the program's guidelines.

Through the personal pages of their diaries, five RDs describe the experiences that gave them a new appreciation for families who are food insecure.

For many dietitians, whether they're employed with a hospital, WIC, supermarket, or outpatient clinic, helping people feed their families nutritious food within their budget can be one of the most important—and rewarding—achievements of their career.

Currently, one in six people in the United States struggles with hunger. In 2012, 49 million Americans (33.1 million adults and 15.9 million children)[1] were food insecure, defined as reduced food intake or disrupted eating patterns in a household due to lack of money or other resources.

Battling food insecurity has long been a primary goal of the Academy of Nutrition and Dietetics (the Academy). The Academy states that it's committed to improving the health of Americans by ensuring they have access to a healthful, safe, and adequate food supply through protecting and strengthening the Supplemental Nutrition Assistance Program (SNAP),[2] a key initiative in our nation's nutrition safety net. SNAP, WIC, the National School Lunch Program, and the School Breakfast Program form the core of a network of national nutrition assistance programs designed to increase food security.

A Snapshot of SNAP

Formerly known as the Federal Food Stamp Program, SNAP is the largest program in the domestic hunger safety net, offering nutrition assistance to millions of eligible low-income individuals, families, and communities. The first Food Stamp Program, which allotted stamps to purchase agricultural surpluses, dates back to 1939 and is credited to its first administrator, Milo Perkins, who was quoted as saying, "We got a picture of a gorge, with farm surpluses on one cliff and undernourished city folks with outstretched hands on the other. We set out to find a practical way to build a bridge across that chasm."[3]

Since then, the Food Stamp Program slowly has evolved to what it is today. Recipients can use the benefits to buy food, from authorized stores, that will be consumed at home. In 2012, 82 percent of benefits were redeemed in supermarkets and superstores. Nationwide, there were 3,214 farmers' markets and farmers who sold directly to consumers with food stamp benefits.[4]

The amount in benefits a household receives is called an allotment, the household's net monthly income multiplied by 0.3, which is subtracted from the maximum allotment for the household size. The calculation is based on the projection that SNAP households are expected to spend about 30 percent of their resources on food. For a household of four, for example, the maximum monthly allotment is $632.[5]

Since November 1, 2013, SNAP has been in the news because of the elimination of the temporary increase in benefits included in the American Recovery and Reinvestment Act of 2009. Ultimately, Congress did not continue that $11 billion increase. The recently passed farm bill that funds SNAP also included an additional $8 billion in cuts over 10 years, according to the *Wall Street Journal.* Together those reductions will result in an estimated drop of $90 in SNAP benefits per month for a family of four, according to *Mother Jones Earth News.*

Studies have shown that SNAP helps reduce food insecurity. An August 2013 USDA study found that participating in SNAP for six months was associated with a decrease in food insecurity of about 5–10 percentage points. SNAP was associated with lower percentages of households that were food insecure, that experienced very low food security, and that had children who were food insecure.[6]

"As RDs, we know that enough healthful food at all stages of development keeps people healthy and prevents chronic diseases. SNAP helps to improve diets," says Karen Ehrens, RD, LRD, past chair of the Academy's Legislative and Public Policy Committee who also works with the North Dakota Department of Health to coordinate the Creating a Hunger Free North Dakota Coalition.

Getting Acquainted with SNAP

It's important for dietitians to understand this nutrition program even though they may not work directly with SNAP recipients. "All RDs can and should be mindful of how we can advocate for a healthy food system," says Brooke Nissim-Sabat, MS, RD, LD, an assistant professor of foods and nutrition at Pierpont Community and Technical College in West Virginia. "Working to alleviate hunger is an undeniable part of our profession, and RDs are poised to work toward solutions. Food is at the heart of our profession, and promoting access to nutritious choices for our vulnerable populations is some of the most important work an RD can do."

"Every day, in any job an RD has, we make recommendations about what people should eat to be healthiest," Ehrens says. "We all need to understand how easy, difficult, or even impossible our recommendations might be based on a client's background, which includes their health status, personal preferences, motivation, living circumstances, and ability to access healthful food. Helping people access the healthiest foods within the limits of their resources I hope is a goal that each of us works toward. Understanding SNAP can help us understand how to help people make food choices."

Five RDs Take the SNAP Challenge

To understand SNAP firsthand, Ehrens, Nissim-Sabat, and many other dietitians have taken what's called the SNAP challenge to find out what it's like to live on a limited food budget of about $4.50 per person per day as both a hunger awareness statement and a way to better appreciate the challenges that food-insecure clients and patients face every day. Others, from restaurant CEOs and congressman to journalists, have tried it, too.

Today's Dietitian shares real-life stories of five RDs who took the SNAP challenge last fall through the encouragement of the HEN DPG. If you're interested in taking a SNAP challenge, you can find out more information on the Food Research and Action Center website (www.frac.org).

Lisa Dierks, RD, LD

A mother of three, Dierks is nutrition manager at the Mayo Clinic and lives in Wanamingo, Minnesota. Here's an excerpt from Dierks' SNAP challenge diary.

Day 1: For ease of writing, I'm going to use some Twitter abbreviations for family members: DH = darling husband, DS14 = darling son 14-year-old, DS11 = darling son 11-year-old, and DS5 = darling son 5-year-old.

After working a full day, I hopped on my commuter bus for the 45-minute ride home. DH and DS11 called me to ask what's for supper because basketball practice was at 6 P.M. I told them they'd have to eat a peanut butter sandwich, yogurt, or fruit for a snack to hold them over. I was greeted at the door by DS5 tossing a half-eaten apple into the garbage and DS14 complaining about wanting supper and "why do we have to eat like poor people?" (He is a good kid, just your typical teenager.)

For breakfast and an after-school snack, DS11 and DS5 helped me make peanut butter/banana/oatmeal muffins. The batch made 22. I thought I could get by with eating one muffin per day, but after going to the gym this morning, I had to eat two to fill up. We have oatmeal for when the muffins run out.

For lunch, DH and I will either take leftovers from the evening meal or a peanut butter sandwich. To round out the meal, we can have yogurt, fresh fruit, and raw veggies.

Our decision for what to prepare for supper was based on the desire to dispel comments we've heard from both sides of the SNAP argument, such as "People on SNAP only buy processed junk" and "People on SNAP can buy only beans and rice." It was our goal to see if we could have a healthful meal that included fruits and vegetables, and everyone would leave the table satisfied.

Tonight's meal was chili beef cornbread bake, green beans, and unsweetened applesauce. I also had some carrot and celery sticks left from my lunch that I put on the table rather than throwing them away. DS14 had this evening's parting comments: "Wow, Mom, this was really good. I thought when you said we were doing this that we had to eat ramen noodles, Hamburger Helper, and TV dinners. I didn't know it would be real food. I also thought I couldn't have seconds and would have to be hungry. And I was really surprised that there were fresh vegetables on the table; I thought we were eating canned veggies."

Isn't it interesting how experience can change our perceptions?

Day 3: DH, DS14, and DS11 had Boy Scouts at 6:30, so they ate a bowl of cold cereal and will eat supper when they get home. I think they were hoping for pizza.

For tonight's menu, I chose fish for a couple of reasons: The 2010 Dietary Guidelines recommend we increase our consumption of fish to 8 oz per week, but could we afford it? And I wanted to get DH more involved in this week's challenge. I scanned the grocery ads and found cod at $6.98/lb. If I bought one pound and cut it into five pieces, we'd have a little more than 3 oz each. It seemed that we could afford one meal of cod, but two meals were out of the question.

What would it take to meet the guidelines for our family if we chose local fish? After all, we live in the "Land of 10,000 Lakes." Here are some of DH's thoughts: Fishing is free in Minnesota state parks, but the closest one to us with good fishing is more than one hour away. A license costs $22, and we still need to drive about 30 minutes to get to a good spot. Bait would be about $3 per trip. There are daily limits and possession limits for every kind of fish. You can't fish all year long, and many waterways are closed from one to three months in the spring for spawning. Then there's the time factor; DH and I both work full-time, and the kids are busy with activities. Needless to say, the avid fisherman thought I was crazy to think that we could catch enough local fish to sustain our fish intake and meet the guidelines. So what did I do? I made Curried Tomato Cod with barley and sweet potato. Everyone also had a fresh pear. Total bill: $14.68.

Day 6: I asked everyone what they were thankful for after doing the challenge. Responses included having enough food to eat for the week; creative recipes from basic ingredients; peanut butter sandwiches (that's from DS5); having enough food to eat all the time, and that the food was better than I thought it was going to be; a family to share meals with, that when I ask my mom if a friend can stay for supper the answer is always yes and that we don't worry about having enough; being able to share our story with friends; and making new friends through our storytelling.

Brooke Nissim-Sabat, MS, RD, LD

Living in the community of Fairmont, West Virginia, Nissim-Sabat took the SNAP challenge with her husband. Here's what she recalls from her experience.

We devoted one week to eating on about $4.50 per person per day and found ourselves counting pennies as the day wore on into evening. The protein-rich foods and fresh produce were some of the more costly; it would be very easy to fall back on nutrient-poor, energy-dense choices. It's clear to me how, when money is limited, families can think in terms of total calories rather than nutritional quality. I found myself much more cognizant of food waste and acutely aware of hunger and satiety. Even as an RD with hundreds of low-cost recipes at my fingertips, I still was preoccupied with having enough money to last the whole week and stretching out my meals.

I did little snacking and consumed only about 1,200–1,300 kcal/day, which isn't enough for me to maintain a healthful weight and is difficult to meet my nutrient needs. I normally take great pleasure in eating and enjoying meals with loved ones; this week felt much more utilitarian. Eating local and sustainable foods became quite difficult. For example, one egg as part of a dozen from the farmers' market might work out to be $0.29, while one egg from the discount grocery store might cost $0.11—less than half as much. Many people don't bat an eye at paying $3.50 per dozen for fresh eggs from hens who live on pasture, but when money is this tight and you can't keep your own chickens, it's a different perspective. Luckily, dried beans and lentils always are in heavy rotation in our household, and for this week, we barely strayed from legumes at all.

Here's a sample day's menu:

Breakfast: plain yogurt, one banana, one boiled egg, and coffee with a splash of half and half (a complete splurge)

Lunch: 1/2 can of tuna with a squirt of mayo, 1 slice of whole wheat bread, 1 cup of baby carrots

Dinner: 1 cup of cooked black beans (from dried), 1 cup of cooked brown rice (from dried), 1 1/2 cups of spinach cooked with one pat of butter

Snack: 1 small apple

Total cost: $4.04

My analysis of this day indicates I consumed approximately 1,250 kcal, which is much lower than the amount I require to maintain my weight. I exceeded my Dietary Reference Intake for protein, coming in at about 67 g, and had about 183 g of carbohydrates with 32 g of fiber; the beans went a long way toward helping me meet many of my nutrient goals. I met my needs for vitamin A thanks to the carrots, and had plenty of folate and magnesium, again because of the liberal plant proteins. On the other hand, on this day, I was very low in vitamins C and E as well as calcium and iron.

Because my husband is very active, he fell short of many of his nutrient needs. He toughed it out though, going to bed hungry rather than staying awake and ruminating on what to eat that might cut into the next day's budget. At this point, I tried to talk him out of it, but he took the challenge seriously.

When the challenge was over, we had the luxury of going back to our eating habits: purchasing organic ingredients, dining out, preparing new dishes that require an investment of ingredients. Individuals and families who qualify for SNAP don't have these prospects; rather, their experience in poverty may run generations deep with no sign of letting up.

This experience strengthened my resolve to not only make individualized recommendations that are sensitive to my clientele but also to continue working to improve access to a healthful, sustainable food supply for everyone.

Kristina DeMuth, RD

DeMuth, a University of Minnesota MPHN candidate, chronicled her experience on her blog http://for-i-was-hungry.blogspot.com. Here are some highlights.

I decided to take the SNAP challenge because hunger and poverty are at the core of the work I do. I spent one year living in Haiti and came home wanting to learn more about the hunger that not only exists in other parts of the world but also here in my home country.

Doing the SNAP challenge for one week will never equate with the experience of people who live on SNAP benefits day to day. However, engaging in the week-long activity provided me a window of insight to various challenges people may face living on tight budgets here in America. I also wanted to see if it was possible to consume an entire whole, plant-based diet on fewer than $4 per day.

For the first few days of the challenge, I felt extremely hungry. I was afraid of running out of food by the end of the week, so I didn't eat as much as I could have and should have. Surprisingly, however, I ended up with leftover food at the end of my challenge and only ended up consuming about $25 worth of food for the week.

Shopping for the challenge was exciting when I found great deals, but it also was mentally exhausting as I tried to decide which foods to buy, determine whether I had enough money, and prioritize my food list. I realized that while shopping, I had the luxury of going to three different locations to get my food for the week. I also had the luxury to shop at a farmers' market. These are situations that people living on a budget may have to face: what stores to shop at, how to be savvy with coupons and deals, and even consider the transportation to get to various stores.

I also realized on the second day of the challenge that I needed to give up coffee to incorporate peanut butter into my meal plans. Originally, I avoided purchasing peanut butter because the ingredient list on the cheapest peanut butter had ingredients I usually avoid (added sugar, palm oil). I caved in on the second day and decided that I'd just eat the cheap peanut butter to meet my dietary needs.

Also, I chose to eat entirely from scratch, which can save an extraordinary amount of money; however, it does require some basic cooking and baking skills, resources for preparing and storing foods, and the confidence to try new things. I realize that not everyone is like me. Not everyone feels confident in the kitchen, and not everyone likes to be creative with food.

The following are foods I ate throughout my challenge:

Breakfast: oatmeal banana pancakes with peanut butter, oats cooked in a slow cooker overnight with banana and peanut butter, and a sweet potato oatmeal casserole.

Snacks: Almost daily, I ate carrots, an apple, and pumpkin seeds (saved those from my pumpkin). I also used leftover frozen pumpkin to make pumpkin ice cream, and I made homemade air-popped corn.

Lunch and dinner: Lunch consisted of leftovers from the night before. I made creamy tomato soup (made with tofu), pumpkin soup, veggie burgers with sweet potato and roasted vegetables, lentil-oat meatballs, carrot-ginger soup, lentil apple and sweet potatoes with vegetables, and peanut butter.

I ate incredibly healthy and at a very low cost. The cost of plant proteins vs. organic animal-based proteins was much more economical. A serving of lentils costs $0.10 (13 g of protein); organic quinoa costs $0.30 per serving (6 g of protein); and edamame costs $0.50 per serving (13 g of protein). Eating less expensive protein increases the amount of money you can spend on fruits and vegetables.

Recently, I spoke with a few parents who use SNAP benefits. Some of them don't think they'd be able to eat as healthfully without the SNAP program. I was surprised by how many of the parents said they cook from home because it's cheaper. Perhaps there are many misconceptions about what people's lives are like on a tight budget.

Elizabeth Lee, MS, RD

Working in Orange County, California, as an outpatient dietitian and blog writer at HEALing Foodie, Lee shares a glimpse of her experience during the SNAP challenge.

I took the SNAP challenge for one week because I thought it'd give me a glimpse into some of the food struggles that millions face each day.

For the most part, I was able to manage the week on the SNAP budget because I have basic cooking skills, time, and a functional kitchen. For some low-income families, those three essentials may not be available to them. Unprocessed whole foods often are cheaper than convenience foods, such as microwavable meals and fast foods. To say that it costs much to eat well may not be true. However, not everyone has the ability to turn fresh ingredients into meals.

Not being able to afford certain organic produce while knowing they belong to the Dirty Dozen list or organic ground turkey when conventional was found to contain the highest amount of antibiotic-resistant bacteria was difficult. Shopping for the week required either lots of arm strength and strong walking legs or a car. It would have been nearly impossible for me to buy everything I needed if I was taking public transportation. I felt that I ate healthfully on the budget, perhaps even more so than usual because I didn't have extra money to spend on prepackaged snacks. Here's a sample of what I ate:

Breakfast: chia oatmeal topped with 1/2 banana
Lunch: leftovers from the night before
Afternoon snack: apple
Dinner: two-bean and yam turkey chili

Karen Ehrens, RD, LRD

Ehrens, past chair of the Academy's Legislative and Public Policy Committee, shares a few pages from her diary during the SNAP challenge, which she took with her husband and 15-year-old daughter in North Dakota.

Day 1: Feeling humbled and grateful for the food skills and knowledge we have. We've been blessed and have had the opportunity to work toward having many resources, such as a well-stocked pantry, cooking tools, pots and pans, a great stove, and refrigerator. Many in our country don't start out with nearly this much.

Grocery shopping takes a long time when you need to budget down to the penny. We spent our dinner conversation planning. More time afterwards discussing. Went to two stores and tried to guess which one would have the lower prices on certain items; I lost a couple of bets. We saved $0.10 by bringing our own bags to Target. Small victories. Tired from making so many choices. Fully recognizing that our choices were small potatoes compared to really hard choices others face day in and day out.

Honestly, the hardest thing to deal with during this challenge was not being able to access the food in our pantry and recognizing how hard it could be to build a pantry on a very limited budget. How can you purchase for the future while trying to meet today's needs first? I could have blown my day's worth of resources on one jar of spices that I might need to make a delicious recipe.

We groaned when we cut into the pear and found half of it bad, leaving less to eat at supper. My husband returned the pear to the grocery store, and they gave us double our money back. Because we weren't working, have a reliable car, and live just under one mile from the store, we could do this. Not the case for many others relying on SNAP benefits.

Day 2: Preoccupied by thoughts of food. Can't sleep. Trying to make sure there will be enough food for the short five days of this challenge. We convinced our 15-year-old daughter to join in, so we have her share of $4.25/day as well. For her, we're getting by with a modified version. We'll run out of milk by the end of the challenge, so I'll make sure she has milk each day. I can't knowingly shortchange my growing daughter with food.

Day 4: As of this morning, my daughter, Emily, finished off the milk. There's more in our fridge, so she'll have that. But for those other parents out there who don't have more milk in their fridges or bread in the breadbox, what do they do? Eat less? Not pay a bill? Ask a neighbor? Visit a food pantry?

Day 5: So glad to report that although we ran out of some foods, we still have some left. Our family will be using peanut butter to hold together our last day of the challenge. Emily is so glad. She and my husband will be having peanut butter for breakfast, and I'll have a peanut butter/banana tortilla roll-up for lunch. For supper, it'll be a mishmash of what's left: a couple of eggs, two small zucchinis, a small bit of chicken lunchmeat, two slices of bread, and yogurt.

The fifth and last day of our challenge was a roller coaster ride. It started in the morning after I posted the recording of the interview about our SNAP challenge experience online. I went to the Facebook page of the television station where the link was posted and started reading the comments that started to pour in. I should have put on a flak jacket first. The comments judged, derided, and attempted to shame people who accept assistance: "Those people have cell phones and fancy jeans." "They fill up their carts with soda and chips." "I pulled myself up by my bootstraps." These sent my stomach churning; 83 percent of the households receiving SNAP benefits have a child, a senior, or a disabled person living in them.

We did it. We pulled it together. But to anyone who says that this is "taking the easy way out," I encourage you to try it yourself. It will change how you think about how people access what's necessary for all human life: food.

Notes

1. Hunger and poverty statistics. Feeding America website. http://feedingamerica.org/hunger-in-america/hunger-facts/hunger-and-poverty-statistics.aspx. Accessed December 20, 2013.
2. Academy of Nutrition and Dietetics. Priorities for the 2012 Farm Bill. Maryland Academy of Nutrition and Dietetics website. http://www.eatwellmd.org/docs/Congressional Materials/Farm Bill recommendations313.pdf. Accessed December 15, 2013.
3. Supplemental Nutrition Assistance Program: a short history of SNAP. US Department of Agriculture Food and Nutrition Service website. http://www.fns.usda.gov/snap/short-history-snap. Accessed December 20, 2013.
4. The facts about SNAP benefits and where they are used. US Department of Agriculture Food and Nutrition Service website. http://www.fns.usda.gov/sites/default/files/Fact Sheet_011613.pdf. Accessed December 21, 2013.
5. Supplemental Nutrition Assistance Program: how much could I receive? US Department of Agriculture Food and Nutrition Service website. http://www.fns.usda.gov/snap/how-much-could-i-receive. Accessed December 28, 2013.

6. Measuring the effect of Supplemental Nutrition Assistance Program (SNAP) participation on food security (summary). US Department of Agriculture Food and Nutrition Service website. http://www.fns.usda.gov/sites/default/files/Measuring2013Sum.pdf. Accessed August 2013.

Critical Thinking

1. Design a one-month meal plan for a family of four that can be purchased by a SNAP allotment.
2. Explain why the Food Stamp program was renamed the "Supplemental Nutrition Assistance Program."

Create Central

www.mhhe.com/createcentral

Internet References

Academy of Nutrition and Dietetics
www.eatright.or

Feeding America
www.feedingamerica.org/hunger-in-america/

Food Action and Research Letter
http://frac.org/

U.S. Department of Agriculture
www.usda.gov

Sharon Palmer, RD, is a Los Angeles-based foodie, the author of *The Plant-Powered Diet*, the editor of the *Environmental Nutrition* newsletter, and a contributing editor at *Today's Dietitian.*

Article

Prepared by: Janet Colson, *Middle Tennessee State University*

More College Students Battle Hunger as Education and Living Costs Rise

TARA BAHRAMPOUR

Learning Outcomes

After reading this article, you will be able to:

- Explain why food insecurity among college students has increased since 2008.
- Describe ways colleges are trying to assist students who experience hunger or food insecurity.

When Paul Vaughn, an economics major, was in his third year at George Mason University, he decided to save money by moving off campus. He figured that skipping the basic campus meal plan, which costs $1,575 for 10 meals a week each semester, and buying his own food would make life easier.

But he had trouble affording the $50 a week he had budgeted for food and ended up having to get two jobs to pay for it. "Almost as bad as the hunger itself is the stress that you're going to be hungry," said Vaughn, 22, now in his fifth year at GMU. "I spend more time thinking 'How am I going to make some money so I can go eat?' and I focus on that when I should be doing homework or studying for a test."

A problem known as "food insecurity"—a lack of nutritional food—is not typically associated with U.S. college students. But it is increasingly on the radar of administrators, who report seeing more hungry students, especially at schools that enroll a high percentage of youths who are from low-income families or are the first generation to attend college.

At the same time that higher education is seen as key to financial security, tuition, and living expenses are rising astronomically, making it all the more tempting for students to cut corners on food.

"Between paying rent, paying utilities and then trying to buy food, that's where we see the most insecurity because that's the most flexible," said Monica Gray, director of programs at the College Success Foundation-District of Columbia, which helps low-income high school students go to college.

Growth in college food banks

The number of food pantries on college campuses has increased rapidly in the past six years—especially at colleges with a lot of low-income or first-generation students.

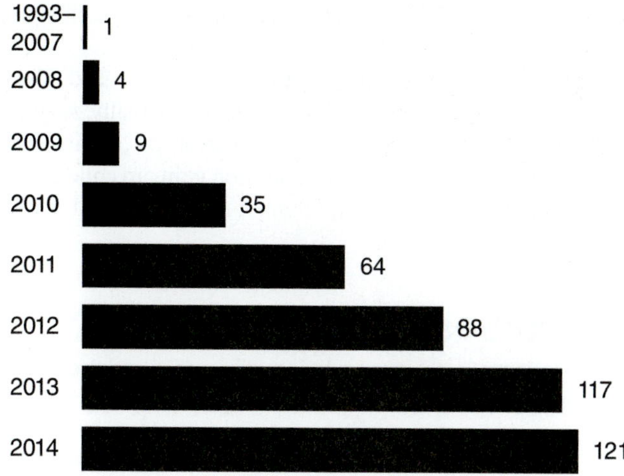

Growth in college campus food banks

Source: The Washington Post/Source: Michigan State University Student Food Banks.

As campuses look for solutions, the number of university food pantries has shot up, from four in 2008 to 121 today, according to the Michigan State University Student Food Bank, which has advised other campuses on starting them. Trinity Washington University in the District opened one in September, and the University of Maryland at College Park is looking into opening one.

In the fall, GMU started a voucher program, using donations from the campus food service and others, to provide food coupons to needy students. And this year, Feeding America, a national hunger-relief charity, will for the first time include in its quadrennial survey a breakdown of college students seeking food assistance.

Although there are no comprehensive nationwide surveys of student hunger, experts said, there is evidence that it is rising and may be much higher than the national average for all age groups.

A University of Oregon survey this year found that 59 percent of students at Western Oregon University had recently experienced food insecurity. The figure was 21 percent in a 2009 report on students at the University of Hawaii at Manoa. The Centers for Disease Control and Prevention estimates that 14.5 percent of U.S. households fall into that category, which is associated with lower academic achievement.

"Campuses across the country are starting to realize that there is that sector of people who don't know where their next meal is coming from," said Nate Smith-Tyge, director of the MSU Student Food Bank. "It's not only a moral issue but also a curricular and academic issue."

At College Park, where the most common meal plan costs $2,065 a semester, campus dietitian Jane Jakubczak has in the past two years seen a sharp rise in students who can't afford proper nutrition—a shift she attributes to changing demographics.

"In the past, not everyone went to college," she said. "Now our society is realizing that a college degree is really essential in terms of getting anywhere in your career. . . . A few have mentioned that they're the first generation going to college, and that, mixed with the economy, I think it may just be that perfect storm of what's going on."

Difficulties of Budgeting

When students try to save by living off campus and eschewing the meal plan, they often find that budgeting for food can be difficult.

"If you have only $10 a day, how do you keep within that budget and make sure you're getting your nutritional needs met?" asked Karen Gerlach, vice president for student affairs at Trinity, where an increasing number of students come from low-income households and some also support families.

Sometimes, Gerlach said, "it is a choice between whether they buy a book for class or they put food on the table for their family."

Full-time students generally do not qualify for food stamps unless they are the sole supporters of a child younger than 12, said Alex Ashbrook, director of D.C. Hunger Solutions, an organization that seeks to reduce hunger among District residents.

"A lot of people tend to think that when you go to college you're on the meal plan or the university is taking care of you, but for millions of students attending college, that is not the case . . . and with groceries rising and D.C. being a particularly expensive city, you'll see that magnified," she said.

Stigmas about Seeking Help

Sometimes students don't know about campus programs that offer help. But many are also reluctant to ask.

"We've had kids who've called us and said, 'I haven't eaten for two days,'" Gray said. "Often they're pretty humiliated because it's not an ask they want to make. It's easier to talk about the cost of books or tuition."

Joe Bradley, 22, another GMU student, couldn't ask his parents for help. He moved out of his family's house after a fight with his father and spent a semester homeless and hungry while eating friends' leftovers and trying to keep up with school.

"Going to sleep hungry, it's kind of a lonely feeling," he said. "I felt weak a lot." He eventually dropped out and now lives with his brother in Nevada.

Counting hungry students is hard because the issue is often shrouded in shame. On a Facebook page called GMU Confessions, an 18-year-old student with three part-time jobs confided anonymously last month that "I send my parents 50 dollars every month just so that they can manage to buy groceries, I have a 5 meal per week plan and I'm like REALLY REALLY hungry all the time."

The student said she was considering suicide, prompting other students to offer her meals from their plans. Yara Mowafy, a senior there, said she had tried a couple of years ago to start a program that would redistribute unused meals from student plans to needy students, but the university had told her that it did not have the budget for it.

Instead, she and another student founded the voucher program, which has helped 12 students, with four or five more showing interest. "We expect more are out there," Mowafy said, adding that the program is planning an ad campaign to spread awareness.

But the stigma remains. A 21-year-old student from Gray's program who graduated from Ballou High School and is studying visual arts and graphic design at Penn State thought he would save money by moving off campus his junior year.

He works at Home Depot and cooks at home, with a grocery budget of $100 every three to four weeks. "Right now, I don't have enough food in my house till the next paycheck," he said.

His best friend sometimes treats him to meals, and when he is desperate, he borrows from relatives. But as the first in his family on track to graduate from college, he doesn't like to ask.

"I like to provide for myself," he said. "It's the worst feeling you can think of to ask for somebody's help in your time of struggle."

Instead, he said, he plans to move back on campus next year.

Critical Thinking

1. Calculate the amount you spend on foods and beverages in a week. List three ways you can reduce the cost.
2. If your college or university has a food bank, describe who began the bank, which office currently sponsors it, and the types of foods provided to students.
3. Other than campus food banks, describe food assistance programs that are available to students in your area.

Create Central

www.mhhe.com/createcentral

Internet References

College and University Food Bank Alliance
www.cufba.org

Feeding America
www.feedingamerica.org

Food Action and Research Letter
http://frac.org/

U.S. Department of Agriculture
www.usda.gov

Tara Bahrampour, a staff writer based in Washington, D.C., writes about aging and mental health.

Article

Prepared by: Janet Colson, *Middle Tennessee State University*

The Food Crisis and the Deregulation of Agriculture

BILL WINDERS

Learning Outcomes

After reading this article, you will be able to:

- Summarize the impact of weather, oil prices, the expansion of agrofuels, the financial crisis of 2008–2009, increases in meat consumption, and population growth impact global food prices.
- Describe how the U.S. policies to manage its food supply have impacted world food trade and prices.

Food prices began to climb throughout the world in 2007. World wheat prices climbed from an average of $127 per ton in 2004–2005 to $397 per ton in the spring of 2008—an increase of more than 200 percent—and rice prices rose by more than 250 percent to $962 per ton in 2008.[1] Prices for corn, meat, oils, and dairy products saw similar though less dramatic increases at this time as well.[2] Not surprisingly, world hunger and malnutrition rose along with food prices. The Food and Agriculture Organization (FAO) estimates that more than one billion people were undernourished in 2009, representing a dramatic increase from 15 years before when fewer than 800 million people were hungry.[3]

As food prices rose and the threat of hunger spread in 2007 and 2008, protests struck dozens of countries, including Argentina, Mexico, India, Italy, Bangladesh, Egypt, Somalia, and Morocco. These protests contributed to political instability in a number of countries. In Haiti, for example, the prime minister was removed after a week of food riots in April 2008.[4] Although rising food prices did not lead to disruptive protests in every nation, reduced access to food was undoubtedly a destabilizing political force in many.

Though food prices declined in 2009 and protests faded, prices began to increase again in 2010 and continued rising in early 2011. In fact, the FAO's food price index (a composite look at real food prices) was higher in February, March, and April of 2011 than at any other point in the previous 20 years. Wheat prices, for example, rose to $336 per ton in April.[5] Also, of course, protests rocked the Middle East in the first three months of 2011. This "Arab Spring" began in January with food riots in Tunisia, which were soon followed by protests in Algeria, in which rising food prices also played a role.

The food crisis, then, has entailed not only rising food prices and increasing world hunger, but also greater political instability and change. Food crises hold the potential to destabilize existing political alliances, mobilize masses against regimes, and prompt some people to begin questioning economic systems. Given the possibility of such significant scenarios, how can we explain this food crisis in the world economy? Why did it come about? We might start by putting the factors behind this crisis into two categories: immediate (or proximate) causes and secular (or systemic) causes.[6] The immediate or proximate factors are those current elements and conditions surrounding the rise in food prices, while the secular or systemic causes are more long-term trends and changes that are not as immediately visible.

While most public attention is paid to the immediate context of the food crisis—issues such as weather conditions and ethanol production—I argue that deregulation in agriculture in both national policies and the level of the world economy set the stage for the crisis. Over the past 40 years, regulations that had helped stabilize agricultural prices and production were eroded or eliminated altogether. Recognizing the role of long-term deregulation also reveals an important insight about the recent food crisis: the instability and volatility of prices is as important as the existence of high prices. Before we explore this point, however, I will first turn briefly to the factors commonly cited as contributing to the food crisis.

Immediate Causes of Rising Food Prices

Observers tend to point to several factors in explaining recent increases in food prices: inhospitable weather and climate, the proliferation of agrofuels, rising oil prices, commodity speculation, greater meat consumption, and population growth. There should be little doubt that most of these factors played a role in rising food prices in the past four years, and certainly these factors receive the most public attention. While this immediate context is not my central focus, acknowledging the part that these factors played in the food crisis is important nonetheless.

First, harsh or inhospitable weather clearly affects crop harvests and result in higher prices due to unexpected decreases in the supply of food. Leading up to the 2007–2008 food crisis, Australia suffered from a drought, which affected wheat and rice production, and a cyclone hurt rice production in Thailand—the world's leading rice exporter.[7] Then in the summer of 2010, Russia and parts of Europe experienced a severe drought that reduced wheat harvests and pushed the Russian government to ban wheat exports. A *New York Times* article on the drought noted, "Wheat prices have soared by about 90 percent since June because of the drought in Russia and parts of the European Union, as well as floods in Canada, and the ban pushed prices even higher."[8] Food prices are likely to rise if weather patterns depress agricultural production.

Second, the shift from food grains to agrofuels undermined food supply and drove prices up. In particular, observers have highlighted the increased use of corn for ethanol production in 2006–2008, especially in the United States and European Union. As Fred Magdoff and Brian Tokar note, "Close to one-third of the entire 2008 United States corn crop was used to produce ethanol to blend with gasoline to fuel cars."[9] In 2007, Congress tried to encourage the use of corn for ethanol production by passing the Energy Independence and Security Act, which "mandates the increase of agro-fuels production [...] from 4.7 billion gallons in 2007 to at least 36 billion gallons in 2022."[10] To encourage agrofuel production, the United States has also created a number of subsidies.[11] This push to increase agrofuel production reduced the supply of food in the world economy.

This push to increase agrofuel production reduced the supply of food in the world economy.

Third, rising oil prices can contribute to higher food prices. Agricultural production, especially grain production, in developed countries relies heavily on oil as industrial agriculture employs heavy machinery as well as petroleum-based chemical fertilizers. The food crisis of 1973, for example, was exacerbated by the historic rise in oil prices. Oil prices began to rise in 2007 and peaked in 2008 (when gasoline in the United States rose above $4 per gallon).[12]

Fourth, the financial crisis of 2008–2009 contributed to rising food prices. As real estate markets began to falter, investors sought alternative outlets such as commodities futures markets. Farmers and others use futures markets to lock in a price for a commodity, allowing them "some protection from price fluctuations and allow[ing] them to plan their business effectively."[13] The financial crisis, however, increased the level of speculation, which is basically a "bet on the probability that the price of a commodity will rise or fall in order to profit from changes in prices."[14] This influx of money into the futures market drove up commodity prices, increasing the price of food.[15]

Fifth, rising meat consumption in the world contributed to higher food prices. Though meat consumption has increased in the past 20 years in the United States and Europe, it has risen much more in countries such as China and India. In the latter, growth in the middle class and rising per capita income have helped to fuel increased per capita meat consumption. And as meat consumption increases, more land is used for pasture or to grow feed grains, such as corn and soybeans. This reduces the land devoted to food crops to be consumed directly by people. In addition, meat production is a less efficient way to feed people since it "takes seven to eight kilos of grain to produce one kilo of beef."[16]

Though it was cited as an important factor in the 1970s, population growth has rarely been singled out as a significant contributor to the recent food crisis. Nonetheless, *The Economist* recently published a special report titled, "The 9 billion-people question," which focused on the implications of population growth. The world's population is projected to reach 9 billion by 2050. This report asked: Will there be enough food?[17]

This immediate context undoubtedly contributed in varying degrees to recent increases in food prices. Yet focusing on these factors really remains at the surface and leaves fundamental trends and processes unexplored. The broader political-economic context was such that these trends could come together. Understanding how this context came about is central to understanding the fundamental processes leading to this crisis.

Secular Causes of Rising Food Prices

The commonly cited factors are not the only forces contributing to rising food prices, nor are high food prices the only concern. Greater instability in agricultural prices and production is also an important problem. In the past five years, food prices have fluctuated dramatically. For example, wheat prices rose by about 200 percent, then fell by 55 percent, then rose again by almost 100 percent—all within the span of a few years. This volatility is linked to policies of deregulation in the United States and elsewhere over the past 40 years. This instability in prices and production was central to rising food prices and the food crisis.

Importantly, food prices have historically been a function of international food regimes—the institutions, rules, and norms that shape food and agricultural production, trade, and consumption in the world economy. Therefore, the ebb and flow of food prices and the degree to which prices are volatile are functions of the changes in food regimes, which are shaped by national policies and agrarian politics.[18]

To put this process into proper context, we need to begin with the mid-twentieth century, when the United States created global institutions to support its position as the dominant economic and political power in the world economy. At that time, the United States food regime came to stress regulation in agriculture with the aim of stabilizing prices and production.

Regulating Food and Agriculture, 1945–1970

Following the Great Depression and World War II, the United States set out to liberalize the world economy. In particular, the United States sought to tear down many of the trade barriers and regulations created during the Depression. The General Agreement on Tariffs and Trade (GATT) was the primary vehicle for trade liberalization. Coming into effect in 1948, GATT set forth rules for trade and aimed to reduce trade barriers in the world economy through multilateral trade agreements. It was effective at reducing trade barriers, as the average tariff rate on dutiable imports fell from about 40 percent when GATT was formed to five percent by 1990. GATT had one important caveat, however: it exempted agriculture from liberalization. As a result, nations could still regulate agricultural production, prices, and trade.

The exemption of agriculture from GATT was, of course, due to the United States' desire to protect its policy of supply management, which rested on three programs: price supports, production controls, and export subsidies. Price supports provided a minimum price for agricultural goods, thereby protecting farmers from severe downturns in the market. Production controls restricted the amount of acreage that farmers could devote to particular commodities (e.g., corn, wheat, cotton), but also regulated production in a manner that helped to guarantee a steady production of these commodities.[19] Export subsidies, including international food aid, were created to help lower the price of agricultural exports, which had been artificially inflated because of price supports. Together, these programs aimed to stabilize the market for agriculture.

In part because agricultural regulations were exempt from GATT, many other nations adopted similar agricultural policies including France, Canada, Mexico, Germany, Australia, and Japan. These nations adopted supply management not simply because GATT allowed it, but also because they faced competition from United States agriculture concerns, which were subsidized and extensively regulated. This competition prompted many farmers around the world to push their respective governments for protections from United States agriculture. United States agricultural policy, then, encouraged other nations to extensively regulate agriculture. Thus, supply management was a widespread national policy in the world economy.[20]

Just as importantly, the regulation of agriculture existed at the level of the world economy beyond GATT. Indeed, while GATT merely allowed—and encouraged—the national regulation of agriculture, a variety of international organizations and agreements were created to oversee extensive regulations of agriculture, in effect instituting supply management policy at the international economic level.

For example, the International Wheat Agreement (IWA) brought wheat-exporting and wheat-importing nations together to coordinate the market to ensure supply and prices. The first IWA went into effect in 1949 and was "a long-term, multilateral commodity contract, which specifies the basic maximum and minimum prices at which 'guaranteed quantities' of wheat will be offered by designated exporting countries or purchased by designated importing countries."[21] IWA-exporting countries included the United States, Canada, and Australia, which combined accounted for more than 75 percent of world wheat exports at the time. The International Wheat Council oversaw the terms of the IWA, which was renegotiated seven times over the next two decades. While not all world wheat exports went through the IWA, the agreement nonetheless offered significant stability in terms of world wheat prices and production between 1949 and 1970.[22]

Other commodities had similar institutions and agreements. The International Coffee Agreement (ICA) set export quotas and prices, overseen by the International Coffee Organization. Created in 1962, the ICA governed the international coffee market until 1989, when the agreement broke down. Like the IWA, the ICA had a significant stabilizing effect on world coffee prices, which fluctuated between $1.00 and $1.50 per pound during this period.[23] Sugar, cocoa, wool, cotton, and rubber also had international agreements and organizations that helped to stabilize prices, production, and trade.

Of course, not all agricultural commodities had international agreements regulating trade, production, and prices. The world corn market, for instance, did not have such regulation. This was in part because market stability existed without regulation since the United States dominated world corn exports and regulated corn prices and production domestically. Between 1957 and 1970, for example, the United States accounted for roughly 57 percent of world corn exports.[24] This dominance helped to stabilize the market for corn.

Did these national policies and international agreements regulating prices and production help to stabilize agriculture? Yes and no. We should first recognize that because agricultural production is so dependent on the weather, some fluctuations in production and, hence, prices are bound to occur. Some years bring good weather and large harvests, while other years see bad weather and crop shortfalls. Also, of course, prices and farm income do not necessarily vary with production; when good harvests abound, prices and income may drop. When crops fall short of expectations, prices may rise but farmers may not have the crop to take advantage of high prices. Such fluctuations in fortunes occur in agriculture with or without state intervention.

Nonetheless, national agricultural policies that rested on supply management policies used price supports to help prevent market collapses by instituting a minimum price. Furthermore, price supports generally involved buying excess commodities with the aim of eliminating oversupply and low prices. The government-held stocks could then be released during periods of unexpected crop shortfalls. Such price support programs helped to stabilize production, as well as prices, by removing excess commodities during times of surplus and adding previously purchased and stored commodities during shortages. Thus, national policies of supply management helped to smooth out the vagaries of the market on prices and of nature on production, thereby creating greater stability in agriculture.

Fluctuations in fortunes occur in agriculture with or without state intervention.

In addition, international commodity agreements had similar effects: they helped to reduce market instability by setting a minimum price, or at least a range in which prices could vary. These agreements also worked to regulate production, trade, or both. This kind of coordination helped to prevent some of the steep fluctuations in prices that we have seen recently.

During the mid-twentieth century, agriculture was regulated at both the level of national policy and world economy. These policies helped to stabilize agriculture prices and production. In the 1970s, however, deregulation began and marked a significant shift in agriculture.

Deregulating Agriculture, 1970s–Present

The United States food regime, with its extensive economic regulation, was gradually dismantled during the last quarter of the twentieth century. This process of deregulation was apparent at three levels: the breakdown of international commodity agreements, the incorporation of agriculture into GATT, and the retrenchment of national agricultural policies emphasizing supply management.

First, international agreements such as the IWA and ICA began to weaken during this period, resulting in greater instability in commodity markets. The last wheat agreement was approved in 1967 and lasted only three years. Though there were two subsequent attempts to establish another agreement in 1970 and 1971, no deals regulating prices or exports were approved.[25] The ICA lasted until 1989, when the United States withdrew from the International Coffee Organization. Disagreements between producing and consuming nations about quotas and prices were generally at the core of these collapses. After the failure of these international agreements, the markets for these commodities demonstrated much more price volatility.

Second, the Uruguay Round of GATT talks began in 1986 and included agriculture for the first time, thus starting the process of incorporating that sector in GATT's general push toward liberalization. This same round of GATT talks led to the creation of the World Trade Organization (WTO) in 1995. The WTO replaced GATT as the locus of trade rule negotiations, implementation, and dispute settlement, including agriculture. Consequently, international pressure increased on nations to reduce regulations in agriculture. This pressure was central enough to the WTO's trade policies that it led several ministerial meetings to collapse as many nations resisted liberalizing agriculture.[26]

Other international organizations, including the International Monetary Fund (IMF) and World Bank also pushed nations to liberalize their agricultural policies. The IMF and World Bank often made agricultural liberalization a condition of loans.

Third, individual nations—most notably the United States—began to weaken their policies of agriculture supply management. This tended to happen after the elements of supply management at the level of the world economy had been washed away. For example, although the IWA effectively ended in 1970, the national regulation of wheat prices and production remained (at least in the United States) until the 1990s. In this way, the end of the international commodity agreements was the first phase of liberalization in agriculture, followed later by the retrenchment of national policies of supply management.

In 1996, the United States passed the Federal Agriculture Improvement and Reform (FAIR) Act, which eliminated production controls and decoupled farm subsidies from market prices. By removing production controls, in particular, it essentially ended supply management policy after almost 60 years. While the United States eliminated production controls, it reinstituted income supports for farmers in response to the decline in prices precipitated by the passage of the FAIR Act.[27]

Not all nations, however, were in a position to continue subsidizing farmers. Some simply did not have the national budget resources to do so, while others were limited by IMF or World Bank restructuring agreements. With the creation of NAFTA, for example, Mexico agreed to end its long-standing policy protections of corn and open its market to corn from the United States. Consequently, Mexican imports of corn increased substantially, depressing prices and flooding the Mexican market.

The elimination of stabilizing policies signaled fundamental shifts in agricultural and food production, trade, and prices. The safeguards against market volatility were weakened or eliminated beginning in the 1970s. What were the effects of this deregulation? How exactly did this contribute to the food crisis?

The Consequences of Liberalization

The elimination of price supports and production controls made agriculture more vulnerable to market vagaries. First, this deregulation destabilized production and prices. Consequently, the supplies of grains and other foods that poorer countries had come to depend on between 1945 and 1975 were no longer reliable. Following the passage of the FAIR Act, between 1996 and 2005, United States corn production increased by about 20 percent. By contrast, wheat production fell slightly by about five percent. Without regulations on production, farmers could more easily shift between crops, resulting in less stable supply of various commodities.

The collapse of international agreements had similar effects on agricultural production in the Global South. When the ICA broke down in 1989, for example, coffee production shifted dramatically. Vietnam went from being a small producer of Robusta coffee (about 400,000 60-kilogram bags annually) in the mid-1980s to being the dominant producer (almost 11 million bags) by 2000. Consequently, Vietnam alone increased total world production of Robusta coffee by about 50 percent in less than ten years.[28] This dramatic shift in production would not have been possible under the stricter arrangements of the mid-twentieth-century ICA. With the collapse of the coffee agreement, however, a nation could emerge as a top coffee producer and add enough coffee to flood the market.

Second, this deregulation made markets for commodities originating from the Global South less stable. Fluctuating commodity prices, especially price collapses, can endanger the incomes of producers and raise the poverty level in developing countries. Falling incomes inevitably reduce access to food and food insecurity rises.

Returning to the example of coffee, a crisis plagued the world coffee market for about two decades. When the ICA broke down in 1989, coffee production and prices became much less stable. The ICO's composite price fell from $1.15 per pound in 1988 to $0.63 in 1993. After rising again between 1994 and 1998, the composite price fell further to $0.47 per pound in 2002. While coffee prices rose between 2003 and 2008, the peak in this was still below the average price of $1.31 for 1982–1988.[29] As the gourmet coffee market (e.g., Starbucks) took off and American consumers paid more for their daily cup of coffee, world production increased and prices to producers fell. As Daniel Jaffee notes, "The share of the purchase price kept by coffee-producing nations, then, plunged from between 30 and 33 percent to less than 8 percent in a little more than a decade."[30] Higher prices paid by American coffee drinkers have not necessarily meant higher incomes for coffee farmers around the world.

Higher prices paid by American coffee drinkers have not necessarily meant higher incomes for coffee farmers around the world.

Instability in the price of a central commodity produced in the Global South, such as coffee, has important implications for income and poverty in that part of the world.[31] These commodities are important sources of income for nations and individuals, and the prices of the commodities do not necessarily vary with prices for commodities that are imported, such as rice, wheat, or other grains. Therefore, the collapse in the price of coffee had the effect of increasing poverty in coffee-producing nations such as Brazil, Kenya, Ethiopia, India, and Vietnam. Increasing poverty contributes to the likelihood of a food crisis because food is a commodity that must be purchased. When incomes fall while the prices for basic foodstuffs rise, people lose adequate access to food. The deregulation in agriculture over the past 40 years contributed to the food crisis by undermining incomes around the world and contributing to spikes in food prices. The food crisis, then, is merely exacerbated poverty and hunger.

Conclusion

The immediate context certainly helped to create the recent food crisis. Bad weather, the diversion of crops to biofuel and livestock feed, oil prices, and financial speculation all played a role in increasing prices. But to focus on these short-term trends at the expense of understanding the secular effects of liberalization over the past 40 years is a mistake. The shift toward deregulated agriculture between 1970 and the 1990s played a fundamental role in creating the context that allowed for the recent extreme volatility seen in food prices.

From the 1940s to the 1970s, agricultural production, prices, and trade were regulated at the level of national policy and the world economy. These regulations attempted to manage the supply of various commodities, and in doing so they also worked to stabilize prices. This food system was by no means perfect, but it nonetheless helped to eliminate some of the worst excesses of the market economy, smoothing out the sharp fluctuations in prices and shifts in production. The push for deregulation beginning in the 1970s removes these stabilizing policies.

The current food crisis has revealed how precarious the underlying system has become. The food regime is increasingly susceptible to sharp changes in prices as the buffers that had been in place for decades are now either severely weakened or eliminated. This change has left many people and nations throughout the world more vulnerable to extreme market swings in prices and production. The food crisis occurred at least in part because of that vulnerability.

What does such a food crisis mean? What are the implications of being more susceptible to sharp fluctuations in prices? First, such crises affect individuals, and those most vulnerable are the poor in developing countries. A high proportion of their budget is devoted to food, and they generally have few resources to absorb sudden and sharp increases in food prices.[32] This is, at its root, a very personal side of food crises as food is a basic need that every one of us has. When food is a commodity that becomes swept up in a wave of economic crisis, it often means even tougher times for those who are already struggling.

Second, food crises bring the possibility of political and economic instability. Food riots, political shifts, economic downturns, increased debt and financial problems, and other potential troubles can accompany food crises—particularly for food-importing and developing countries. As with individuals, food crises can exacerbate the financial, economic, or political difficulties that countries may face, especially in a global context in which buffers against extreme volatility have been significantly weakened.

Nonetheless, we should remember that political decisions construct the market and build the parameters of international regimes. The long-term movement between regulation and deregulation in food regimes is an ongoing process that can be traced back to the mid-1800s, when Britain established a food regime based primarily on free trade. The ebb and flow of regulations will continue. The question now is: How can we move toward a food regime that offers more food security to people around the world?

Notes

1. Based on monthly world prices from FAOSTAT. See: Food and Agriculture Organization of the UN, *International Commodity Prices Database,* www.fao.org/es/esc/prices/PricesServlet .jsp?lang=en.
2. Food and Agriculture Organization of the UN, *FAO Food Price Index,* August 2011, www.fao.org/worldfoodsituation/ wfs-home/foodpricesindex/en/.
3. Food and Agriculture Organization of the UN, *The State of Food Insecurity in the World: Addressing Food Insecurity in Protracted Crises,* 2009.

4. Joseph Guyler Delva and Jim Loney, "Haiti's Government Falls after Food Riots," *Reuters,* April 12, 2008.
5. While the food price index was higher in early 2011 than in 2008, the prices of rice and wheat were not. Wheat and rice prices in 2011 were still notably higher than the average for 2004–2005, but they did not reach the heights of 2008. This, of course, means that other food prices are higher than in 2008 See: FAO, *Food Price Index.*
6. Others use this or a similar distinction. For example, see: Eric Holt-Gimenez and Raj Patel, *Food Rebellions! Crisis and the Hunger for Justice* (Oakland, CA: Food First Books, 2008); Walden Bello, *The Food Wars* (London: Verso Books, 2009).
7. Keith Bradsher, "A Drought in Australia, a Global Shortage of Rice," *New York Times,* April 17, 2008; "Cyclone fuels rice price increase," *BBC News,* May 7, 2008.
8. Andrew E. Kramer, "Russia, Crippled by Drought, Bans Grain Exports," *New York Times,* August 5, 2010.
9. Fred Magdoff and Brian Tokar, "Agriculture and Food in Crisis: An Overview," in *Agriculture and Food in Crisis,* edited by Fred Magdoff and Brian Tokar (New York: Monthly Review Press, 2010), 9–30, 11.
10. Walden F. Bello, *The Food Wars* (New York: Verso Books, 2009), 107.
11. Saturnino M. Borras, Jr., Philip McMichael, and Ian Scoones, "The Politics of Biofuels, Land and Agrarian Change," *Journal of Peasant Studies* 37, no. 4 (2010): 575–92.
10. From June 9 to July 24, average retail gas prices were above $4 per gallon. United States Energy Information Administration, *Weekly Retail Gasoline and Diesel Prices (Dollars per Gallon, Including Taxes),* www.eia.gov/dnav/pet/pet_pri_gnd_dcus_nus_w.htm.
13. Holt-Gimenez and Patel, *Food Rebellions,* 16.
14. Ibid.
15. Jayati Ghosh, "The Unnatural Coupling: Food and Global Finance," *Journal of Agrarian Change* 10, no. 1 (2010): 72–86.
16. Holt-Gimenez and Patel, *Food Rebellions,* 14.
17. "The 9 billion-people question," *The Economist,* February 26, 2011.
18. For food regimes, see: Harriet Friedmann, "The Political Economy of Food: A Global Crisis," *New Left Review* 197 (1993): 29–57.
19. In the United States, production controls and price supports rested on "base acreage," which restricted eligibility for subsidies and acreage allotments for particular commodities based on the farm's historical production patterns. To maintain a steady base acreage for wheat, for example, a farm generally had to continue growing wheat. This helped to ensure fairly stable production levels.
20. For a more extensive discussion of agriculture in GATT, see: Bill Winders, "The Vanishing Free Market: The Formation and Spread of the British and US Food Regimes," *Journal of Agrarian Change* 9, no. 3 (2009): 315–44.
21. Helen C. Farnsworth, "International Wheat Agreements and Problems, 1949–56," *The Quarterly Journal of Economics* 70, no. 2 (1956): 217–48.
22. C. D. Harbury, "An Experiment in Commodity Control—The International Wheat Agreement, 1949–1953," *Oxford Economic Papers* 6, no. 1 (1953): 82–97. See also: Ian McCreary, "Protecting the Food Insecure in Volatile International Markets: Food Reserves and Other Policy Options," *Canadian Foodgrains Bank Occasional Paper,* March 2009, Figure 4.
23. Daniel Jaffee, *Brewing Justice: Fair Trade Coffee, Sustainability, and Survival* (Berkeley, CA: University of California Press, 2007): 42.
24. Bill Winders, *The Politics of Food Supply: U. S. Agricultural Policy in the World Economy* (New Haven: Yale University Press, 2009), Figure 6.4, 152.
25. There have since been several wheat agreements, but they have not entailed the kind of regulations seen before 1970.
26. This was most apparent in the ministerial meeting in Cancun, Mexico, in 2003. See: Gimenez and Patel, *Food Rebellions,* 50–52.
27. For an extensive discussion of the history and politics of US agricultural policy, including the FAIR Act, see: Winders, *Politics of Food Supply.*
28. United States Department of Agriculture: Foreign Agricultural Service, *Production, Supply and Distribution Online Database,* www.fas.usda.gov/psdonline/.
29. International Coffee Organization, ICO Indicator Prices, www.ico.org/.
30. Jaffee, *Brewing Justice,* 45.
31. For example, see: Jaffee, *Brewing Justice.*
32. Food and Agriculture Organization of the UN, *The State of Food Insecurity in the World* (Rome: FAO, 2011): 13–20.

Critical Thinking

1. Differentiate between the immediate (short-term) and secular (long-term) causes of increases in global food prices.
2. Explain how unpredictable weather, oil prices, the expansion of agrofuels, the financial crisis of 2008–2009, increased meat consumption, and population growth impact global food prices.
3. Summarize the methods by which the United States controls its food supply.

Create Central

www.mhhe.com/createcentral

Internet References

Food and Agriculture Organization of the United Nations (FAO)
www.fao.org

National Institute of Food and Agriculture
www.csrees.usda.gov

World Health Organization (WHO)
www.who.int/en

Bill Winders is an associate professor of sociology in the School of History, Technology, and Society at the Georgia Institute of Technology. His publications include *The Politics of Food Supply: United States. Agricultural Policy in the World Economy.*